Physical Therapy: A Clinical Handbook

Physical Therapy: A Clinical Handbook

Editor: Adelaide Holbrook

MURPHY & MOORE
www.murphy-moorepublishing.com

Murphy & Moore Publishing,
1 Rockefeller Plaza,
New York City, NY 10020, USA

Visit us on the World Wide Web at:
www.murphy-moorepublishing.com

ISBN: 978-1-63987-429-3 (Hardback)

Cataloging-in-Publication Data

Physical therapy : a clinical handbook / edited by Adelaide Holbrook.
p. cm.
Includes bibliographical references and index.
ISBN 978-1-63987-429-3
1. Physical therapy. 2. Therapeutics, Physiological. 3. Medicine, Physical.
I. Holbrook, Adelaide.
RM700 .P49 2022
615.82--dc23

Table of Contents

Preface

The main aim of this book is to educate learners and enhance their research focus by presenting diverse topics covering this vast field. This is an advanced book which compiles significant studies by distinguished experts in the area of analysis. This book addresses successive solutions to the challenges arising in the area of application, along with it; the book provides scope for future developments.

Physical therapy, also called physiotherapy, is an area of medicine that provides services which help develop, maintain and restore the movement and functional abilities of people. It can be provided to people of any age, whose movements or functions are threatened by ageing, injury, diseases, disorders, conditions or environmental factors. Physical therapy helps maximize the quality of life by improving the physical, psychological, emotional and social wellbeing of people. It is used in health promotion, prevention, treatment and rehabilitation. Massage, heat treatment and exercise are some of the treatment methods used within this field. Physical therapy can be provided in hospitals, nursing homes, private practices and outpatient clinics. This book discusses the fundamentals as well as modern approaches of physical therapy. It elucidates the concepts and innovative models around prospective developments with respect to this field. This book aims to equip students and experts with the advanced topics and upcoming concepts in this area.

It was a great honour to edit this book, though there were challenges, as it involved a lot of communication and networking between me and the editorial team. However, the end result was this all-inclusive book covering diverse themes in the field.

Finally, it is important to acknowledge the efforts of the contributors for their excellent chapters, through which a wide variety of issues have been addressed. I would also like to thank my colleagues for their valuable feedback during the making of this book.

Editor

1

Pelvic Movement in Aging Individuals and Stroke Patients

Hitoshi Asai

Additional information is available at the end of the chapter

Abstract

The mobility of the lumbar spine (anteversion and retroversion) may be reflected in seated pelvic mobility. When sitting with the soles of the feet in contact with the floor, friction may restrict the flexion of the knees and, consequently, the pelvic anteversion. In general, joint mobility declines with advancing age. Lumbar spine mobility in anteversion and retroversion also decreases with advancing age. The first half of this chapter is based on a study that investigated the relationship between age and the maximum pelvic anteversion and the retroversion angles in healthy volunteers. The measurements were performed with the subject in a sitting position with free knee movement. On the other hand, the sit-to-stand movement is one of the most mechanically demanding tasks undertaken during daily activity. The sacral sitting posture, which is a characteristic posture of stroke patients, is not ideal for smoothly executing the sit-to-stand movement. Stroke patients may adopt this posture due to the need to increase sitting stability. The second half of this chapter discusses a study that investigated the relationship between the pelvic anteversion and retroversion angles and the ability of stroke patients to perform the sit-to-stand movement.

Keywords: pelvic movement, anteversion, retroversion, aging, stroke, sit-to-stand

1. Introduction

Maintaining sagittal balance is important to both sitting and standing. Sagittal balance, or "neutral upright sagittal spinal alignment," is a postural goal of surgical, ergonomic, and physiotherapeutic intervention [1]. Kyphotic curvature of the spine negatively impacts the quality of life (QOL) in elderly people [2]. Kasukawa et al. reported that the sagittal balance was well maintained in subjects who had both a good thoracic range of motion (ROM) and good lumbar ROM and back muscle strength, which indicates that these factors are also related in maintaining sagittal balance [2]. The clarification of the relationship between the QOL and abnormal posture in elderly individuals may help to improve the QOL through preventive methods and exercises [3]. Although the degree of lumbar lordosis when sitting has been shown to be weakly associated with age, lumbar lordosis was not found to be affected by lifestyle, the level of physical activity, or an individual's type of work [4]. Little is known about the sitting posture of elderly individuals in comparison with young individuals [5]; thus, investigating the effects of aging on the sagittal spinal and pelvic alignment in the sitting position is important for clarifying the relationship between pelvic movement and the QOL. Sitting positions are generally categorized into two types: the quiet sitting position and the functional sitting position. A person sits in the functional sitting position during (or when anticipating) physical activity. The functional sitting position therefore requires control in various sitting postures.

Multiple movements of the spine and pelvis are needed to maintain the various sitting positions. The relationship between the movements of the lumbar spine and pelvis has been investigated [5, 6]. The relationship between the pelvic inclination angle and lumbar spine lordosis was more distinct in the sitting position than in the standing position [5, 7]. Thus, lumbar spine mobility (kyphosis and lordosis) may be reflected in seated pelvic mobility. However, it has been reported that joint mobility is generally reduced by aging. The trunk mobility of elderly individuals is inferior to that of young people [8–10]. In particular, lumbar spine mobility in both lordosis and kyphosis decreases with aging [1, 11, 12]. In addition, Keorochana et al. suggested that the degeneration of the interspinous ligaments with aging is one of the factors that contributes to the low mobility of the lumbar spine [13]. Hence, the movement patterns of elderly individuals may be restricted when they are seated because there is less variety in their sitting positions in comparison with young subjects.

The pelvic tilt in the sagittal plane may be affected by flexion and the extension mobility of the hip joints, because the pelvis moves forward and backward around the hip joint as a pivotal axis in the seated position. Since the hamstring muscles originate at the ischial tuberosity of the pelvis, the tension in the hamstring muscles has an effect on the pelvic inclination angle in the sitting position [14, 15]. Thus, a forward pelvic tilt may increase the tension in the hamstring muscles when sitting with a fixed knee angle and the sole of the foot in contact with the floor. Connective tissue compliance is considered a major factor in musculoskeletal flexibility [16]. Muyor et al. [17] reported that the forward pelvic tilt angle increased after hamstring muscle stretching, and Feland et al. [16] confirmed that pelvic mobility in the sagittal plane increased in elderly people after hamstring muscle stretching. The increase in the tension in the hamstring muscles when sitting with the soles of the feet in contact with the floor may restrict the pelvic forward tilt. Thus, the free movement of the knees should be possible during pelvic movement when sagittal plane pelvic mobility is investigated with a subject in a sitting position. However, some sitting pelvic mobility studies have not clearly described foot contact with the floor or the knee joint positioning [6, 18].

On the other hand, the recovery of sitting balance is commonly assumed to be essential for obtaining independence in other vital functions such as reaching, sit-to-stand, and sitting down [19–21]. The early assessment and management of trunk control should be emphasized after stroke [22]. Many researchers have suggested that the trunk control or sitting balance of early stage stroke patients can predict a late stage activities of daily living (ADL) outcome [19, 22, 23]. The sit-to-stand task is frequently performed and this ability is considered a prerequisite for upright mobility and therefore, for performing other important daily activities such as locomotion [24, 25]. Riley et al. suggested that the sit-to-stand movement is the most mechanically demanding task undertaken during daily activity [26]. The sit-to-stand movement represents a common functional movement that is practiced in the early stage of rehabilitation [27].

Stroke patients have less stability in the sitting position in comparison with age-matched healthy subjects [28–30]. The reason for this is explained in a number of reports. In stroke patients, the activity of the rectus abdominis and latissimus dorsi muscles on the affected side of the body is reduced and delayed in comparison to both the unaffected side and control subjects [31]. Moreover, the temporal synchronization between the pertinent muscular pairs in stroke patients is lower in comparison to healthy subjects [32]. The following factors can also be considered to be related to the sitting position: firstly, stroke patients cannot adequately flex the hip when the trunk extensor muscles are contracted; secondly, it is difficult to maintain the trunk in a vertical position when the subject is seated due to the insufficiency of the abdominal muscles [33]. Thus, when stroke patients attempt to perform the sit-to-stand movement with a retroverted pelvis and kyphotic trunk, the standing up action is affected due to the insufficiency of pelvic anteversion and trunk extension. In addition, Campbell et al. suggested that deficits in the muscle strength and trunk amplitude of stroke patients result in reduced pelvic mobility, apparently as a strategy to protect against a potential risk of loss of balance when reaching in the sitting position [34].

Numerous studies investigating trunk movement have considered the supine position as one segment, ignoring the complexity of intervertebral movement [35]. Campbell et al. indicated that little attention has been paid to how elderly persons coordinate the head, pelvis, and trunk during movement [34]. Studies on the sitting posture of stroke patients have a similar tendency. Few studies have investigated the movement of the spine and pelvis separately. Verheyden et al. reported on pelvic movement during lateral reach movements in the sitting position [36], and Messier et al. described the movements of the upper trunk and pelvis when subjects touched a target placed in front of them with the forehead [37]. To execute the sit-to-stand movement smoothly, the pelvis must be leaned forward to flex the hip joint, and the trunk must be flexed in order to: (1) use the hip extension moment; (2) reduce the knee extension moment; and (3) project the center of gravity within the base of support [38–43].

Pelvic mobility plays an important role in the sit-to-stand movement in elderly people and stroke patients.

This chapter first discusses the age-related changes in the maximum anteversion and retroversion of the pelvic angles in the sitting position [44] and then explores the relationship between the ability to perform the sit-to-stand movement and the maximum pelvic anteversion and retroversion angles in stroke patients [45].

2. The age-related changes in the pelvic angles during sitting

The first section investigated the relationship between age and the maximum pelvic anteversion and retroversion angles, as well as the associated pelvic range of motion, which is measured based on the knee movement in the sitting position [44]. The pelvic range of motion was defined as the difference between the maximum pelvic anteversion and retroversion angles. The hypothesis of the present study was that pelvic range of motion would be affected by aging.

The participants included 132 healthy volunteers (female, $n = 74$; male, $n = 58$) of 20–79 years of age (**Table 1**). The participants were recruited from a university, two workplaces, and the community near the university. The participants were free from neurological and orthopedic impairments. After the experimental protocol was explained to all of the participants, they gave their informed consent.

All measurements were taken with the participants seated on a chair with a 50 cm × 50 cm seat face. The height of the seat face was 65 cm from the floor to allow the free movement of the knee joints. The participants sat on the chair. The front edge of the seating face was aligned with the point 66% along the length of the thigh from the greater trochanter.

The pelvic angles were measured based on the sacral inclination angle [46]. An inclinometer with a resolution of 1° was used to measure the pelvic angles. The pelvic tilt angle was defined as the angle between the longitudinal axis through the midline of the dorsal sacral surface and the anterior horizontal line (**Figure 1**).

The subjects were instructed to maintain the same anteroposterior shoulder position throughout the movements of pelvic inclination to avoid anteroposterior movement of the trunk. The

Age group	*n*	Maximum pelvic anteversion angle (°)	Maximum pelvic retroversion angle (°)	Pelvic range of motion (°)
20–29 years	*n* = 48	84.5±3.4	123.1 ± 6.1	38.7 ± 6.0
30–39 years	*n* = 13	87.8±4.1	125.7 ± 6.8	37.6 ± 9.2
40–49 years	*n* = 13	90.1±5.4[a]	124.1 ± 8.9	34.0 ± 8.7
50–59 years	*n* = 23	88.8±4.6[a]	118.2 ± 9.8	29.4 ± 8.4[a,b]
60–69 years	*n* = 19	92.6±6.5[a,b]	117.1 ± 8.7[b]	24.3 ± 6.3[a,b,c]
70–79 years	*n* = 16	9.39 ± 4.0[a,b,d]	117.8 ± 9.3	23.8 ± 8.6[a,b,c]

[a] Significant difference from 20 to 29 years of age.
[b] Significant difference from 30 to 39 years of age.
[c] Significant difference from 40 to 49 years of age.
[d] Significant difference from 50 to 59 years of age.

Table 1. The mean and standard deviation of the pelvic angles in each age group [44].

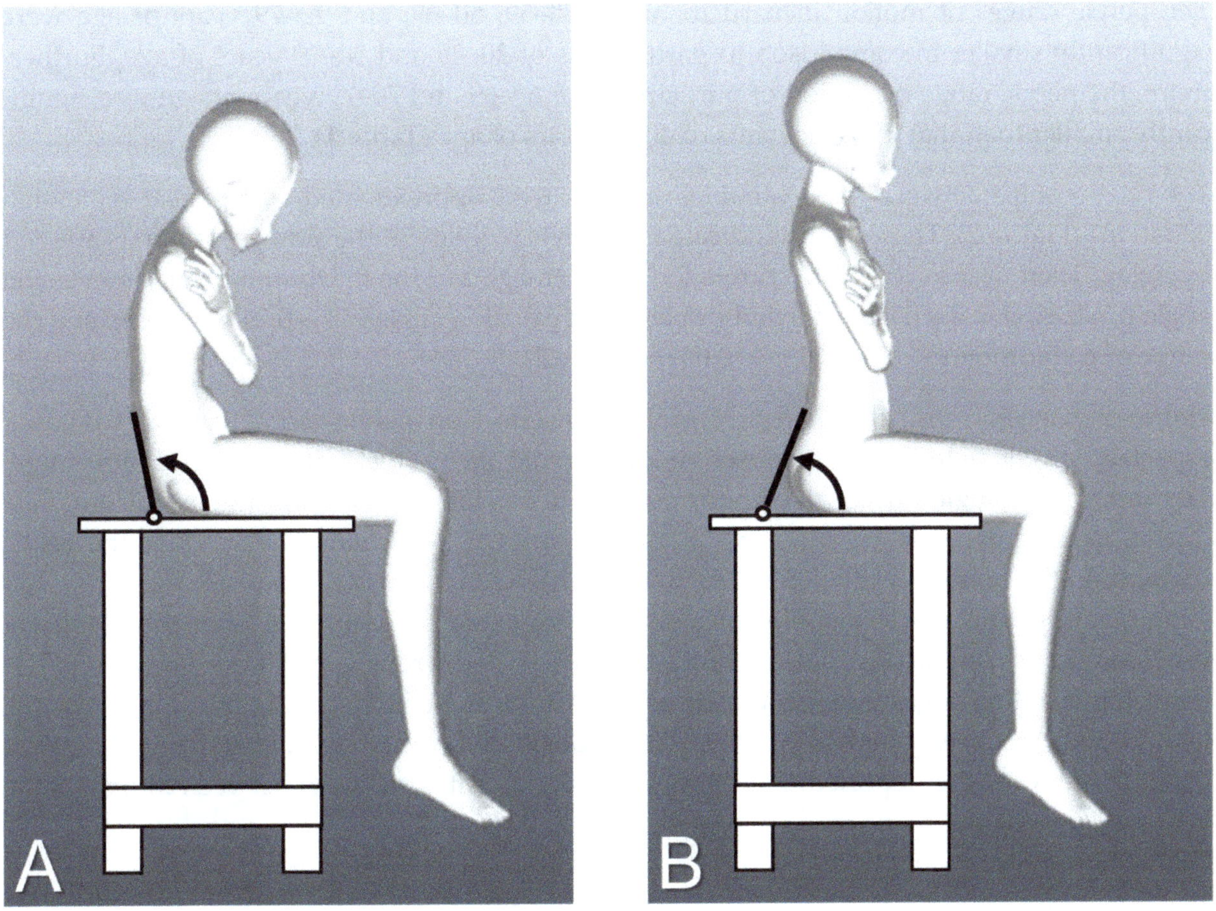

Figure 1. A schematic illustration of the procedure for measuring the pelvic inclination angle: (A) the pelvic retroversion angle, (B) the pelvic anteversion angle [44].

instruction to the subjects was, "Please maintain your shoulder position during pelvic movement." Participants assumed alternating maximum pelvic anteversion and retroversion positions five times. The maximum and minimum angles were excluded, and the mean of the three remaining values was calculated. The pelvic range of motion was defined as the difference between the average maximum pelvic anteversion and retroversion angles.

The maximum pelvic anteversion angle, maximum pelvic retroversion angle, and the range of pelvic motion were significantly affected by aging (**Table 1**).

The maximum pelvic anteversion angles in participants of 40–49, 50–59, 60–69, and 70–79 years of age were significantly smaller than those in participants of 20–29 years of age. The maximum pelvic anteversion angles in participants of 60–69 and 70–79 years of age were significantly smaller than those in participants of 30–39 years of age, and the maximum pelvic anteversion angles in participants of 70–79 years of age were significantly smaller than those in participants of 50–59 years of age (**Table 1**).

With regard to the maximum pelvic retroversion angle, none of the age groups showed a significant difference in comparison to the 20–29 year age group. The maximum pelvic retroversion angle in the participants of 60–69 years of age was significantly smaller than that in the participants of 30–39 years of age (**Table 1**).

The pelvic ranges of motion in participants of 50–59, 60–69, and 70–79 years of age were significantly smaller in comparison to participants of 20–29 and 30–39 years of age. Furthermore, the pelvic range of motion of participants of 60–69 and 70–79 years of age was significantly smaller than that in participants of 40–49 years of age (**Table 1**).

The relationships between these variables and age were approximated using linear regression equations (**Figure 2**). These results indicate that pelvic mobility in the sitting position is affected by aging. There was a significant correlation between age and the maximum pelvic anteversion angle ($r = 0.61$, $p < 0.001$), the maximum pelvic retroversion angle ($r = -0.29$, $p < 0.05$), and the range of pelvic motion ($r = -0.63$, $p < 0.001$) (**Figure 2**).

Hamstring tension probably had an insignificant effect on pelvic mobility in this dataset, especially on the anterior tilt, because the knees could move freely during pelvic movement. The hip flexion angle during maximum pelvic anteversion was 87° and the extension angle during maximum retroversion was 57° in participants of 70–79 years of age. Thus, the pelvic mobility in the present study did not seem to be affected by hamstring muscle tension or hip joint mobility. The pelvic mobility measured in this study was in line with the results of previous studies on lumbar spine mobility, which reported strong correlations between pelvic tilt or the sacral tilt angle, and the lumbar spine lordosis angle in the sitting position [5, 46, 47]. In addition, the pelvic mobility in the sitting position is larger than that in the standing position [6]. Kuo et al. reported that there was a significant correlation between lumbar spine

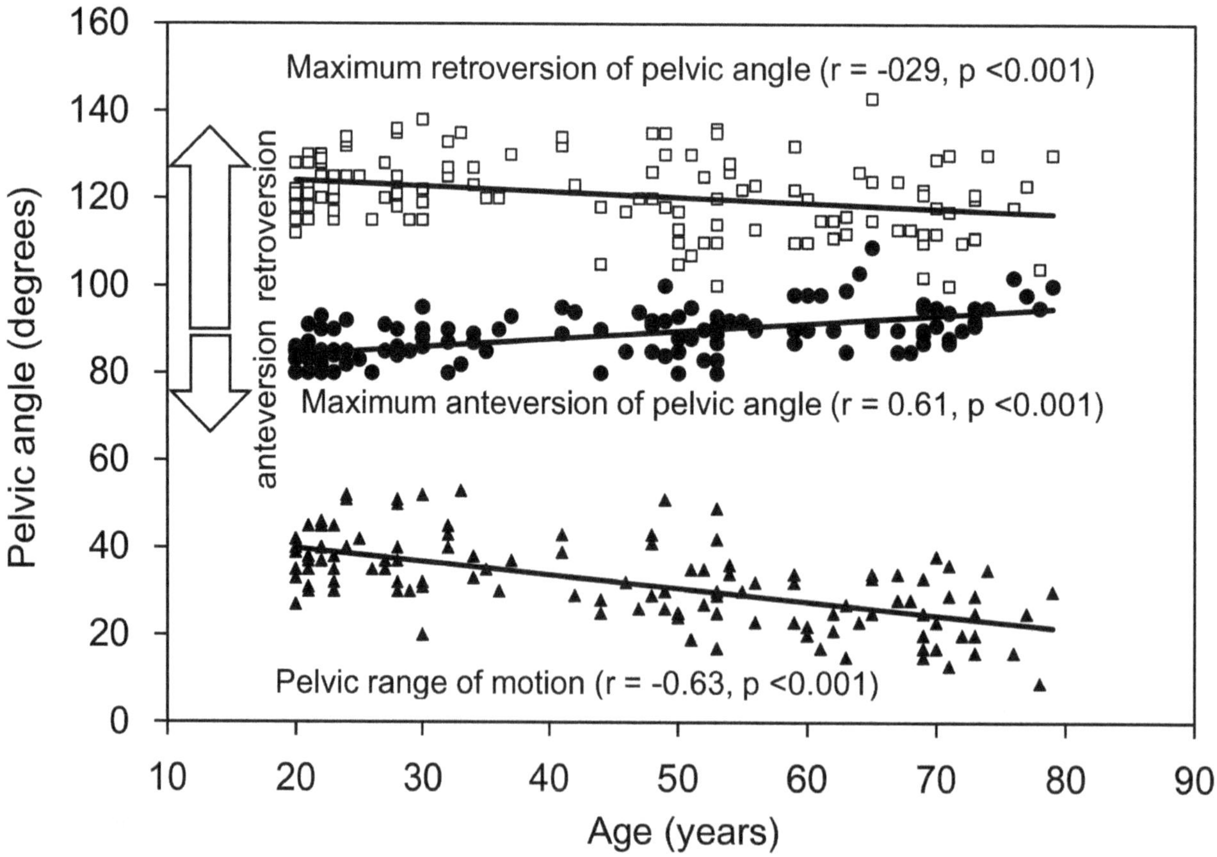

Figure 2. The correlations between age and the maximum pelvic anteversion angle (black circles), the maximum pelvic retroversion angle (white squares), and the pelvic range of motion (black triangles) [44].

mobility and the pelvic tilt angle (r = 0.67) in the sitting position [5]. Thus, changes in the maximum pelvic anteversion and retroversion angles that occur with aging might be directly affected by the changes in lumbar spine mobility that occur with aging [11]. When sitting, the angle between the lumbar spine and the pelvis is reduced when leaning forward, especially in elderly individuals. It is considered that thoracic kyphosis becomes more pronounced and that the thoracic and the lumbar spines almost act as one segment to compensate for this reduced lumbar mobility [5].

However, due to the aging-related shortening of the hamstring muscles, the maximum pelvic anteversion angle may be more restricted when performing this movement without the free mobility of the knees.

The pelvic range of movement was approximately 40° in participants of 20–29 years of age and approximately 24° in participants of 60–69 and 70–79 years of age. The rate of pelvic mobility limitation that occurred with aging in this study (approximately 30%) was larger than that previously reported for hip extension (approximately 20%), which is considered to be the joint in the lower extremities that is most limited by aging [48]. Thus, sagittal plane pelvic mobility may be an important factor that is associated with mobility limitation during the sit-to-stand movement in elderly adults.

3. The relationship between the ability to perform the sit-to-stand movement and the pelvic angles in patients with stroke

The sacral sitting posture, which involves a high degree of trunk flexion and neck extension, is frequently observed in stroke patients. This sitting posture is not the ideal posture for smoothly performing the sit-to-stand movement. Maintaining the sitting position with pelvic retroversion may be necessary to increase the sitting stability of stroke patients. However, the ability to achieve anteversion of the pelvis is necessary to perform the sit-to-stand movement.

The second section investigates the relationship between the pelvic anteversion and retroversion angles and the ability to perform the sit-to-stand movement [45]. The hypothesis of this study was that stroke patients who are able to stand from sitting in a chair have a larger maximum pelvic anteversion angle than patients who are unable to stand from a chair.

Thirty-two hemiparetic subjects (female, n = 15; male, n = 17; age, 66.7 ± 7.6 years) and 50 age-matched healthy control subjects (female, n = 40; male, n = 10; age, 64.2 ± 8.2 years) participated in this study. The inclusion criteria were predetermined as follows: (1) a poststroke period of more than 3 months and (2) the ability to maintain the sitting position without the use of aids. The hemiparetic subjects were classified into two groups according to their performance in the sit-to-stand movement test (described later): a group with the ability to stand up (the stand-able group; n = 18 persons) and the group that was unable to stand up (the stand-unable group; n = 14 persons). Patients with a history of low back pain or surgery, hemispatial neglect, bilateral stroke, visual deficit, comprehension impairment, cognitive and/or communication deficits that precluded cooperation, as well as neurological or musculoskeletal disorders that were not related to the current stroke, were excluded. The exclusion criteria for healthy subjects included known vestibular dysfunction, a history of neurological disease, or orthopedic conditions that had the potential to interfere with the experiment.

The participants sat on the chair, with the front edge of the seat aligned with the point corresponding to 66% of their thigh length from the greater trochanter. The subjects sat with their feet in the parallel position with both arms crossed on their chest and with no support for the trunk or upper extremities. The chair seat height was adjusted to 100% of the subject's lower leg length (the distance from the lateral femoral condyle to the ground); the knee flexion angle was 90°.

The pelvic angles were measured according to the sacral inclination angle (**Figure 3**). Pelvic anteversion was reported as a positive angle and pelvic retroversion was reported as a negative angle. The subjects were instructed to maintain the initial acromion anteroposterior position during the movements to avoid trunk anteroposterior movement. The stroke patients (barefoot) were then asked to stand up at a self-selected speed while keeping the arms folded across the chest. Three trials were performed with no restrictions on the position of the feet. Stroke patients who could independently perform all three trials were classified into the stand-able group. The remaining patients were classified into the stand-unable group.

The maximum pelvic anteversion angle in the stand-able, stand-unable, and control groups ranged from 5 to −4°, −5° to −22°, and 10° to −13°, respectively (**Figure 4**). In the stand-able

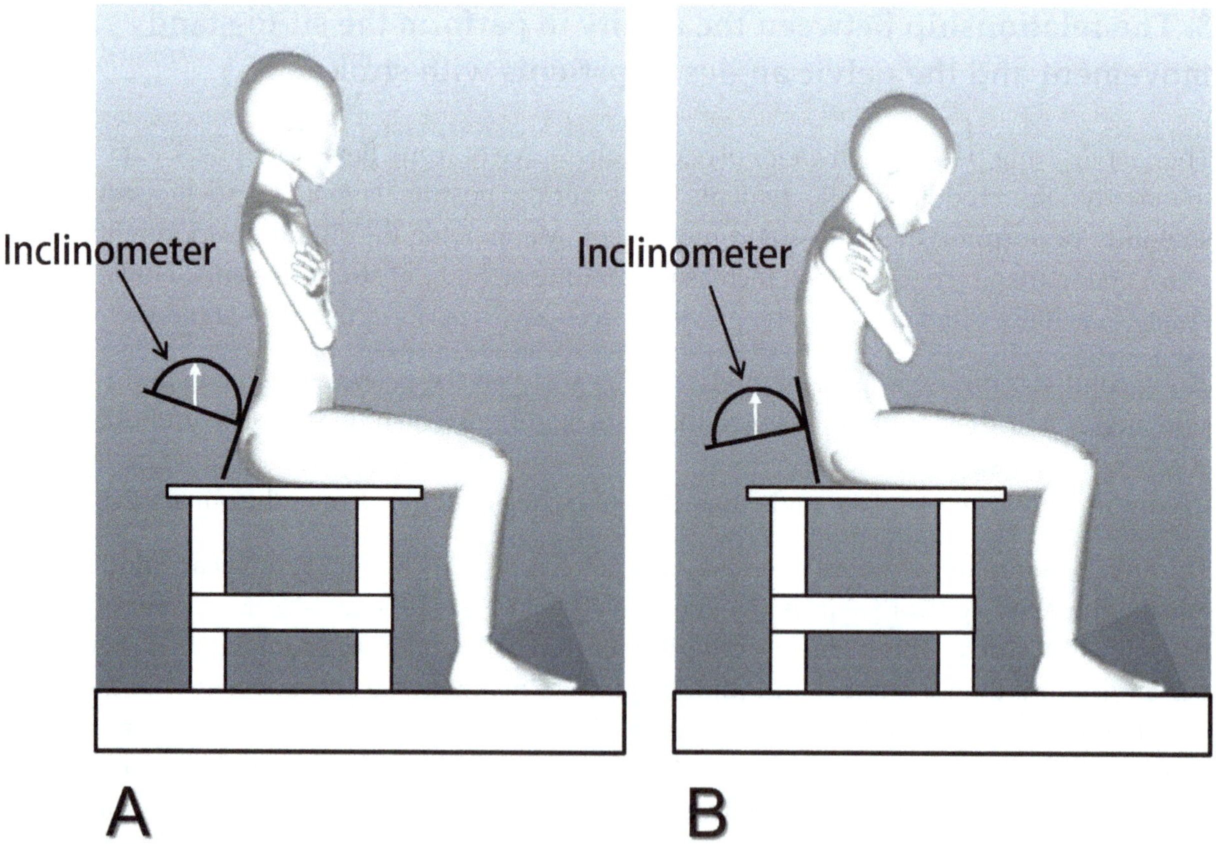

Figure 3. A schematic illustration of the procedure for measuring the pelvic inclination angle: (A) the pelvic retroversion angle, (B) the pelvic anteversion angle [45].

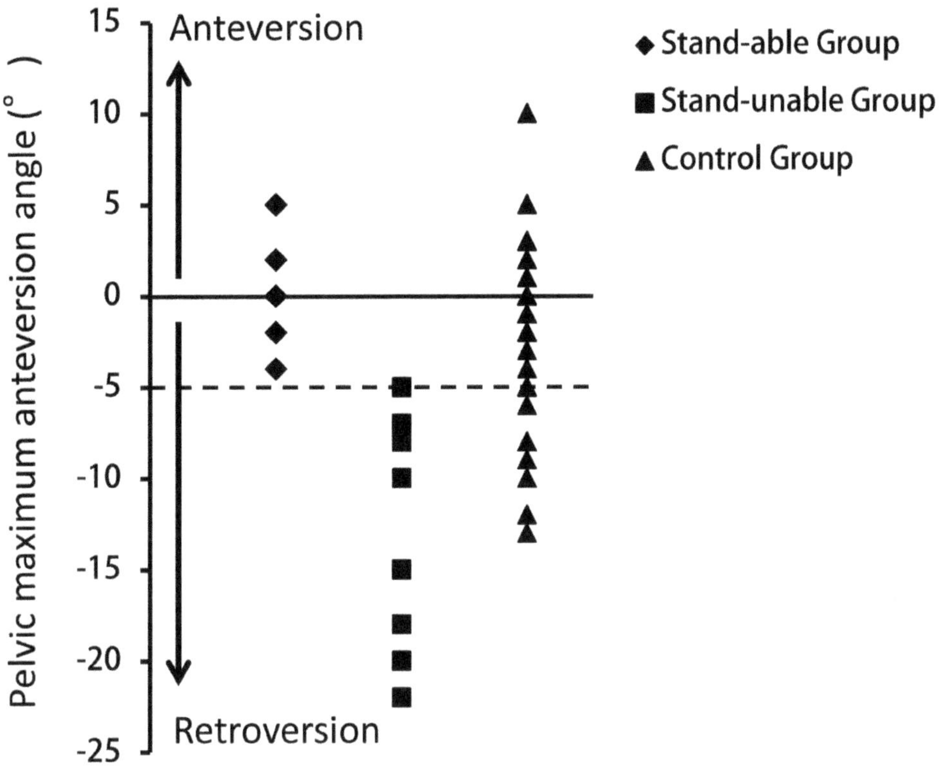

Figure 4. The distribution of the pelvic angles in the stand-able, stand-unable, and control groups.

group, the maximum pelvic anteversion angles were all above −5°; in contrast, to the angles in the stand-unable group were all below −5° (**Figure 4**). The mean and standard deviation of the maximum pelvic anteversion angles in the stand-able, the stand-unable, and control groups were 1.2 ± 2.8°, −12.4 ± 6.1°, and −1.6 ± 5.0°, respectively. The group was found to have a significant main effect ($p < 0.001$). The maximum pelvic anteversion angle in the stand-unable group was significantly smaller than that in the stand-able and control groups (**Table 2**). Thus, it became clear that the maximum pelvic anteversion angle and the range of pelvic motion in the stand-able group were significantly larger in comparison to the stand-unable group.

The maximum pelvic retroversion angles in the stand-able, stand-unable, and control groups ranged from −10° to −30°, −10° to −27°, and −10° to −46°, respectively (**Table 2**). The mean and standard deviation of the maximum pelvic retroversion angles in the stand-able, stand-unable, and control groups were −18.5 ± 5.6°, −19.6 ± 4.6°, and −27.6 ± 8.1°, respectively (**Table 2**). The group was found to have a significant main effect. Significant differences were found between the control group and the stand-able group, and between the control group and the stand-unable group (**Table 2**). The maximum pelvic retroversion angle in the control group was significantly larger than that in both groups of stroke patients (**Table 2**). The maximum pelvic retroversion angles of the stand-able and stand-unable groups did not differ to a statistically significant extent (**Table 2**).

The range of pelvic motion in the in the stand-able, stand-unable, and control groups ranged from 10 to 28°, 0 to 15°, and 9 to 49°, respectively (**Table 2**). The mean and standard deviation of the range of pelvic motion in the stand-able, stand-unable, and control groups was 19.7 ± 5.1°,

		Stand-able group (n = 18)	Stand-unable group (n = 14)	Control group (n = 50)
Maximum pelvic	Mean ± SD	1.2 ± 2.8	−12.4 ± 6.1[a,b]	−1.6 ± 5.0
anteversion angle (º)	Range (max–min	5 to −4	−5 to −22	10 to −13
Maximum pelvic	Mean ± SD	−18.5 ± 5.6[b]	−19.6 ± 4.6[b]	−27.6 ± 8.1
retroversion angle (º)	Range (max–min)	−30 to −10	−27 to − 10	−46 to −10
Range of pelvic motion	Mean ± SD	19.7 ± 5.1[b]	7.2 ± 5.1[b]	25.9 ± 7.6
(º)	Range (max–min)	28 – 10	15 – 0	49 – 9

[a] Significant difference from the stand-able group.
[b] Significant difference from control group.

Table 2. The mean and standard deviation of the pelvic in the stand-able, stand-unable, and control groups [45].

7.2 ± 5.1°, and 25.9 ± 7.6°, respectively (**Table 2**). The range of pelvic motion in the stand-unable group was significantly smaller in comparison to the stand-able and control groups (**Table 2**).

The hypotheses that the maximum pelvic anteversion angle and the range of pelvic motion in the stand-able group would be significantly larger in comparison to the stand-unable group were confirmed. It is noteworthy that there was a cut-off value maximum pelvic anteversion angle that could divide stroke patients into the stand-able and stand-unable groups. The data suggest that, in order for stroke patients to perform the sit-to-stand movement, the maximum pelvic anteversion angle should be greater than −5°.

To smoothly execute the sit-to-stand movement, the pelvis is anteverted to flex the hip joint and the trunk to perform the hip extension moment, reduce the knee extension moment, and project the center of gravity into the base of support [38–43]. The sitting position stability of stroke patients has been shown to be worse than that in age-matched healthy subjects [5, 11, 12]. It has been shown that stroke patients cannot sufficiently flex the hip joint when it is necessary to activate the trunk extensor muscles during sitting [33]. Stroke patients usually sit with kyphosis and pelvic retroversion to avoid falling backward due to insufficient function of the abdominal muscles. Thus, when performing the sit-to-stand movement, stroke patients may need to lean the trunk further forward to shift the center of gravity into the base of support using their feet due to the increased kyphosis and pelvic retroversion. Lecours et al. observed that, when performing the sit-to-stand movement, the trunk angle during forward leaning in stroke patients was larger than that in healthy subjects [35]. Hesse et al. reported that the average center of gravity projection in the base of support in stroke patients was 3 cm behind that of healthy subjects during the seat off phase in the sit-to-stand movement [49]. In addition, when the trunk is flexed, the hip extension moment becomes insufficient due to the lack of pelvic anteversion; thus, stroke patients may depend primarily on the knee extension movement to stand up.

Some studies have reported a high correlation between pelvic inclination in the sitting position and the degree of lumbar lordosis [5] and a strong relationship between the sacral angle of inclination and the degree of lumbar lordosis [46, 47]. Hence, pelvic inclination (anteversion and retroversion) reflects lumbar movement (lordosis and kyphosis). The range of pelvic motion in the stand-unable group was extremely limited, reaching merely 28% of the control group and 36% of the stand-able group. Accordingly, in the stand-unable group, the lumbar spine movement in the sagittal plane (lordosis and kyphosis) was probably limited in comparison to the control group and the stand-able group.

The pelvic angle measurements were conducted in the sitting position while the subject maintained 90° of knee flexion with their feet in contact with the ground. In the sitting position, the hip joints work as pivotal axes in pelvic anteversion and retroversion. One factor that should influence the range of motion of the hip is the extensibility of the hamstrings, which drive the hip and knee as biarticular muscles. Hamstring stretching was shown to improve the pelvic anteversion angle [17] and the mobility of the hip in elderly individuals [16]. The sitting position in this study fixed the knee flexion angle at 90°, which should have increased hamstring tension during the measurement. Thus, it is likely that pelvic anteversion was restrained by the increased tension of the hamstrings.

Cheng et al. reported the following three characteristics of the sit-to-stand movement of stroke fallers, the stroke nonfallers, and healthy subjects: stroke patients, especially fallers, required a significantly longer time to perform the sit-to-stand movement; the rate of increase in vertical force (%BW/sec) in stroke fallers was significantly lower in comparison with nonfallers and healthy subjects; and the overshoot of vertical force (%BW) in stroke fallers was significantly lower than that in nonfallers and healthy subjects [50]. These characteristics of stroke fallers may be associated with their limited pelvic anteversion during the sit-to-stand movement. Messier et al. suggested that, to execute the trunk flexion task, stroke patients used a compensatory strategy that consisted in using mainly the upper trunk flexion because they were unable to tilt their pelvis anteriorly [37]. Thus, our data, which showed that the maximum pelvic anteversion angle of the stand-unable group was significantly smaller than that of the stand-able and control groups, were supported by these reports. Another point of view that should be mentioned is that Prudente et al. suggested that neuromuscular coordination abnormalities occurred in both of the lower limbs of stroke patients during the sit-to-stand movement [51].

On the other hand, since there was no significant difference in the maximum pelvic retroversion angle of the two stroke groups, it becomes clear that this angle does not affect the patient's ability to perform the sit-to-stand movement. However, it was also demonstrated that the range of pelvic motion in stroke patients was markedly restricted in comparison to healthy subjects. In stroke patients, pelvic anteversion appears to be an important factor for regaining the ability to perform the sit-to-stand movement.

4. Relevance to physical therapy

This session demonstrated that the pelvic range of motion was affected by aging, particularly in the anteversion angle, and that the maximum pelvic anteversion angle and the range of pelvic motion in the stand-able group were significantly larger than those in the stand-unable group. Notably, if these patients are to be able to perform the sit-to-stand movement, it is important that they acquire a pelvic anteversion angle of greater than −5°.

The mobility of the lumbar spine, which is associated with the strength and coordination of the trunk and the lower limbs, should be considered as the background of these results. The physical therapy program described below would help as an initial step for improving the physical function of elderly individuals and stroke patients—especially with regard to improving their sit-to-stand movement.

For elderly individuals: (1) pelvic anteversion and retroversion—the patient should maintain a seated position with their feet contacting the floor in a parallel position and move slowly, alternating the pelvis from maximum anteversion to maximum retroversion. They should maintain the same shoulder anteroposterior position throughout the pelvic inclination movements in order to avoid anteroposterior movement of the trunk. (2) Leaning the trunk forward with pelvic anteversion—the patient should lean their trunk forward maintaining pelvic anteversion in a seated position with their feet contacting to the floor. This movement should be performed slowly and repeated. It is important to perceive the increasing load to the lower limb during the leaning of the trunk.

For stroke patients: as soon as the stroke patient has obtained an independent sitting position, the treatment should focus on the mobility of the trunk and weight transfer to the lower limbs, using the same methods as for elderly individuals.

Author details

Hitoshi Asai

Address all correspondence to: asai@mhs.mp.kanazawa-u.ac.jp

Department of Physical Therapy, Graduate Course of Rehabilitation Science, School of Health Sciences, College of Medical, Pharmaceutical and Health Sciences, Kanazawa University, Kanazawa, Japan

References

[1] Been E, Kalichman L: Lumbar lordosis. Spine J. 2014;**14**:87–97. DOI: 10.1016/j.spinee.2013.07.464.

[2] Kasukawa Y, Miyakoshi N, Hongo M, Ishikawa Y, Noguchi H, Kamo K, et al.: Relationships between falls, spinal curvature, spinal mobility and back extensor strength in elderly people. J Bone Miner Metab. 2010;**28**:82–87. DOI: 10.1007/s00774-009-0107-1.

[3] Imagama S, Matsuyama Y, Hasegawa Y, Sakai Y, Ito Z, Ishiguro N: Back muscle strength and spinal mobility are predictors of quality of life in middle-aged and elderly males. Eur Spine J. 2011;**20**:954–961. DOI: 10.1007/s00586-010-1606-4.

[4] Nourbakhsh MR, Moussavi SJ, Salavati M: Effects of lifestyle and work-related physical activity on the degree of lumbar lordosis and chronic low back pain in a Middle East population. J Spinal Disord. 2001;**14**:283–292.

[5] Kuo YL, Tully EA, Galea MP: Video analysis of sagittal spinal posture in healthy young and older adults. J Manipulative Physiol Ther. 2009;**32**:210–215. DOI: 10.1016/j.jmpt.2009.02.002.

[6] Endo K, Suzuki H, Nishimura H, Tanaka H, Shishido T, Yamamoto K: Sagittal lumbar and pelvic alignment in the standing and sitting positions. J Orthop Sci. 2012;**17**:682–686. DOI: 10.1007/s00776-012-0281-1.

[7] Youdas JW, Grarrett TR, Harmsen S, Suman VJ, Carey JR: Lumbar lordosis and pelvic inclination of asymptomatic adults. Phys Ther. 1996;**76**:1066–1081.

[8] Kienbacher T, Paul B, Habenicht R, Starek C, Wolf M, Kollmitzer J, et al.: Age and gender related neuromuscular changes in trunk flexion-extension. J Neuroeng Rehabil. 2015;12:3. DOI: 10.1186/1743-0003-12-3.

[9] Lee ES, Ko CW, Suh SW, Kumar S, Kang IK, Yang JH: The effect of age on sagittal plane profile of the lumbar spine according to standing, supine, and various sitting positions. J Orthop Surg Res. 2014; 9(1):11. DOI: 10.1186/1749-799X-9-11.

[10] Sung PS: Different coordination and flexibility of the spine and pelvis during lateral bending between young and older adults. Hum Mov Sci. 2016;**46**:229–238. DOI: 10.1016/j.humov.2016.01.001.

[11] Intolo P, Milosavljevic S, Baxter DG, Carman AB, Pal P, Munn J: The effect of age on lumbar range of motion: a systematic review. Man Ther 2009;**14**: 596–604. DOI: 10.1016/j.math.2009.08.006.

[12] Sullivan MS, Dickinson CE, Troup JD: The influence of age and gender on lumbar spine sagittal plane range of motion. A study of 1126 healthy subjects. Spine. 1994;**19**:682–686.

[13] Keorochana G, Taghavi CE, Tzeng ST, Morishita Y, Yoo JH, Lee KB, et al.: Magnetic resonance imaging grading of interspinous ligament degeneration of the lumbar spine and its relation to aging, spinal degeneration, and segmental motion. J Neurosurg Spine. 2010;**13**: 494–499. DOI: 10.3171/2010.4.SPINE09515.

[14] Congdon R, Bohannon R, Tiberio D: Intrinsic and imposed hamstring length influence posterior pelvic rotation during hip flexion. Clin Biomech (Bristol, Avon). 2005;**20**:947–951.

[15] López-Miñarro PA, Muyor JM, Belmonte F, Alacid F: Acute effects of hamstring stretching on sagittal spinal curvatures and pelvic tilt. J Hum Kinet. 2012;**31**:69–78. DOI: 10.2478/v10078-012-0007-7.

[16] Feland JB, Myrer JW, Schulthies SS, Fellingham GW, Measom GW: The effect of duration of stretching of the hamstring muscle group for increasing range of motion in people aged 65 years or older. Phys Ther. 2001;**81**:1110–1117.

[17] Muyor JM, López-Miñarro PA, Casimiro AJ: Effect of stretching program in an industrial workplace on hamstring flexibility and sagittal spinal posture of adult women workers: A randomized controlled trial. J Back Musculoskelet Rehabil. 2012;**25**:161–169. DOI: 10.3233/BMR-2012-0323.

[18] O'Sullivan K, O'Sullivan P, O'Sullivan L, Dankaerts W: What do physiotherapists consider to be the best sitting spinal posture? Man Ther. 2012;**17**:432–437. DOI: 10.1016/j.math.2012.04.007.

[19] Franchignoni FP, Tesio L, Ricupero C, Martino MT: Trunk control test as an early predictor of stroke rehabilitation outcome. Stroke. 1997;**28**:1382–1385.

[20] Pollock AS, Durward BR, Rowe PJ, Paul JP: The effect of independent practice of motor tasks by stroke patients: A pilot randomized controlled trial. Clin Rehabil. 2002;**16**:473–480.

[21] Tessem S, Hagstrøm N, Fallang B: Weight distribution in standing and sitting positions, and weight transfer during reaching tasks, in seated stroke subjects and healthy subjects. Physiother Res Int. 2007;**12**:82–94.

[22] Hsieh CL, Sheu CF, Hsueh IP, Wang CH: Trunk control as an early predictor of comprehensive activities of daily living function in stroke patients. Stroke. 2002;**33**:2626–2630.

[23] Loewen SC, Anderson BA: Predictors of stroke outcome using objective measurement scales. Stroke. 1990;**21**:78–81.

[24] Bohannon RW, Barreca SR, Shove ME, Lambert C, Masters LM, Sigouin CS: Documentation of daily sit-to-stands performed by community-dwelling adults. Physiother Theory Pract. 2008;**24**:437–442. DOI: 10.1080/09593980802511813.

[25] Dall PM, Kerr A: Frequency of the sit to stand task: An observational study of free-living adults. Appl Ergon. 2010;**41**:58–61. DOI: 10.1016/j.apergo.2009.04.005.

[26] Riley PO, Schenkman ML, Mann RW, Hodge WA: Mechanics of a constrained chair-rise. J Biomech. 1991;**24**:77–85.

[27] Brunt D, Greenberg B, Wankadia S, Trimble MA, Shechtman O: The effect of foot placement on sit to stand in healthy young subjects and patients with hemiplegia. Arch Phys Med Rehabil. 2002;**83**:924–929.

[28] Genthon N, Vuillerme N, Monnet JP, Petit C, Rougier P: Biomechanical assessment of the sitting posture maintenance in patients with stroke. Clin Biomech (Bristol, Avon). 2007;**22**:1024–1029.

[29] Perlmutter S, Lin F, Makhsous M: Quantitative analysis of static sitting posture in chronic stroke. Gait Posture. 2010;**32**: 53–56. DOI: 10.1016/j.gaitpost.2010.03.005.

[30] van Nes IJ, Nienhuis B, Latour H, Geurts AC: Posturographic assessment of sitting balance recovery in the subacute phase of stroke. Gait Posture. 2008;**28**:507–512. DOI: 10.1016/j.gaitpost.2008.03.004.

[31] Dickstein R, Shefi S, Marcovitz E, Villa Y: Anticipatory postural adjustment in selected trunk muscles in post stroke hemiparetic patients. Arch Phys Med Rehabil. 2004;**85**:261–267.

[32] Dickstein R, Shefi S, Marcovitz E, Villa Y: Electromyographic activity of voluntarily activated trunk flexor and extensor muscles in post-stroke hemiparetic subjects. Clin Neurophysiol. 2004;**115**:790–796.

[33] Davis PM: Problems associated with the loss of selective trunk activity in hemiplegia. In: Right in the middle. New York: Springer-Verlag; 1990. pp. 31–65.

[34] Campbell FM, Ashburn AM, Pickering RM, Burnett M: Head and pelvic movements during a dynamic reaching task in sitting: Implications for physical therapists. Arch Phys Med Rehabil. 2001;**82**:1655–1660.

[35] Lecours J, Nadeau S, Gravel D, Teixera-Salmela L: Interactions between foot placement, trunk frontal position, weight-bearing and knee moment asymmetry at seat-off during rising from a chair in healthy controls and persons with hemiparesis. J Rehabil Med. 2008;**40**:200–207. DOI: 10.2340/16501977-0155.

[36] Verheyden G, van Duijnhoven HJ, Burnett M, Littlewood J, Kunkel D, Ashburn AM: Kinematic analysis of head, trunk, and pelvis movement when people early after stroke reach sideways. Neurorehabil Neural Repair. 2011; **25**: 656–663.

[37] Messier S, Bourbonnais D, Desrosiers J, Roy Y: Dynamic analysis of trunk flexion after stroke. Arch Phys Med Rehabil. 2004;**85**:1619–1624.

[38] Fujimoto M, Chou LS: Dynamic balance control during sit-to-stand movement: An examination with the center of mass acceleration. J Biomech. 2012;**45**:543–548. DOI: 10.1016/j.jbiomech.2011.11.037.

[39] Nikfekr E, Kerr K, Attfield S, Playford DE: Trunk movement in Parkinson's disease during rising from seated position. Mov Disord. 2002;**17**:274–282.

[40] Tully EA, Fotoohabadi MR, Galea MP: Sagittal spine and lower limb movement during sit-to-stand in healthy young subjects. Gait Posture. 2005;**22**:338–345.

[41] Janssen WG, Bussmann HB, Stam HJ: Determinants of the sit-to-stand movement: A review. Phys Ther. 2002;**82**:866–879.

[42] Schenkman M, Berger RA, Riley PO, Mann RW, Hodge WA: Whole-body movements during rising to standing from sitting. Phys Ther. 1990;**70**:638–651.

[43] Ishigaki N, Kimura T, Usui Y, Aoki K, Narita N, Shimizu M, et al.: Effect of ageing on quadriceps muscle strength and on the forward shift of center of pressure during sit-to-stand movement from a chair. J Phys Ther Sci. 2005;**17**:23–28. DOI: 10.1016/j.jbiomech.2011.04.016.

[44] Asai H, Tsuchiyama H, Hatakeyama T, Inaoka PT, Murata K: Age-related changes in maximum pelvic anteversion and retroversion angles measured in the sitting position. J Phys Ther Sci. 2014;**26**:1959–1961. DOI: 10.1589/jpts.26.1959.

[45] Asai H, Tsuchiyama H, Hatakeyama T, Inaoka PT, Murata K: Relationship between the ability to perform the sit-to-stand movement and the maximum pelvic anteversion and retroversion angles in patients with stroke. J Phys Ther Sci. 2015;**27**:985–988. DOI: 10.1589/jpts.27.985.

[46] Kobayashi T, Atsuta Y, Matsuno T, Takeda N: A longitudinal study of congruent sagittal spinal alignment in an adult cohort. Spine. 2004;**29**:671–676.

[47] Amonoo-Kuofi HS: Changes in the lumbosacral angle, sacral inclination and the curvature of the lumbar spine during aging. Acta Anat. 1992;**145**:373–377.

[48] Roach KE, Miles TP: Normal hip and knee active range of motion: The relationship to age. Phys Ther. 1991;**71**:656–665.

[49] Hesse S, Schauer M, Malezic M, Jahnke M, Mauritz KH: Quantitative analysis of rising from a chair in healthy and hemiparetic subjects. Scand J Rehabil Med. 1994;**26**:161–166.

[50] Cheng PT, Liaw MY, Wong MK, Tang FT, Lee MY, Lin PS: The sit-to-stand movement in stroke patients and its correlation with falling. Arch Phys Med Rehabil. 1998;**79**:1043–1046.

[51] Prudente C, Rodrigues-de-Paula F, Faria CD: Lower limb muscle activation during the sit-to-stand task in subjects who have had a stroke. Am J Phys Med Rehabil. 2013;**92**:666–675. DOI: 10.1097/PHM.0b013e318282c87a.

2

Therapeutic Ultrasounds: Physical Basis and Clinical Assessment

Elisa Edi Anna Nadia Lioce, Matteo Novello and Caterina Guiot

Additional information is available at the end of the chapter

Abstract

Improving quality in US physiotherapeutical treatments is mandatory in order to get 'evidence-based' clinical results. This implies quality assurance protocols for the equipment, as well as some tentative dosimetrical approaches to predict local heating in joints following US parameter setting and operative modality. Finally, the possibility of 'personalized therapy' with multimodal (by qualitative and quantitative, e.g. based on sonography) assessment is discussed.

Keywords: ultrasound, physiotheraphy, quality, assessment, dosimetry, phantom

1. Introduction

Therapeutic ultrasound (US) is performed in physiotherapy to treat a variety of inflammatory and post-traumatic diseases. Most of their effects depend on the induction of local thermal increases, which elicit local vasodilatation and toxic substances washout; however, specific and quantitative effects are often misconsidered in physiotherapy units. Moreover, despite its widespread use in rehabilitative practice and a large number of studies, low scientific, statistically assessed evidences of therapeutic US effectiveness are available. As a matter of fact, details about the treatment modalities and the way in which the patients' feedback was collected are often missing. The chapter will be focused on the following points:

(1) Physical bases, technical approach and quality assurance of ultrasonic equipment: technological development and wide use of US within the patient's rehabilitation program

led to the need for a thorough understanding of the interaction between ultrasonic waves and biological matter. Scientific evidence of US therapeutic effectiveness in rehabilitation fields requires more attention on the technical specifications of devices used, and the exact parameters applied in the treatment of selected patients in order to avoid standardized US treatments using 'protocols' and non-specific parameter settings.

(2) Towards physiotherapeutic US dosimetry: treatment planning by the assessment of thermal and mechanical effects. Quantitative assessment of thermal and mechanical effects, and their dependence on the US parameters (frequency, emitted power, pulsed or continue waves) and the treatment modalities (fixed field or massage, duration of the treatment) may be quantitatively investigated on joint mimicking phantoms made of muscle-equivalent agar-based material and bone disks. '*In vitro*' temperature increases can be predicted, which are the 'asymptotical values' in the absence of blood perfusion and other heat dissipation mechanisms.

(3) Customized 'in-patient' assessment of clinical effects: clinical, functional and sonographycal evaluation can/should be performed before and at the end of the US therapy using Numeric Rating Scale, Constant Score, DASH questionnaire and sonographic images supporting clinical and functional data.

2. Main body

2.1. Physical bases, technical approach and quality assurance of ultrasonic equipment

Ultrasound (US) is a mechanical non-ionizing radiation, which propagates in a medium transferring energy from one particle to another by molecular oscillation. The longitudinal waves (compression) can propagate in any medium, while the transverse waves are observed only in solids, because of the weak links that are established between atoms and molecules in the tissue fluids. The ultrasonic wave is mainly longitudinal in biological tissues and characterized by alternating compression and rarefaction of the medium in which it propagates, with variations in pressure within it. Related to the pressure amplitude, which describes the degree of compression and rarefaction and thus the strength per unit area to which the material is subjected in unit of Pascal (Pa = N/m^2) and its multiples (e.g. MPa), also the concept of power of an ultrasound beam, i.e. the energy transmitted in the time unit measured in Watt and that of wave intensity, that is the amount of energy flowing in the time unit through a surface of unit area, perpendicular to the direction of wave propagation (measured in W/cm^2) are important. The intensity varies over time both in the case of continuous wave (CW) or pulsed wave (PW): in particular, the presence of a pulsed field introduces a temporal variation, defining a duty cycle (DC) as the ratio between the pulse duration ultrasound (in time units) and the length of the period, calculated as a percentage. Therapies that employ the US can be divided into two groups: 'high power' and 'low power' [1]. The high power applications include HIFU (high-intensity focused ultrasounds) and lithotripsy, while low-power applications include physical therapy, sonophoresis, sonoporation and gene therapy. When a US wave proceeds from one medium to another, it is partly reflected and partly transmitted, according to the laws of classical mechanics. Each medium is inherently characterized by a complex quantity, the impedance Z, which synthesizes the acoustic characteristics of the medium and quantifies the resistance that the medium itself opposes the passage of sound waves. The acoustic impedance is defined as the product of the density ρ of the medium (kg/m^3) for the propagation velocity c (m/s)

$$Z = \rho c \tag{1}$$

Its unit of measure is Pa s/m or Rayl, named after the famous British scientist Lord Rayleigh, which is equivalent to kg/m^2 s. Propagating in a medium, the acoustic wave is subject to a progressive loss of energy and, more properly, it causes a decrease in the intensity as a function of distance from the source. This is due both to the absorption, where the mechanical energy of the waves is partially converted into heat, and to the scattering, where the interaction between the wave and any inhomogeneous structure in the medium determines a partial diffusion of energy along directions different from that of direct wave propagation.

The overall effect, in a homogeneous medium, is such that a field of wave initial intensity I_0 after a certain distance z, has an intensity, which decreases exponentially according to the equation:

$$I = I_0 \exp(-2\alpha z) \tag{2}$$

where I_0 is the initial intensity I α and the absorption coefficient of the medium (cm^{-1}).

The energy absorption of ultrasound within the medium (and the biological tissues as well) depends on the frequency of the waves, being the coefficient of attenuation α inversely dependent on the square of the frequency. This is responsible for the fact that most of the tissues crossed by US exhibit an increase in the absorption coefficient of at least three times when the frequency is increased from 1 to 3 MHz (e.g. from 0.14 to 0.42 cm^{-1} in fat, from 1.12 to 3.36 cm^{-1} in tendons, from 0.76 to 2.28 cm^{-1} in muscle).

Lower absorption (and therefore higher penetration) of the ultrasonic wave is observable in water and in fact as tissue rich in water, and therefore the local heating is not significant. On the contrary, the absorption is much higher in the bone tissue and tendons [2]. In general, soft tissues absorb about 10–20% of the emitted power per centimetre, while adult bone completely absorbs the ultrasound beam in short distances. US at the frequency of 1 MHz is mainly absorbed by tissues that are 3–5 cm from the probe, and precisely for this property they are recommended for deeper lesions and in patients with subcutaneous fat [3].

Note that 3 MHz frequency is instead recommended for more superficial lesions, e.g. 1–2 cm deep [3, 4]. All the above parameters contribute to the effects of US in biological tissues, which are normally accounted for as 'thermal' and 'non-thermal' effects.

(i) Thermal effects: When US loose energy and the beam is attenuated due to the absorption and dissipation of the ultrasonic energy, heat is produced by vibration, shock, and friction with the cellular and intercellular structures of the crossed tissues. The temperature increase that occurs in the medium can cause chemical or structural changes in biopolymers.

This phenomenon is influenced by both the characteristics of the ultrasound beam (intensity and frequency), the duration of exposure and the characteristics of the crossed tissues (acoustic impedances). Heating is established quickly; however, a thermal equilibrium due to the heat dissipation due to blood flow is reached in longer times.

The thermal effect is most evident at the interface between tissues and in particular at the interface between fat and muscle and at the level of the periosteum. The periosteum, for its anatomical structure and for the continuity with the bone, absorbs a large amount of energy and is therefore easily heated. The thermal elevation generates, as secondary effects, increase in cellular metabolism and vasodilation; in particular, the latter property is important in the use of therapeutic US in physiotherapy, promoting the wash-out of pro-inflammatory substances and pro-algogenic tissues.

(ii) Non-thermal effects: They include cavitation, which consists in the formation, growth and implosion of gas bubbles within the fluid subjected to an ultrasonic field. In general, the cavitation can be seen as the 'break' of a liquid and the consequent formation inside the same of 'cavities' (bubbles) of the liquid containing dissolved gas or vapour itself. This phenomenon occurs in many situations, for example, in boiling water or in proximity to the propeller in rotation of a ship, and in any case when liquids are subject to high and rapid changes in pressure and can occur in the use of therapeutic US or in Doppler ultrasound [5].

The almost instantaneous variations of density, pressure and temperature of the fluid in which propagates the ultrasonic wave can also produce the so-called shock waves or pressure waves which can also be extremely intense. The ultrasonic irradiation of water leads to the formation of the hydroxyl radical and hydrogen radical, which give as the main final products H_2O_2 (hydrogen peroxide) and H_2.

At the cellular level, the production of radicals induced by exposure to the US can also produce biological effects on DNA; theoretical models and experimental studies have shown that the effects of the US on biopolymers especially relate to the degradation pattern of structures [6].

The specificity of the effects stresses the need for accurate quality assessment, by specific acoustic measurements on the clinical equipment.

The performances of the equipment have been investigated, especially on a local basis, by many authors (see Refs. [7–10]), and recommendations have been proposed [11]. For example, the Italian National Institute of Metrological Research (INRIM) settled a protocol [12] for evaluating the ultrasonic power produced by clinical equipment using the Radiation Force Balance (RFB) method. The ultrasonic power is actually determined by the measurement of the force exerted on a target by the sound field generated from an ultrasonic source. The absorbing, connected to the load cell, measures the apparent mass variation due to the ultrasonic field when the source is alternately switched on and off.

2.2. Towards therapeutic US dosimetry: treatment planning by *'in vitro'* parameter evaluation

Most of the therapeutic applications of US induce heating in insonated tissues to obtain some beneficial effect. By increasing temperature a few degrees above the normothermic levels, it is possible to induce temporary vasodilation and increase blood inflow in the affected area, performing a sort of 'thermotherapy'. This mechanism has been proposed as the principal one to explain the therapeutic effects obtained in physiotherapy applications: the analgesic effect in the joints and muscles is mediated by vasodilation and by the subsequent wash-out of pro-algogenic substances and pro-inflammatory with local edema reduction. In addition, the increase of tissue temperature promotes a higher extensibility of soft tissue, and a relaxing effect on the muscles; the increase of cell activity and of the local metabolism caused by the heat stimulates the accelerated wound healing and repair of tendon injuries, ligament, muscle, etc.

Even non-thermal effects (cavitation, emulsion, streaming and sonoporation) may play a role in the physiotherapy field: they, in fact, generate a sort of 'micro-massage' in tissues, promote the increase of local blood flow; furthermore, at cellular and intracellular level, US induces an increase of membrane permeability, calcium uptake, protein synthesis, mast cell degranulation, production of growth factors, angiogenesis, increased fibroblast motility and orientation modification of the fibres collagen and shift the type of collagen (type III to type I) in tissue repair [13].

Controindications to the therapeutic US are possibly due to interference with other electronic devices (e.g. cardiac pacemaker) or are related to the possible effects induced from heat and cavitative phenomena.

US can cause damage to eyes, gonads, encephalon and ears, and the presence of growing cartilage remains the most substantial downside.

It is also recommended not to use the US in body regions where there are implants or metallic synthesis; in fact, given the large difference in impedance between these materials and human tissues, areas of friction and heat accumulation can be formed, with unpredictable consequences.

It is also not recommended for any kind of treatment with US in the presence of malignancies, to avoid the spread in a circle of pathogenic cell lines. In order to get the therapeutic effects described above, it is mandatory to know how US may increase local temperature depending on the setting of the main parameters (frequency, power, etc.) and the modality of treatment (CW, PW, etc.). Although in living tissues many biological mechanisms may dissipate heat, preliminary investigations on '*in vitro*' phantoms may help in finding the 'asymptotic' values of the thermal increase locally induced by the US. Many approaches have been proposed in the literature [see 14–16], based on different test materials exhibiting the same mechanical and thermal properties of homogeneous tissues. Also, numerical simulations have been proposed [17].

The use of 'tissue-mimicking phantoms', coupling different tissues (e.g. muscle-equivalent and bone), as the two presented in **Figure 1** to simulate a superficial (A) and a deep (B) joint, respectively, may be useful to evaluate the temperature at different depth depending on the choice of the parameter values of the equipment and the different treatment protocols [18].

A cartoon cylinder filled with homemade agar-based gel, prepared using bi-distilled water (86.5%), glycerine (5.5%), graphite (2%), agar (2.5%) and salicylic acid (traces) was produced.

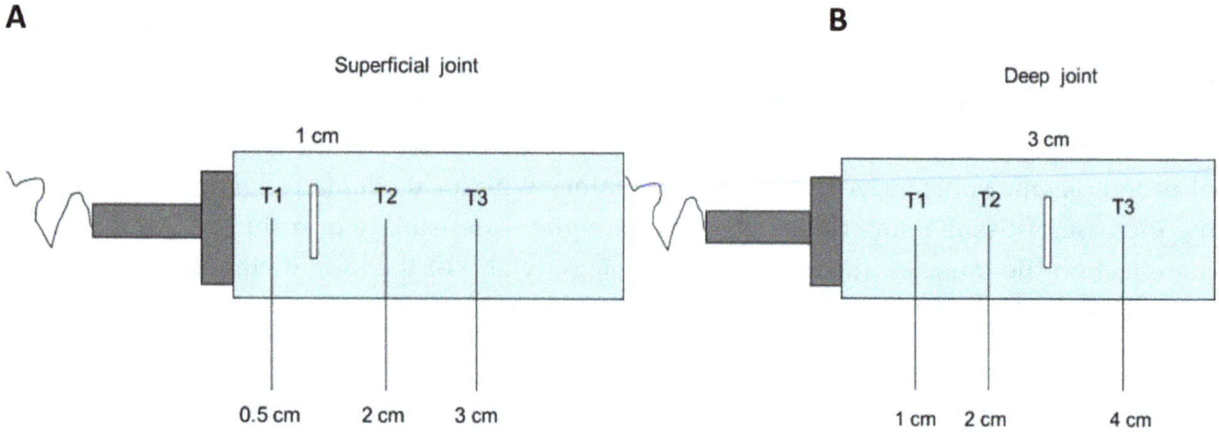

Figure 1. Scheme of the phantoms mimicking a superficial (A) and a deep (B) joint indicating the position of the bone insert and of the temperature probes.

The phantom contains at one end a bovine bone disk 2 (±1) mm thick inserted at 3 (±0.5) cm depth (simulating a 'deep joint') and at the other end a bovine bone disk 1 (±0.5) mm thick inserted at 1 (±0.5) cm (simulating a 'superficial joint') (see **Figure 1A** and **B**). The two disks were always fixed approximately in the centre of the phantom, and their diameter was always smaller than one-half of the phantom diameter. Deep and superficial 'joints' were treated at 1 and 3 MHz, respectively, using the equipment Enraf Nonius SonoPlus. Thermal probes, inserted at different depth, perform temperature measurements before, during and after sonications lasting 5 min and performed using the most diffused clinical treatment modalities (e.g. selecting 'continuous' (CW) or 'pulsed' (PW) wave on the apparatus and keeping fixed or massaging the probe on the phantom surface). Such massaging is performed by small circular movements where the probe is freely and randomly moved on the phantom cross section. The temperature increases detected into the phantoms are different in superficial and deep joints, and mainly depends on the operating mode (CW or PW) and on the fixed or massage modality selected for the probe application. The (min-max) temperature increases detected at different positions (see **Figure 1**) and with different modalities are given in **Table 1**.

3 MHz		
T1	T2	T3
CW: (5–10)	CW: (10–12.5)	CW: (5–15)
PW: (0–2.5)	PW: (0–2.5)	PW: (2.5–5)
1 MHz		
T1	T2	T3
CW: (5–7.5)	CW: (5–7.5)	CW: (2.5–5)
PW: (0–2.5)	PW: (0–2.5)	PW: (0–2.5)

Table 1. (Min-max) temperature increase (in °C).

PW modality is always safer, while CW can induce temperature peaks (hot-spots) at different depth inside the joint.

The local characteristics of the thermal field are not easily predictable based only on wave attenuation, because the bone insertions influence the temperature distribution. In Ref. [18] also the mechanical effects may be detected by inserting contrast agents (e.g. nanobubbles [19]), which can be exploded when the US pressures exceed some threshold values, but no significant differences could be detected in the nanobubbles diameter distribution before and after US sonication. As a consequence, very accurate and anatomically based experimental and numerical models are required to predict the thermal field inside any particular joint or non-homogeneous body region. The starting points should be joints which most benefit from physiotherapeutic US [20, 21], and in particular, shoulders, which often suffer from muscle-skeleton diseases treated with US [22]. On any specific pathologies, such specifically those affecting the shoulders, the previous investigations on phantoms may be useful to perform some 'treatment planning' based on the different anatomical and functional features [23], as shown in **Table 2**.

Clinical diagnosis	US parameters selected (intensity (W/cm^2); frequency (MHz); modalities; duration (minute)
Impingements and tendonitis BBLC	1.5; 3; pulsed (DC 25%); massage; 10
Frozen shoulder	1.5; 1; continuos; massage; 5
Rotator cuff tendinopathy	1.5; 1; pulsed (DC 25%); massage; 10
Suvraspinal tendonitis and bursitis SAD	1.5; 3; pulsed (DC 25%); massage; 10
Impingement syndrome	1.5; 3; pulsed (DC 25%); massage; 10
Tendonitis BBLC	1.5; 1; pulsed (DC 25%); massage; 10
Tendonitis BBLC and rotator cuff	1.5; 3; pulsed (DC 25%); massage; 10

Table 2. 'Treatment planning' based on the different anatomical and functional features in shoulders.

3. 'Customized' 'in-patient' assessment of clinical effects

Very often physiotherapeutic US is applied by using 'protocols' which sets the same treatment parameters values (e.g. duration and treatment modalities) for all patients and all kind of diseases [22, 24]. In everyday clinical practice, it is uncommon to give a definite and quantitative clinical evaluation of the therapeutic results. Whenever it is done, the effectiveness of the US treatment is often evaluated only by using clinical tests and pain scores such as VAS or NRS, which give a subjective rather than quantitative and objective measure. It is therefore necessary, in order to obtain an objective assessment of the US treatment effectiveness, a multimodal evaluation of patients, including clinical, functional and pain scores, and also including a sonographic quantitative investigation of the local phlogosis before and after the treatment and of the final edema resolution. In a pilotal study [23] performed at the Department of Physical Therapy and Rehabilitation Medicine at Turin University from May to September 2015, 10 patients with shoulder pain and functional limitation, due to biceps brachii long head muscle or rotator cuff tendonitis, bursitis, intra-articular effusion, without indication for surgical treatment were enrolled. After a preliminary physiatric evaluation, each patient underwent the US and other successive rehabilitative treatments. The US therapeutic protocol is based on 10 sessions in consecutive days for an overall period of 2 weeks. US treatments were then designed and performed by selecting the specific US parameters values and the treatment modalities for each patient in consideration of their specific clinical, functional and sonographic findings. A preliminary sonographic study was performed in order to quantify edema, phlogosis or effusion. Relevant images were saved and transferred on PC for further elaboration. As far as the other US parameter values are concerned, a careful evaluation of the estimated depth of the lesion suggested the choice of the frequency of 1 MHz for deep and of 3 MHz for more superficial treatment sites. Moreover, depending on the expected therapeutic increase in temperature at the lesion, the 'continuous' modality was selected to induce more heat deposition (for a shorter time) while the 'pulsed' modality, with a Duty Cycle (i.e. the US emitting time related to the total time length of the cycle) selected at 25% was preferred for longer time (10 min) treatments. A multimodal assessment (clinical, functional and sonographic) of the actual pathology was performed before the US treatment, recording shoulder pain, ROM, strength, functional parameters and sonographic imaging. Pain was estimated using the Numeric Rating Scale (NRS), Constant Score and DASH scale were used for shoulder's function evaluation [25, 26]. The same procedure for result assessment was followed at the end of the US treatment. The sonographic examination was performed following a standardized procedure for the shoulder imaging named muskuloskeletal ultrasonographic exam (MSUS) which satisfactorily detects the main findings of the phlogosis process [27]. MSUS exam was performed before the US treatment session and at the end of the last US session by a rehabilitation medical specialist, using an Edge Ultrasound System (Sonosite, USA) connected to a 7.5 MHz frequency probe. To each alteration, a semi-quantitative score from 0 to 3 was given (0: no alterations; 1, 2, 3: low, mid and high inflammatory alterations). Single scores were added to give a total value (total score), indicating the global index of phlogosis of the shoulder in each patient [28]. All patients enrolled in the study showed a significant reduction of shoulder pain and functional limitations with NRS and DASH scores significantly improved. Sonographic imaging supports clinical data, showing a considerable reduction of bursa or tendon's area of phlogosis. The previous experience obtained in monitoring temperatures in a realistic model (phantom) heated with US with different modalities have been useful in defining more precisely which values of the US parameters and which treatment modalities would be optimal to induce the expected thermal effects for each specific patient.

4. Conclusions

Paying attention to the equipment efficiency, the '*in vitro*' and '*in vivo*' investigations of the thermal field induced by any specific US probe working at different modalities and to the specific characteristics of the joint to be treated, US physiotherapy may dramatically improve its quality and possibly show evidences of effectiveness which are nowadays lacking.

Author details

Elisa Edi Anna Nadia Lioce[1], Matteo Novello[2] and Caterina Guiot[2*]

*Address all correspondence to: caterina.guiot@unito.it

1 School of Physical Medicine and Rehabilitation, University of Torino, Torino, Italy

2 Department of Neuroscience, University of Turin, Corso Raffaello, Torino, Italy

References

[1] Ter Haar G. Therapeutic applications of ultrasound. Progress in Biophysics and Molecular Biology. 2007;93(1–3):111–129.

[2] Gann N. Ultrasound: current concepts. Clin Manage. 1991;11(4):64–69.

[3] Dyson M. Mechanisms involved in therapeutic ultrasound. Physioterapy. 2017;93:116–20.

[4] Ziskin M, McDiarmid T, Michlovitz S. Therapeutic ultrasound. Thermal agents in rehabilitation.1st ed. Philadelphia: F. A. Davis; 1990.

[5] Langton N, Vaugan P. Cavitation and the ultrasonic degradation of high polymers. Br J Appl Phys. 1962;13:478–482.

[6] Fuciarelli A, Sisk E, Ronald M, Miller D. Induction of base damage in DNA solutions by ultrasonic cavitation. Free Radic Biol Med. 2017;18(2):231–238.

[7] Allen KBattye C. Performance of ultrasonic therapy instruments. Physiotherapy. 1978;64(6): 173–4.

[8] Rivest M, Quirion De Girardi C, Seaborne D, Lambert J. Evaluation of therapeutic ultrasound devices: performance stability over 44 weeks of clinical use. Physiother Can. 1987;39(2):77–86.

[9] Hekkenberg R, Oosterbaan W, Beekum W. Evaluation of ultrasound therapy devices. Physiotherapy. 1986;72(8):390–395.

[10] Pye S, Milford C. The performance of ultrasound physiotherapy machines in Lothian Region, Scotland, 1992. Ultrasound Med Biol. 1994;20(4):347–59.

[11] National Council on Radiation Protection and Measurements. Exposure Criteria for Medical Diagnostic Ultrasound, I: Criteria based on Thermal mechanisms. 1st ed. Bethesda: MD: National Council on Radiation Protection and Measurements; 1992.

[12] Durando G, Fernicola V. Technical Report 16/2012. 1st ed. Istituto Nazionale di Ricerca Metrologica; Torino, 2012.

[13] Nadler N, Weingand K, Kruse. The physiologic basis and clinical applications of cryotherapy and thermotherapy for the pain practitioner. Pain Physician. 2017;3(7):395–399.

[14] Browne J, Ramnarine K, Hoskins P. Assessment of the acoustic properties of common tissue-mimicking test phantoms. Ultrasound Med Biol. 2017;(7):1053–1060.

[15] Shaw A, Pay N, Preston R. Proposed standard thermal test object for medical ultrasound. Ultrasound Med Biol. 1999;(1):121–132.

[16] Sun, Pye, Moran. The speed of sound and attenuation of an IEC agar-based tissue-mimicking material for high frequency ultrasound application. Ultrasound Med Biol. 2012;38(7):1262–1270.

[17] Teixeira C, Pereira W, Ruano A, Ruano M. On the possibility of non-invasive multilayer temperature estimation using soft-computing methods. Ultrasonics. 2010;50(1):32–43.

[18] Lioce E, Novello M, Durando G, Bistolfi A, Actis M, Massazza G et al. Therapeutic ultrasound in physical medicine and rehabilitation: characterization and assessment of its physical effects on joint-mimicking phantoms. Ultrasound Med Biol. 2014;40(11):2743–2748.

[19] Cavalli R, Bisazza A, Giustetto P, Civra A, Lembo D, Trotta G et al. Preparation and characterization of dextran nanobubbles for oxygen delivery. Int J Pharm. 2009;381(2):160–165.

[20] Van Der Windt D, Van DerHeijden G, Van DerBerg S, Ter Riet G, De Winter A, Bouter L. Ultrasound therapy for musculoskeletal disorders: a systematic review. Pain. 1999;81(3):257–271

[21] Loyola-Sánchez A, Richardson J, MacIntyre N. Efficacy of ultrasound therapy for the management of knee osteoarthritis: a systematic review with meta-analysis. Osteoarthritis Cartilage. 2010;18(9):1117–1126.

[22] Desmeules F, Boudreault J, Roy J, Dionne C, Frémont P, MacDermid J. The efficacy of therapeutic ultrasound for rotator cuff tendinopathy: a systematic review and meta-analysis. Phys Ther Sport. 2015;16(3):276–284.

[23] Lioce ECG. Personalized Therapeutic Ultrasound in Shoulder Disease: Multimodal Assessment and Results. J Nov Physiother. 2016;06(02):2743–2748.

[24] Analan P, Leblebici B, Adam M. Effects of therapeutic ultrasound and exercise on pain, function, and isokinetic shoulder rotator strength of patients with rotator cuff disease. J Phys Ther Sci. 2015;27(10):3113–3117.

[25] Constant CMurely A. A clinical method of functional assessment of the shoulder. Clin Orthop Relat Res. 1987;214:160–164.

[26] Hudak P, Amadio P, Bombardier C. Development of an upper extremity outcome measure: the DASH. Am J Ind Med. 1996;(29):602–609.

[27] Schneebeli A, Egloff M, Giampietro A, Clijsen R, Barbero M. Rehabilitative ultrasound imaging of the supraspinatus muscle: intra- and interrater reliability of thickness and cross-sectional area. J Bodywork Movement Ther. 2014;18(2):266–272

[28] Iagnocco A, Perella F, Magrini L, Valesini G. Ultrasonographic assessment of the response to Etanercept treatment in patients with rheumatoid arthritis. Reumatismo. 2006;58(3): 233–238.

3

Special Rehabilitation Treatment Methodology: INFINITY method®

Michaela Tomanova

Additional information is available at the end of the chapter

Abstract

The INFINITY method® is a special rehabilitation method developed at the Rehabilitation Institute in Brandys nad Orlici, Czech Republic. It is a kinesitherapy approach based on neurophysiology, biomechanics, and anatomy. The method is employed during rehabilitation of patients with functional and/or structural changes of the musculoskeletal system. It allows adjustment of the postural control system of the body, which gradually improves balance and symmetrization of the whole body in space, thus creating a precondition for better quality and more efficient movement. Specifically, therapy movements can be active and/or passive, and great variability of active movements is a perfect advantage for autotherapy. Now, the corrective therapeutic movement and posture can be conscious, meaning there is an increased awareness and control of the patient's whole body, and/or subconscious, which is based on a reflex therapy. In both cases, straightening and balancing of the patient's body are increased. This method positively affects the musculoskeletal system and quality of the soft tissue, such as the muscle and connective tissue. Thanks to its well-crafted methodology, easily practiced active exercises, and passive therapy performed with the help of a therapist, the method works well for patients with painful disorders of the spine and joints.

Keywords: INFINITY method®, low back pain, rehabilitation, musculoskeletal model, plantography, posturography

1. Introduction

Traditional physical therapy or fitness training has emphasized strengthening of individual muscles. It has been proposed that the skill or the quality of the movement pattern that is used could be more important than achievement of muscle strength [1]. We have observed a demand for rehabilitation treatment based on the knowledge of modern science in our clinical practice. Therefore, a new rehabilitation technique has been developed with emphasis on simple comprehensible principles, allowing a wide range of variations in therapy and exercises. The new method is applicable for patients with a limited range of motion, for patients after surgery, as well as for patients sustaining moderate diseases of the musculoskeletal system like low back pain (LBP). The new method can also be preventative, keeping people healthy and fit. The specific aim was to develop a large series of autotherapeutic exercises. The method has been developed, and we keep on improving it by incorporating original theoretical knowledge and experience gained in everyday clinical practice.

Our special rehabilitation method is called the INFINITY method®. Its name comes from the English word *infinity* because it utilizes movement in a figure of eight as a key segment of the exercises. The INFINITY method® is a special rehabilitation method developed at the Rehabilitation Institute in Brandys nad Orlici, Czech Republic.

The method has been verified in several clinical studies. We hypothesized that there would be certain differences in all measured values of patients before and after rehabilitation treatment with the INFINITY method®. The aim of one study was to confirm the relationship between the values of the center of force (COF) that were measured and the pain perceived by low back pain patients using a visual analogue scale (VAS), before and after therapy. The results were then used to assess the effectiveness of the INFINITY method® for treatment of patients with LBP [2]. This clinical study of 331 patients showed considerable improvement in all measured parameters. Characteristics of individual groups are described in **Table 1**.

Gender		
Females	234	(70.7%)
Males	97	(29.3%)
Mean age (SD)		
Females	61.5 ± 13.32	
Males	61 ± 12.46	
SD, standard deviation.		

Table 1. Characteristics of patients with low back pain.

2. INFINITY method®

The INFINITY method® presents a kinesitherapeutic approach based on neurophysiology, biomechanics, and anatomy. It is a unique rehabilitation method used in rehabilitation and movement medicine, and it can be applied in patients with musculoskeletal system diseases. The method is employed during rehabilitation of patients with functional and/or structural changes of the musculoskeletal system. It allows adjustment of the postural control system of the body, which gradually improves balance and symmetrization of the whole body in space, thus creating a precondition for better quality and more efficient movement. Specifically, therapy movements can be active and/or passive. The great variability of active movements is advantageous for autotherapy, thanks to its well-crafted methodology, easily practiced active exercises, and passive therapy performed with the help of a therapist. The method works well for patients with painful disorders of the spine and joints. The corrective therapeutic movement and posture can either be conscious, meaning there is an increased awareness and control of the patient's whole body, and/or subconscious, which is based on a reflex therapy. In both cases, straightening and balancing of the patient's body are increased. This method positively affects the musculoskeletal system and quality of the soft tissue, such as muscle and connective tissue. The INFINITY method® can even be applied in the acute phase when a patient may be suffering from intense pain. Therapy and exercises are based on improvement of stabilization, centering, coordination, perception, and control of the entire body, including the spine. The INFINITY method® is a method of rehabilitation aimed at stabilizing and strengthening the thoracic, back, and abdominal muscles, including deep stabilization system of the spine (DSS) with connection to diaphragmatic breathing. At the same time, it enables increased mobility and flexibility via relaxation, stretching, and mobilization of soft tissues of the musculoskeletal system.

3. Types of movement

The method uses three types of 3D movement. Components of INFINITY method® include visualization, micromovement, and macromovement. Visualization as therapy is especially used by more disabled patients. Micromovement (which is movement in millimeters) can be also used by disabled patients or by patients with a limited range of motion, because of intensive pain or restrictions and other medical indications, for example, patients with discopathy. Micromovement is a fine movement that minimally loads the motor system, improves muscle activity, and trains the higher motor centers in the central nervous system. Macro-movement (which is movement in centimeters similar to tai chi movements) allows this application to be used by less-disabled patients. The macromovement component can also be used as a prevention of low back pain. 3D movements in the continuous figure eight and linear motions are performed from the center of the body and back to stabilize and centralize the whole body and spine, for example, in low back pain patients. The center of the body is identified as the patient's visualization of the body's median. INFINITY method® works in different part of the body. Individual areas of the body targeted by INFINITY include the head, chest, pelvis, spine, and so on. Additionally, the whole body and/or upper and/or lower extremities can be activated by INFINITY. The therapy includes special exercises and training of breathing, which allow both muscle relaxation and activation of several muscle groups, including the deep stabilization system, as well as improving psychological factors.

4. Indications

The method presents many opportunities in the therapy of patients sustaining musculoskeletal system diseases, and it has almost no contraindication if applied well. Patients can visualize exercise in their mind, and in normal patients, this type of visualization activates muscles and the central nervous system with no overload or damage. The same is valid for micromovements where the range of movements is in millimeters.

The method is very effective when applied in patients with muscle imbalance, patients with changes of muscle tonus (e.g. trigger and tender points), and patients with low tissue quality (mainly older patients). We have achieved excellent results in patients with scoliosis, posture malfunction, as well as patients with spinal pain.

Rehabilitation treatment can also be given to patients with degenerative changes of the musculoskeletal system affecting function, structure, and pain (such as spondyloarthritis, spondylosis including root syndromes, and osteoarthritis of other joints), to patients after surgery (orthopedic and trauma surgeries like arthroscopy, joint replacement), and to patients after other traumas.

5. Statistical studies

We evaluated the efficacy of the rehabilitation therapy using the plantar pressure measurement platform, for example, the pressure mat system MatScan (Tekscan, USA). The patients were assessed using plantography and posturography, during both the start and the completion of treatment. During the measurement process, the patients stood up and had their eyes open. The results were compared before and after the INFINITY method® therapy. We compared the values measured before and after the intervention of the INFINITY method® [2]. Several variables were measured such as bilateral pressure on the right and left soles of the feet, gravitational forces between both soles, anteroposterior (A-P), and mediolateral (M-L) displacement of COF [3] (COF being the center of gravity of the body between both soles of the feet). During a 30-second period, we recorded the change in value of the COF and the area defined by the movement of A-P and the M-L of the COF. These data allowed us to calculate the difference in COF and COF area before and after INFINITY method® therapy. A total of six dependent variables were statistically evaluated. Five of these variables were the posturographic measurements and are presented in **Table 2**.

Feet parallel, eyes open			**Feet parallel, eyes closed**		
Parameter	**Mean (cm)**	**SD (cm)**	**Parameter**	**Mean (cm)**	**SD (cm)**
Area before*	2.76	4.88	Area before*	3.09	4.46
Area after*	2.23	3.01	Area after*	2.40	5.47
Dist before	37.72	16.64	Dist before*	50.30	30.56
Dist after	36.97	15.26	Dist after*	46.68	27.50
Var before	0.03	0.02	Var before*	0.04	0.03
Var after	0.03	0.02	Var after*	0.04	0.02
AP Exc before	2.75	1.25	AP Exc before*	3.25	1.61

Feet parallel, eyes open			Feet parallel, eyes closed		
Parameter	**Mean (cm)**	**SD (cm)**	**Parameter**	**Mean (cm)**	**SD (cm)**
AP Exc after	2.67	1.14	AP Exc after*	2.87	1.44
ML before*	1.80	1.39	ML before*	1.77	1.53
ML after*	1.56	1.08	ML after*	1.48	1.41

Feet parallel, eyes open			Feet parallel, eyes closed		
Parameter	**Mean (cm)**	**SD (cm)**	**Parameter**	**Mean (cm)**	**SD (cm)**
Area before*	4.43	3.49	Area before*	9.27	8.12
Area after*	4.03	3.80	Area after*	7.90	6.19
Dist before*	49.92	23.79	Dist before	87.60	45.79
Dist after*	46.85	22.03	Dist after	85.34	41.53
Var before	0.04	0.03	Var before	0.07	0.05
Var after	0.04	0.03	Var after	0.07	0.04
AP Exc before	2.94	1.22	AP Exc before*	4.25	1.82
AP Exc after	2.93	3.32	AP Exc after*	3.94	1.66
ML before*	2.98	1.27	ML before*	4.48	2.27
ML after*	2.76	1.44	ML after*	4.21	1.75

Dist, distance; Var, variability; AP, anteroposterior directions; ML, medial-lateral directions.
*Statistical significance at $p < .05$.

Table 2. Posturographic parameters—results of the paired samples test.

A VAS was used to assess each patient's personal assessment of pain [2]. Given the results, it can be stated that due to the rehabilitation process, there was a statistically significant improvement of the above parameters (**Table 3**). There were significant differences in measurements between pre- and post-rehabilitation treatment.

Measurements in the antero-posterior direction of movement of the COF, medial-lateral movement of the COF, the area covered, the COF distance, and the variation of COF were all reduced. The subjective assessment of pain also showed a statistically significant reduction. The results of this study show that the INFINITY method® rehabilitation treatment resulted

Parameter	Mean (cm)	SD (cm)
VAS before*	5.3	1.78
VAS after*	3.5	1.77

* Statistical significance at $p < .0001$.

Table 3. VAS parameter—results of the paired samples test.

in statistically significant improvements in the observed plantographic and posturographic parameters of stance stability. Subjective pain using VAS was also much lower, which must be considered as being extremely beneficial to overall patient health [2].

There are various rehabilitation techniques employed in clinics that exhibit different success for the given diagnosis. Our empirical evidence initiated further theoretical studies of the musculoskeletal system based on mathematical modeling (**Figure 1**).

The mathematical models can assess muscle activity of various motion patterns and can validate the effectiveness of the motion pattern used in the INFINITY method®. It was hypothesized that a figure of eight motion contributes to the stabilization and the strengthening of trunk muscles, including the deep stabilization system. Advances in mathematical modeling and technology are creating new opportunities that may be able to quantify the effect of physiotherapy on the lumbar spine [4]. The overall aim of one particular study was to compare the effect of a figure of eight movement on deep muscle activation and spinal load with simple movements during rehabilitation.

The spinal muscle and L5/S1 load were assessed using mathematical modeling. The model was designed to study the INFINITY method® that is primarily based on small micromotions [2]. The study indicates that a more complex motion provides higher frequency load to passive structures and requires complex activation of muscles enhancing neural system involvement. The conclusions were that the complexity of motion pattern directly influences the spinal load and muscle activation pattern [5]. Simple pendulum-like or circular-like motions do induce harmonic muscle activation and spinal load. But the results show that the figure of eight pattern (∞) proposed in the INFINITY method® doubles the frequency of spinal loading while conditions complex muscle activation patterns that could induce remodeling in passive structures, strengthen active structures, and effectively train the central neural system (**Figure 2**).

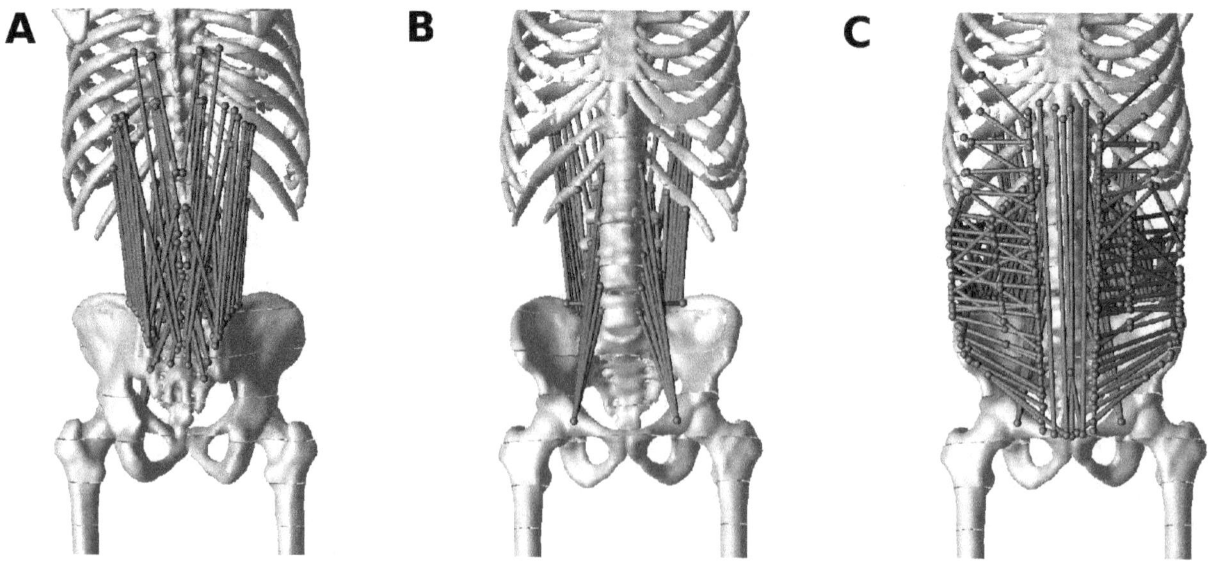

Figure 1. A Rear view, B Front view - spine muscles, C Front view - abdominal muscles.

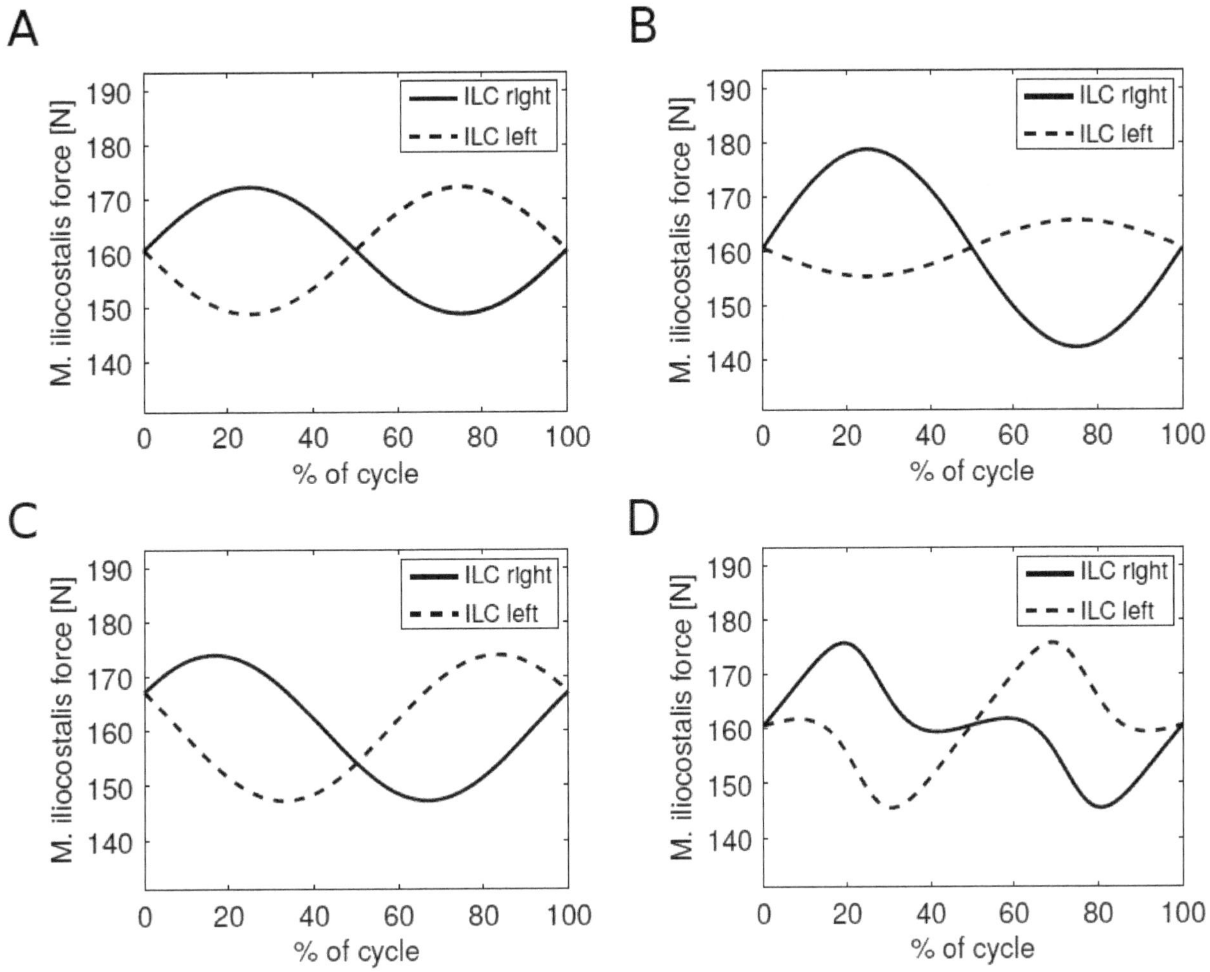

Figure 2. Movement patterns.

6. Conclusions

The INFINITY method® is a rehabilitation therapy and exercises developed by Michaela Tomanová, MD, PhD, who is the head physician and director of a large rehabilitation clinic in the Czech Republic. The clinic has 220 beds. Based on clinical experience gained in the years of practice, Dr. Tomanová has developed a system of diagnosis and therapy for patients with musculoskeletal problems. The basis of INFINITY method® was laid out in the beginning of this century, and the method has been improved and developed since then. The method has been based on knowledge gained in works published already.

The method utilizes motion in all three planes of the body and in all possible directions. The method primarily addresses muscles and connective tissues that are used in an incorrect manner due to our modern lifestyle, that is, muscles that are overloaded or underloaded. Corrective motion patterns similar to daily activities are used. Relaxation and strengthening of individual muscles and muscle groups occur during therapy, and the quality of connective and soft tissues is influenced as well. The muscle tone is normalized. Movements in an upright standing position are necessary to correct the optimal body posture, including neutral positions. Therapy and exercises gradually and automatically lead to improvement in posture. The method also improves body segment positions because it impacts the whole posture and spine stabilization with the help of gravity effects. The emphasis is on proprioception, exteroception, sense of position, and sense of movement, as well as the patient's awareness of his or her own body and its motion.

The considerable advantage of the INFINITY method® is a wide range of autotherapy techniques, well-understood principles, and a wide range of variations. Using these treatments and exercises, the musculoskeletal system is loaded, but not overloaded, and it activates and often relaxes these structures as well. The patient experiences whole-body stabilization after treatment and practices the method with the assistance of a therapist. The treatment also results in biomechanical rebalancing and body symmetrization in a space allowed by structures of the musculoskeletal and central neural system. This should also result in improvement in quality and effectiveness of the motion, and also in improvement in connective and soft-tissue quality and functionality (muscles, ligaments, tendons) as well as a reduction of pain in the musculoskeletal system.

Author details

Michaela Tomanova

Address all correspondence to: sekretariat@rehabilitacniustav.cz

Brandýs nad Orlicí Rehabilitation Clinic, Brandýs nad Orlicí, Czech Republic

References

[1] Janda, V. On the concept of postural muscles and posture in man. Aust. J. Physiother., 1983, 29(3):83–4.

[2] Tomanova, M., Lippert-Grüner, M., Lhotska, L. Specific rehabilitation exercise for the treatment of patients with chronic low back pain. J. Phys. Ther. Sci., 2015, 27(8):2413–7.

[3] Brumagne, S., Janssens, L., Knapen, S., et al. Persons with recurrent low back pain exhibit a rigid postural control strategy. Eur. Spine J., 2008, 17:1177–84.

[4] Daniel, M. Role of optimization criterion in static asymmetric analysis of lumbar spine load. Wien. Med. Wochenschr., 2011, 161(19–20):477–85.

[5] Cadova, M., Vilimek, M., Daniel, M. A comparative study of muscle force estimates using Huxley's and Hill's muscle model. Comput. Methods Biomech. Biomed. Eng., 2012, 17(4):1–7.

4

Conservative Management of Chronic Venous Insufficiency

Özlem Çinar Özdemir and Mahmut Surmeli

Additional information is available at the end of the chapter

Abstract

Chronic venous insufficiency (CVI) is a common medical condition with major socioeconomic impact. Prevalence in adult population is estimated to be 5–30%. Its pathology is based on venous hypertension on the lower extremities. This results in edema, subcutaneous fibrosis, pigmentation, chronic pain and ulceration. The severity of chronic venous disease is closely related to the magnitude of venous hypertension. Treatment options for CVI include medical, interventional, surgical and physical treatments. The initial management of CVI involves conservative approaches to reduce symptoms and prevent development of secondary complications and progression of disease. It includes the elevation of the limb together with the supportive methods, pharmacotherapy and structured exercise program, as well as complex decongestive physiotherapy (CDP), intermittent pneumatic compression (IPC), compression stocking (CS), patient education and kinesio tape. CVI is a chronic disease that needs a lifelong care. In this review, we present a discussion about pathophysiology and risk factors for CVI development and conservative treatment options.

Keywords: chronic venous insufficiency, conservative treatment, compression, exercise

1. Introduction

Chronic venous insufficiency (CVI) is described as the inadequacy of the venous system to return blood to the heart [1]. It is common condition which affects many people around the world [2] and denotes some symptoms ranging from minor reticular veins to serious skin changes such as lipodermatosclerosis or venous leg ulcers [1, 3].

CVI is commonly seen in lower limbs. The prevalence of CVI varies in the populations, but it is reported that the prevalence of CVI ranges between 25 and 40% and 10 and 20% in women and men, respectively [4–6]. Because of its clinical characteristics, it restricts individual's daily activities and has great impact on physical and psychosocial status, as well as socioeconomic status [7].

There are many treatment options such as medical, pharmacological and conservative methods used in CVI. Among these, because of being invasive and causing less adverse effects than other methods, conservative approaches are commonly used to treat CVI [8]. On account of this, we aimed to give information about the conservative approaches used in the treatment of CVI in this chapter. However, due to the different structure of the venous system, to understand the effectiveness of the treatment and how it works, it is necessary to comprehend well the anatomy and pathophysiology of the venous system.

2. Anatomy of the venous system

The venous blood flow in the lower extremity is located at three positions, which are superficial, deep and perforating veins [9].

More than 80% of the blood flow in the lower extremity occurs through the deep veins. The deep veins accompany the arteries and run deep to the muscles and fascia [10, 11]. It includes the posterior tibial vein, anterior tibial vein, femoral vein, profunda femoris vein and common femoral vein in the leg. It also includes the popliteal vein and femoral vein in the thigh, and the external iliac vein, internal iliac vein, common iliac vein and inferior vena cava in the pelvis [12].

The major axial veins are accompanied by matching the venae comitantes in the calf. These veins that accompany the posterior tibial and peroneal veins are particularly large (up to 10 mm in diameter in male) and participate in the muscle pump mechanism for the return of blood from the legs to the heart. In addition, the medial and lateral heads of the gastrocnemius and soleus muscles include vein pairs in these muscles (the calf) that accompany the major arteries. These usually have a large diameter and participate in the calf muscle pump. The calf veins drain into the popliteal vein. Once the popliteal vein has entered the thigh, it is known as the femoral vein. The deep femoral veins which open into the femoral veins derived from the common femoral vein in the inguinal triangle drain the thigh muscles. This drains into the great saphenous vein and is the major point of the venous return in the lower extremity [12].

The superficial compartment lies between the dermis and the deep fascia [12]. Duplex scanning has resulted in recognition of a saphenous subcompartment and saphenous fascia. The vena saphena magna and vena saphena parva are intermediate superficial veins. The VSM is the longest vein in the human body [10, 11].

These veins connect the superficial venous system to the deep venous system. There are approximately 150 perforating veins in each lower extremity and a few of them have clinical significance. The medial calf perforators are very important at this point [12].

The perforating veins are divided into direct and indirect perforating veins. While direct perforating veins provide a connection between the superficial and deep axial veins, indirect perforating veins provide blood drainage from the superficial venous system and join other veins in the muscles [13].

Bicuspid valves in superficial veins provide one-way venous blood flow towards the heart. The frequency of valves is particularly higher below the knee. Valves are large (median 7–10, range 4–13) and placed closer in the small saphenous vein. The frequency of valves increases from proximal to distal in the deep veins. Deep leg veins, peroneal veins and posterior and anterior tibial veins contain plenty of valves which are arranged at approximately 2 cm intervals. However, the common femoral vein usually has one valve. In addition, it must be emphasized that there is only one valve (and sometimes, there is no valve in 37% of the reported cases) in external iliac and common femoral veins, which are proximal to the saphenofemoral junction. The common iliac and vena cava veins have no valves [14].

3. Physiology and hemodynamics of the venous circulation

The primary function of the venous circulation is to return blood to the heart. Effective venous return requires the interaction of a central pump, a pressure gradient, a peripheral venous pump and competent venous valves [14].

Pressures on the vessels are determined by different mechanism. While pressure in arterial vessels is generated mainly by muscular contractions of the heart, the gravity is the main factor that determines the pressure in the venous system. When the body is in a horizontal resting position, pressures in the veins of the lower limb, in the chest, abdomen and arm are similar. On the other hand, when the body goes to the upright position, significant changes occur in the values of these pressures, especially in the venous system. In presence of the upright position, there is an accumulation of approximately 500 ml of blood in the lower extremities. Venous valves play a very important role in the return of blood to the heart from the lower extremities, especially in this position. Direct observation of human venous valves has been made possible by specialized ultrasound techniques [14].

One of the important tasks of the venous valves is to be released during exercise. Supporting the antegrade flow of the venous from the superficial veins to the deep during exercise is the essential part of this important task. Muscle activity through exercise creates volume and pressure changes in the venous system, especially in the calf. While there is no apparent flow in the resting position; with the beginning of the heel strike, the venous plexus under the heel and the plantar surface of the foot (Bejar's plexus) begin to empty from the foot and ankle towards the proximal end of the calf. Then, through calf contraction the blood within the deep veins on the calf is transported into the deep veins of the thigh [14].

In the upright position, the arterial blood pressure is approximately 100 mmHg and the venous pressure is 8 mmHg. The arteriovenous pressure gradient is 92 mmHg. However, this situation changes in the upright position. After 15 min of immobilization, circulating blood volume decreases up to 20% and the velocity of the blood flow decreases. In addition, effective ultrafiltration pressure exceeds effective resorption pressure due to passive hyperemia occurring in blood capillaries. As a result, the flow moves from the blood vessel system to the interstitium in the lower extremities. This situation changes during walking. The venous blood pressure falls up to 25 mmHg in the leg due to the venous leg pump which consists of the calf muscles, joints, skin, fascia and venous valves. The contraction of the calf muscles moves the blood from the subfascial veins into the heart. The venous blood pressure of 25 mmHg is considerably lower than 100 mmHg but higher than 8 mmHg. This is called as physiological ambulatory venous hypertension. However, it can be tolerated by veins under normal conditions [15].

4. Pathophysiology

Clinical manifestations of CVI occur primarily due to ambulatory venous hypertension in the upright position or during ambulation. These result in clinical sign of edema, subcutaneous fibrosis, pigmentation, chronic pain and ulceration. The severity of chronic venous disease is closely related to the magnitude of venous hypertension. Patients with ambulatory venous pressures less than 40 mmHg have had a lower incidence of venous ulceration compared to patients with ambulatory venous hypertension greater than 80 mmHg [16].

The indications of ambulatory venous pressure are complex. Determinants of ambulatory venous pressure include venous reflux and obstruction as well as calf muscle pump function [17]. Studies have shown that calf muscle pump dysfunction occurs early in the development of CVI and it does not worsen with skin changes and ulceration [18].

In the normal case, the lower extremity muscle pumps and valves limit the accumulation of blood in the lower extremity veins. Failure of the lower extremity muscle pump is associated with peripheral venous insufficiency due to outflow obstruction, musculofascial weakness, loss of joint motion or valvular impairment. However, an effective peripheral pump becomes a compensator for some degrees of reflux and obstruction and prevents symptoms of CVI [13].

When the system operates normally, the ambulatory venous pressure in the superficial system is maintained between 20 and 30 mmHg. The superficial venous pressure may increase up to 60–90 mmHg in cases of venous occlusion, venous valve insufficiency or inappropriate muscle contraction. As mentioned above, this level causes venous hypertension. Thus, it shows that anatomic, physiologic and histological changes associated with chronic venous insufficiency begin. Chronic venous hypertension leads to some histological changes in the capillary bed, which is known as venous hypertensive microangiopathy. These changes include the folding and expansion of the capillary bed and increased endothelial surface [19].

Valvular failure is associated with a rapid recovery time after muscle contraction. If deep venous valves are insufficient, blood simply oscillates within the deep veins and there is no reduction in pressure. Chronic venous hypertension or persistent pressure results in pathological effects in the deep subcutaneous tissues such as edema, pigmentation, fibrosis and ulceration [13].

5. Risk factors for CVI

Risk factors for development of CVI include advanced age, female sex, heredity and trauma to the extremities. Lower limb injuries are a risk factor in women. Age is linked at all levels of the disease in both genders. Older age, Hispanic white ethnicity and family history are risk factors for

CVI. For visible disease, CVI is about twice as common in women than in men. It was reported in the Edinburgh study that CVI was observed two-fold more in men than women [20].

Pregnancy is a critical period for the lower extremity venous system [21], and more than 30% of varicose veins develop only in this period [22, 23]. The reason is considered to be increase in the venous pressure due to the increased blood volume. Moreover, the compression of the iliac veins is an important factor in the later stages of pregnancy. Venous function is undoubtedly influenced by hormonal changes. In particular, progesterone which is released by the corpus luteum stabilizes the uterus by causing relaxation of smooth muscle fibers. This directly affects venous function. Although progesterone affects varicosities in pregnancy at first sight, estrogen also has profound effects [24].

Previous pregnancy, less oral contraceptive use, obesity and mobility at work in women, and height and straining at stool in men may be implicated in the development of reflux [25]. HRT duration or parity is positively associated with all levels of functional disease seen in women. Coughlin et al. [26] reported that multiparity was related with varicose veins in pregnant women.

6. Symptoms for CVI

Symptoms and signs of CVI include hyperpigmentation, stasis dermatitis, pain, cramping, chronic edema and venous ulcers. Approximately 3–11% of the adult population has skin changes and edema due to CVI [27]. Edema was about 50% more common in men than women [28]. In the Edinburg study it was reported that there were more edema in women; however, the CVI was much more common in men [29].

Edema begins in the perimalleolar region and ascends up the leg. Sense of discomfort in legs is often referred to as weight or pain after standing for a long time and it is relieved by leg elevation. Cutaneous changes include skin hyperpigmentation with hemosiderin deposition and eczematous dermatitis. This fibrotic process produces lipodermatosclerosis and there are risks of cellulite, leg ulcers and delayed wound healing. In addition, chronic venous insufficiency contributes to the development of lymphedema [6].

7. Prevalence

The prevalence and gender distribution are very variable in venous disorders. Although recent studies have not reported prevalence differences related to age in men and women, most studies demonstrate a higher prevalence in women than men [27].

The prevalence of CVI is lower in African and Asian or Australian aboriginal populations. Changes in lifestyle and eating habits in the industrialized countries (especially a low-fiber diet causing constipation) and abdominal pressure are considered as one of the main causes of this phenomenon [30].

8. Classification

The Chronic Venous Disorders (CVD) Guideline was released for the Clinical, Etiologic, Anatomic and Pathophysiologic (CEAP) classification in 1994 by American Venous Forum, which is an international ad-hoc committee, and was endorsed by the Society for Vascular Surgery. It was incorporated into "Reporting Standards in Venous Disease" in 1995. Nowadays, clinical papers released on CVD use the whole or some parts of CEAP classification to determine features of disease [31].

The purpose of the CEAP classification is to provide an objective classification system that is valid and reliable throughout the world. This classification identifies the clinical symptoms (C), etiologic factors (E), anatomical features (A) and underlying pathophysiological event (P) [32, 33]. Detailed information is given in **Table 1**.

The clinical classification has seven categories (between 0 and 6) and is further categorized by the presence or absence of symptoms. The etiologic classification is based on congenital, primary and secondary causes of venous dysfunction [34]. The anatomic classification describes the superficial, deep and perforating venous systems with multiple venous segments that may be involved. The pathophysiologic classification describes the underlying mechanism resulting in CVI, including reflux, venous obstruction or both [6].

C0: This refers to early the disease stages and there is usually not any visible or palpable sign of venous disease. Despite the fact that sometimes no clinical evidence is found by the physicians during the examination; clinically CVI is manifested by the presence of some symptoms such as aching legs, heaviness, sensation of burning and nocturnal cramps. Depending on the

Clinical	Etiologic	Anatomic	Pathophysiologic
C_0: There is no sign of venous disease	**Ec:** Congenital	**As:** Superficial veins	**Pr:** Reflux
C_1: Telangiectases or reticular veins	**Ep:** Primary	**Ap:** Perforator veins	**Po:** Obstruction
C_2: Varicose veins	**Es:** Secondary (post-thrombotic, post-traumatic)	**Ad:** Deep veins	**Pr,o:** Reflux and obstruction
C_3: Edema	**En:** There is no cause determined	**An:** There is no venous location identified	**Pn:** There is no venous pathophysiology determined
C_4: Pigmentation or eczema on the skin			
C_{4b}: Lipodermatosclerosis or atrophie blanche			
C_5: Healed venous ulcer			
C_6: Active venous ulcer			

Table 1. CEAP classification system.

severity of the symptoms, there may not be a significant change in the patient's daily life or it may cause significant limitations on the patients.

C1: Telangiectasia (dilated intradermal venules up to a size of about 1 mm) and reticular varicose veins (dilated, nonpalpable and subdermal veins up to a size of about 4 mm). These signs which are associated with increased venous pressure and chronic venous insufficiency occur due to the capillary disorder.

C2: There are several dilated and simultaneously elongated varicose veins. Varicose veins according to etiologic origins are classified as primary (idiopathic), secondary (caused by the post-thrombotic syndrome) and other secondary varicose veins of unclear etiology.

C3: Swelling is one of the most frequent signs of CVI. It is characterized by the accumulation of proteins and water in subcutaneous tissues. While in lying position, the swellings tend to disappear; in long-standing position, swelling increases and causes significant limitations in the daily life of the patients.

C4: As CVI progresses, changes on the skin begin to be observed. On this stage pigmentation, eczema and lipodermatosclerosis are common findings.

C5: Venous ulcers, which are defined as a loss of skin tissue, may develop on the skin in the following periods. Skin changes with healed ulcer are seen in this stage. Only healed varicose ulcers are included within the class 5.

C6: This class is defined by the presence of an active varicose ulcer [35].

Qualification	Absent: 0	Mild: 1	Moderate: 2	Severe: 3
Sense of discomfort, Pain, aching, fatigue heaviness	No	Sometimes, it does not reflect in daily activities	Daily, it does not affect daily activities	Daily, it restricts most of activity
Varicose veins	No	Few and scattered	Confined to calf or thigh	Involve calf and thigh
Venous edema	No	Restricted foot and ankle	Spreads above ankle but don not pass the knee	Extends to knee or above the knee
Pigmentation of the skin	No or focal	Restricted in perimalleolar area	Diffuse over lower third of calf	Diffuse more than lower third of calf
Inflammation	No	Restricted in perimalleolar area	Diffuse over lower third of calf	Diffuse more than lower third of calf
Skin induration	No	Restricted in perimalleolar area	Diffuse over lower third of calf	Diffuse more than lower third of calf
Number of active ulcers	0	1	2	>2
Duration of ulcer	Absent	<3 months	Between 3 months and 1 year	Unhealing >1 year
Size of ulcer	Absent	Diameter <2 cm	Diameter 2–6 cm	Diameter>6 cm
Compression therapy	Not used	Intermittent	Most days	Every day, mostly

Table 2. Venous clinical severity scoring.

To complement the CEAP classification and further define the severity of CVI, the venous clinical severity score (VCSS) was developed (**Table 2**) [36, 37]. The revised VCSS provides clarification of the terms and better definition of the descriptors and has further clinical applicability [38].

The VCSS consists of 10 attributes with four grades (absent, mild, moderate and severe). It has been shown to be useful in evaluation of the response to treatment in CVI. To evaluate severity of disease and treatment outcomes in CVI, it is recommended to make use of validated disease-specific quality-of-life questionnaires in clinical evaluations [39].

9. Treatment of CVI

The initial management of CVI involves conservative approaches to reduce symptoms and prevent development of secondary complications and progression of disease. If conservative approaches fail or provide an unsatisfactory response, further treatment methods should be considered on the basis of anatomic and pathophysiologic features [40]. The treatment options of CVI ranges from simple compression stockings to very complicated venous reconstructions, and the most important step includes patient education to obtain better outcomes after treatment [5].

9.1. Conservative treatment

Conservative approaches aim mainly to restore the altered physiological functions of the venous system. It includes the elevation of the limb together with the supportive methods, pharmacotherapy and structured exercise program, as well as complex decongestive physiotherapy (CDP), intermittent pneumatic compression (IPC), compression stocking, patient training [41–44] and kinesio tape [45].

In order to overcome the effects of the gravity, the elevation of the limb in venous diseases has been applied for centuries. The venous pressure in the tissues around the ankle falls to approximately zero when the feet are at/above the heart level (i.e. toes-above-nose position). When the patient is in this position, all the signs and symptoms, which are directly associated with venous hypertension (i.e. ulcers, eczema, swelling, etc.), resolve without the need for any other treatment, particularly, in lower severity of disease [44].

Training the patient about the changes in lifestyle is important side of the total care. The control of weight, care of the limbs and optimum exercises to keep the calf muscles and ankle joint supple are among the strategies [44].

Compression is advised for the purpose of decreasing ambulatory venous hypertension in patients who have CVI. Changes in lifestyle including weight loss, exercise and elevation of the legs during the day whenever possible are also advised for such patients [46].

9.1.1. Complex decongestive physiotherapy

Since CVI includes combined formats of lymphedema, compression therapy (CT) is preferred as treatment method especially for advanced stages of CVI. CDP is a treatment program consisting of two phases. First phase is the phase in which the edema is decreased and lasts for 4 or more weeks and consists of four components as follows: (1) manual lymph drainage (MLD), (2) skin care, (3) compression bandage and (4) therapeutical exercises. The second phase is the one in which the decreased volume is protected with skin care, compression stocking and exercises. The precautions and patient training are emphasized for the extremity care for this program. The participation and harmony of the patient within the program are important for successful results [47].

9.1.1.1. Manual lymphatic drainage

Manual lymphatic drainage (MLD) is defined as a special manual technique stimulating the superficial lymphatic vessels in order to remove the excessive interstitial fluid [48] and to increase the lymph flow [49]. It has been used for more than 50 years as a type of conservative treatment method in CVI for the purpose of removing extremity edema [50]. In the origin of the technique, there is a soft massage for the purpose of stimulating lymphatic vessels and propel fluid through the channels. Since 20% (or more) patients, who have CVI, also have a lymphedema component, manual lymphatic drainage might have a significant role in a compression therapy program intended for CVI [51]. There have been four MLD techniques well known in the literature, up to now. These include the Foldi, Vodder, Casley-Smith and Leduc techniques [46].

In the study conducted by Foldi et al., it was reported that the MLD was inadequate without using compression therapy [52]. Similarly, Ochalek suggested that the use of compression therapy with MLD was necessary to sustain the effects of MLD [53]. In another study conducted by Bakar et al., 62 patients who had chronic venous disease were included and all the patients treated with CDP. According to the results of the study, CDP application decreased the volume and the percentage-volume of CVI-related edema at a significant level and decreased the intensity of the pain, which was caused by this condition, in the elderly [54].

While it is reported in a meta-analysis study conducted by Karki et al. that MLD was not significantly effective in sustaining decreased edema when used alone [55], Szewczyk et al. reported that MLD was effective in decreasing the edema in the lower limbs of the patients with CVD [56].

9.1.1.2. Skin care

Since CVI is a progressive disease, it disrupts the skin integrity. In healthy skin, the hydrolipid mixture consisting of water and lipid in the epidermis cover and protect the skin from external effects. The lipid component in it decreases the vaporization of the water and ensures the flexibility of the skin. Acidic products (pH 4.5–5.7) and microbial CVI may damage the skin integrity at further stages especially in internal malleoli area. There will be cracks and, in the end, inclination to infection occurs. In order to decrease the risk of infection and the disruption on the skin integrity, it is important to keep the skin moist in the affected area. For this reason, natural products that have balanced contents and that are similar to dermal lipids must be used. Normal skin moisture factors and the lipids that form barriers are important to keep the skin in elastic and slippery form. The applications that are healing and protective are important for both phases of the CDT. In Phase 1, the focus is on healing and care of the damaged skin. In Phase 2, the sustaining of the skin care is important [47].

9.1.1.3. Compression

The limb compression descriptions are to be found in *Corpus Hippocraticum* (450–350 BC) and it is known to be a major milestone in venous insufficiency treatment [51]. Compression treatment is an important part of the two phases of the CDP. During Phase 1, it is necessary to use the compression bandages for 23 hours a day. The purpose of the bandages is to have a certain form of the edema, and decrease the volume in the extremity. During Phase 2, compression is ensured with the compression stockings produced considering the size of the person [47].

The constriction of the leg veins is an essential mechanism of Compression Therapy (CT). In the supine position, a reduction in vein diameter accelerates blood flow velocity and also helps to prevent deep vein thrombosis. In the upright position, external compression is supposed to counteract the hydrostatic pressure. Due to the effect of gravity, external high pressures are required to maintain the same effect in standing position. It can be achieved with high pressure bandages to reduce ambulatory venous hypertension in patients with CVI [57].

The external pressure of approximately 30–40 mmHg is required to constrict the leg veins in the upright position. Complete occlusion of the leg veins occurs at a pressure of 20–25 mmHg in the supine position, at a pressure of 50–60 mmHg in the sitting position and at a pressure of approximately 70 mmHg in the standing position [57].

The treatment aims to correct the long-term complications of CVI at the possible highest level. CT increases pressure on the skin and on the underlying structures to react with the gravity force when it is applied in an external manner to the leg, which may help to relieve the symptoms in the lower limbs by affecting the venous and lymphatic systems to improve the removal of the fluid (i.e. the blood and the lymph) from the relevant limb [51].

The aims of CT may be summarized as follows:

1. Decrease the swollen limb to its minimum size as fast as possible.
2. Maintain the limb at its possible smallest size by using the simplest methods that are possible.
3. Allow the patient to participate in the care of the limb in an active manner by avoiding the factors that aggravate the edema.
4. Train the patient on how to modify his/her own therapy method in case of a problem with edema [51].

In order to treat or prevent the adverse effects, the topical CT provides help. Limb compression changes the tissue pressure gradient, which, in return, reduces the formation of the edema and increases the resorption of the edema; reduces the vein caliber and increases venous flow velocity; reduces orthostatic reflux, residual volume and ambulatory venous pressure (partly by re-recruiting venous valves and by reducing reflux in the perforating vessels) and improves the muscle pump effectiveness [51].

There are many methods in the field of providing CT. The four-layer elastic bandaging (4LB) and the short stretch bandaging (SSB) are the most widely used techniques. The introduction of the graded compression stocking in varying degrees of pressures at the ankle area is a major advance in CT. The purpose of these systems is to provide graduated compression to the lower limb for the purpose of improving venous return and to reduce the edema [51]. Different ambulatory compression techniques and devices cover the compression stockings (CS), paste gauze boots (i.e. the Unna boot), multilayer elastic wraps, dressings, elastic and non-elastic bandages and non-elastic garments. Pneumatic compression devices are also used in patients with refractory edema and venous ulcers [58].

9.1.2. Compressionv stocking

Compression stocking (CS) was first developed in the 1950s by Conrad JOBST. CS is available in various forms, force and size. It provides a pressure decreasing towards proximal from the distal and it has become one of the key treatments and standard procedure in the management of venous lymphatic disorders. Compression pressure ranges and the definition of these classes vary among countries. For this reason, using the pressure ranges as mmHg will be beneficial for universal understanding. CS is classified into four classes according to their pressure values (**Table 3**). The pressures of the CS used in CVI depend on the clinical severity; for CEAP second and third classes, 20–30 mmHg and for CEAP fourth to sixth classes, 40–50 mmHg are used. The most-frequently used size is the one that stretched up to the knee, because the patient participation is more and the symptom healing is adequate. The stockings that reach up to the thigh and groin may be compulsory for the patients that have edema on the knee; however, the use of such stockings is difficult. It must be changed every 6 months [5]. CS must be worn in the stages when the veins are at the emptiest stage. The CS that is worn in the early morning when the patient gets up is the most effective one. The patient must walk in the stockings during the day [40].

9.1.3. Intermittence pneumatic compression (IPC)

Wide consensus exists in the literature that compression is a necessary part of all treatments for CVI and venous ulcers. Compression is usually provided by stockings. Most of the elderly patients have reduced strength and skill and therefore it makes these stockings difficult to wear. Compression can also be provided with the Unna's boot or different types of bandages [27].

Extremity compression can be achieved with pneumatic compression tools. Pneumatic compression devices consist of an inflatable garment for the arm or leg and an electrical pneumatic pump that fills the garment with compressed air. The boot is intermittently inflated and deflated and creates a pumping effect [27]. The inflation and deflation cycles mimic the muscle pump. This is one of the key mechanisms to provide proper venous and lymphatic flow [59].

Compression class	**1**	**2**	**3**	**4**
Compression degree	Mild	Moderate	Strong	Very strong
Pressure (mmHg)	18–21	23–32	34–46	49<

Table 3. Compression classes.

First generation pneumatic compression devices consisted of an inflatable single compartment pressure chamber that applied a non-segmented uniform and sustained level of compression to the entire extremity. Later, multi-segment compression devices were developed in order to increase the effectiveness of the devices. Thanks to these devices, technically, the pressure gradient is created between distal and proximal parts of the limb. The pressure of distal chamber is higher than in the proximal chamber and this enables a sequential mechanism of distal to proximal application of pressure. Pneumatic compression devices have further evolved in recent years and allow digital programming to imitate MLD techniques and promote fluid clearance at the proximal trunk and extremities [60] (**Table 4**).

Pneumatic compression device	Distinctive features
Single chamber non-programmable pumps	• The single sleeve inflates to apply pressure on the leg • No manual control on pressure distribution • No pressure gradient • Nowadays it is not an optimal method for lymphedema treatment
Multi-chamber (segmented) non-programmable pumps	• Approximately three or four chambers swell completely from the distal to the proximal segment and then descend • Perhaps a limited pressure programming option can be found but not independently adjustable • Structurally, each chamber is designed to reach the same pressure gradient, with support from the extremity shape • Pumps can use one or both of the same legs or arms
Multi-chamber programmable pumps	• The pressure gradient is set to be higher in the distal segment and lower in the proximal segment • It produces three different pressure zones, and some pumps allow the divider to set the pressure • Manual programmable and pressure-adjustable for the desired zone • Adjustable from 4 to 36 chambers
Advanced pneumatic compression systems	• Digitally programmable • With proper application to adjoining trunk segments, it can provide a uniform distribution of edema by relaxing the proximal and distal limb • Garbage and proximal chambers can open lymphatic pathways • Only 1 and 2.5 compartments can actively simulate manual lymphatic drainage by providing a pressure increase and progression from distal to proximal

Table 4. Pneumatic compression devices.

The most basic definition of the IPC is that it consists in the application of a force on an edema in order to evacuate its components as much as possible towards the physiological ways of drainage (venous—lymphatics—interstitium) [61].

IPC has physiological effects such as increase in capillary perfusion, increase in tissue oxygenation, increase in the fibrinolytic potential of endothelial cells, increased blood-flow in the deep veins, decrease in stasis, decrease in venous hypertension and decrease in interstitial edema [62–64].

There are some contraindications to pneumatic compression [65] (**Figure 1**). Despite the fact that there is no serious complication of pneumatic compression, It has been reported that there are some complications in the literature [27, 66, 67] (**Figure 2**).

In the study of Caprini, it was reported that pneumatic compression applied 4 hours per day provided significant improvement in symptoms [68]. Another study examined the efficacy of pneumatic compression in those with CVI and it was concluded that a single 30-min session per day of pneumatic compression decreased edema, increased venous blood-flow and improved symptoms [69].

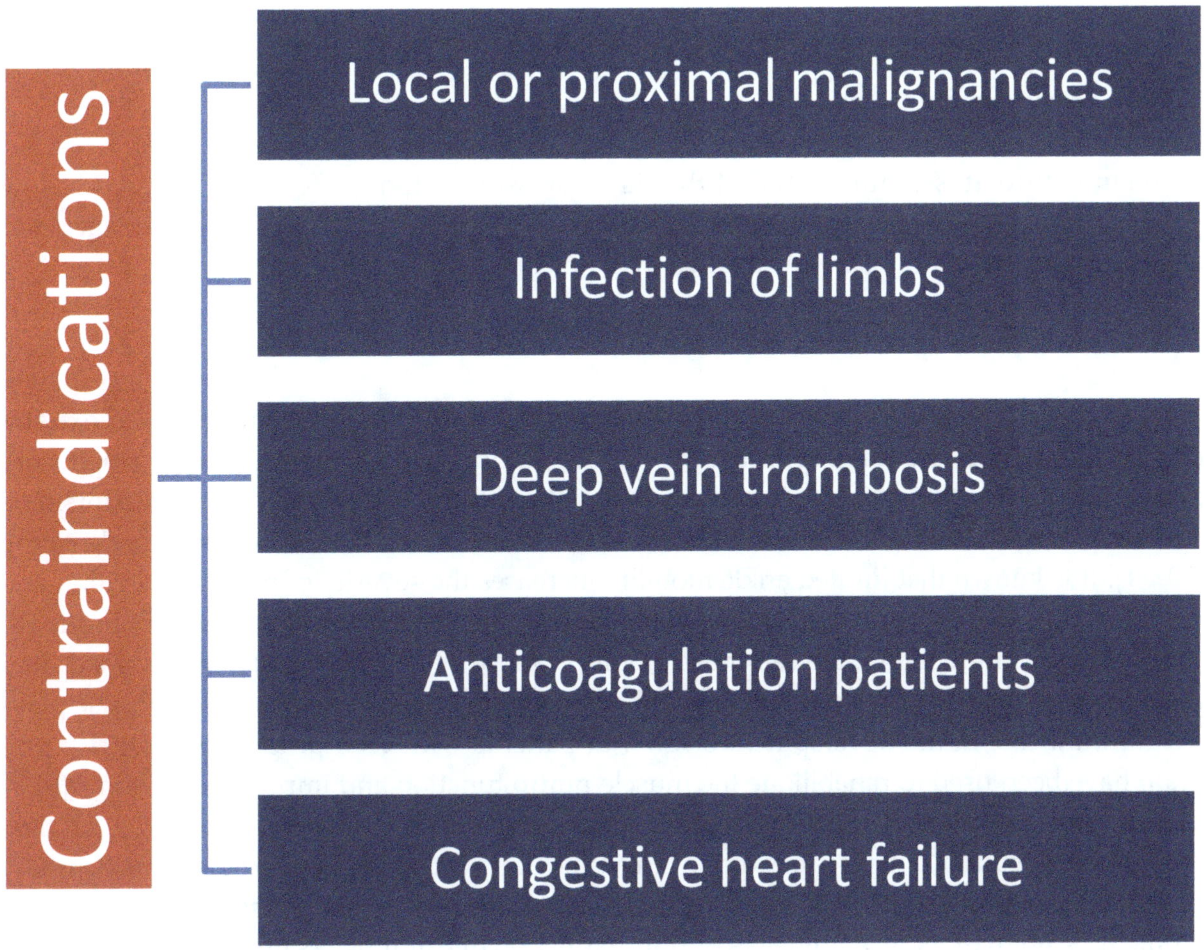

Figure 1. Contraindications of IPC.

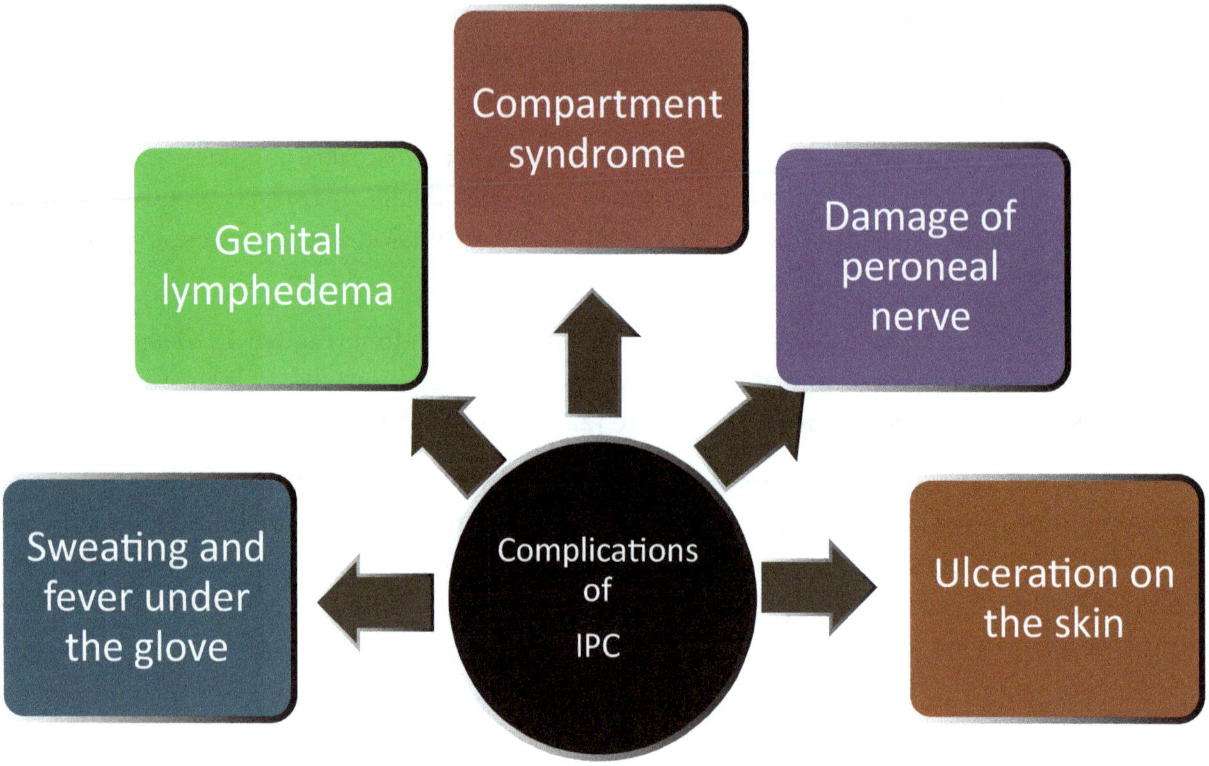

Figure 2. Complications of IPC.

In the literature, it is common in CVI that high pressure is more effective compared to low pressure, multi-layer bandages are more effective compared to single-layer bandages and compression application is more effective than no compression application [63].

9.1.4. Exercise

The calf muscle pump is the basic mechanism in the return of blood from the lower extremity to the heart and also it is supported by the foot pump, the thigh pump and the respiratory pump. The ankle joint is the main component of the calf muscle pump. Therefore, dorsiflexion and plantar flexion of the ankle is the basis for effective function of the calf muscle pump [70, 71]. It is known that limited ankle mobility increases the severity of edema formation and venous reflux in patients with CVI. CVI causes ankle immobility due to storage of fibrotic tissue. Because of immobility, the calf muscle pump cannot be activated and venous blood does not return to the heart [72]. Presence of any abnormality in pump functions of calf muscle plays a significant role in the development of CVI. In patients with CVI, progressive exercise program have been used to rehabilitate the muscle pump function and improve symptoms [6]. A randomized controlled study designated individuals with advance venous disease (CEAP class C4–C6) to structured calf muscle exercise or routine daily activities. To assess venous hemodynamics duplex ultrasound and APG were used, and muscle strength was assessed with a dynamometer. After 6 months, parameters of pump function of calf muscles normalized in patients receiving customized exercise program for calf muscles. However, there was no change in the amount of reflux or severity scores. Although it was found that severity scores of reflux was not changing statistically, it appears that calf muscle pump function could be established by structured exercise in CVI that may prove effective as supplemental therapy to medical and surgical treatment in advanced disease [73].

Research over the past 10–12 years points to ankle joint movement as the key biomechanical element in a functioning calf pump. When artificially restricting the movement of the ankle joint in healthy volunteers, it is demonstrated that a significant decrease occurred in the efficiency of the pump to affect a decrease in venous pressure during exercise [74]. Calf muscle strength may also affect the efficiency of venous return [75]. An improvement in calf muscle strength correlates with improved venous return [76] and loss of muscle strength is seen in patients with long-lasting venous ulcer [75]. Taheri et al. stated that there are three types of atrophy in biopsies of the gastrocnemius muscle in patients with vein insufficiency. These were disuse, denervation and ischemia, which play a role in muscle destruction [77]. How much calf muscle volume contributes to venous insufficiency is unclear [75].

Back et al. stated that a normal walking motion is required for activation of the calf muscular pump and this requires 90 degrees of dorsiflexion [78]. It has been found that exercise program twice a week increased the angle of dorsiflexion and plantar flexion in those with CVI [79].

9.1.5. Kinesio tape

Kinesiology taping (Kinesio Tape) which was developed by Dr. Kenzo Kase in 1996 is a technique that is used to restore muscle function, to increase vascular and lymphatic circulation, to relieve pain or to correct the impaired joint alignment. Kinesio Tape is an elastic, latex-free, adhesive and waterproof tape. Moreover, it is an application that may remain in the skin for 3–5 days. Skin adhesive tape is thicker and more elastic than conventional tape and also it has the ability to stretch up to 120–140% of its normal length. Although there is no definite evidence for its proprioceptive effect, it is thought to act by means of cutaneous mechanoreceptors [80].

Skin-taping increases the circulation in the region by creating convulsions that cause the dermis to rise up. Kinesio Tape, which is frequently used in edema, hematoma and wound healing, has been used as an alternative to compression therapy in patients with venous insufficiency in recent years. Even if it is frequently used, Kinesio Tape has not been proven to have a positive effect on venous insufficiency. In some studies, it has been shown that there was an increase in lymphatic circulation and venous return of individuals who underwent fan technique without strain [81].

10. Conclusion

Chronic venous insufficiency (CVI) is a common disorder. As a result of various pathologies that develop at the lower extremity venous system, venous pressure increases, affecting the whole lower extremity. This could result in valvular insufficiency at superficial or axial deep veins and perforator veins, venous obstruction or a combination of these. These factors worsen with calf muscle pump dysfunction. These mechanisms partially provide grounds for the development of venous hypertension during standing. Patient may not have any symptoms, or they can complain from swelling at legs, discomfort with pain, anxiety, night cramps or pain occurring when standing. There are many treatment options such as medical, pharmacological and conservative methods used in CVI. Among these, conservative approaches because of being invasive with less adverse effects than other methods are commonly used to treat CVI. Conservative treatment of patients with CVI relies on the use of compression therapy, which is considered the "gold standard," provided by means of elastic stockings, bandages and pneumatic compression devices. Patient education is essential. CVI is a chronic disease that needs a life-long care. So patients with CVI should encourage to maintain a normal body weight, exercise daily (a walking program is especially good) and wear compression garment throughout the day.

Author details

Özlem Çinar Özdemir* and Mahmut Surmeli

*Address all correspondence to: ozlemcinar314@hotmail.com

School of Physical Therapy and Rehabilitation, Abant Izzet Baysal University, Bolu, Turkey

References

[1] De Aguiar E, Pinto L, Figueiredo M, Savino N. Diretrizes sobre Diagnóstico, Prevenção e Tratamento da Sociedade Brasileira de Angiologia e Cirurgia Vascular (SBACV). Úlcera de Insuficiência Venosa Crônica. J Vasc Br. 2005;4(Supl 2):S195–200.

[2] Kaplan RM, Criqui MH, Denenberg JO, Bergan J, Fronek A. Quality of life in patients with chronic venous disease: San Diego population study. Journal of Vascular Surgery. 2003;37(5):1047–53.

[3] Marston W. Evaluation and treatment of leg ulcers associated with chronic venous insufficiency. Clinics in Plastic Surgery. 2007;34(4):717–30.

[4] Khan A, Chaudhri R, Ashraf M, Mazaffar M, Zawar-ul-Imam S, Tanveer M. Prevalence and presentation of chronic venous disease in Pakistan: a multicentre study. Phlebology. 2013;28(2):74–9.

[5] Eberhardt RT, Raffetto JD. Chronic venous insufficiency. Circulation. 2005;111(18): 2398–409.

[6] Eberhardt RT, Raffetto JD. Chronic venous insufficiency. Circulation. 2014;130(4): 333–46.

[7] Paul JC, Pieper B, Templin TN. Itch: association with chronic venous disease, pain and quality of life. Journal of Wound, Ostomy, and Continence Nursing: Official Publication of the Wound, Ostomy and Continence Nurses Society/WOCN. 2011;38(1):46.

[8] Castro A, Santos M, ALS CA, Teixeira A. Diagnóstico e tratamento da doença venosa crônica. Jornal Vascular Brasileiro. 2005;4(2):185–94.

[9] Sistem YMAEV. Klinik Anatomisi. İÜ Cerrahpaşa Tıp Fakültesi Sürekli Tıp Eğitimi Etkinlikleri Sempozyum Dizisi. 2007;56:9–17.

[10] Drake R, Vogl W, Mitchell A. Grey's Anatomy. Elsevier/Churchill Livingstone: Philadelphia. 2005.

[11] Bergan JJ, Bunke N. The Vein Book. Oxford University Press: New York. 2014.

[12] Menon RR. Lower limb venous anatomy. In: Vaidyanathan S, Menon RR, Jacob P, John B, editors. Chronic Venous Disorders of the Lower Limbs. Springer: New Delhi, 2015. pp. 9–16.

[13] Meissner MH, Moneta G, Burnand K, Gloviczki P, Lohr JM, Lurie F, et al. The hemodynamics and diagnosis of venous disease. Journal of Vascular Surgery. 2007;46(6):S4–S24.

[14] Ellis H, Logan BM, Dixon AK. Handbook of venous disorders. Annals of The Royal College of Surgeons of England. 2010;92(2):179.

[15] Földi E, Földi M. Chronic venous insufficiency and venous-lymphostatic insufficiency. Földi's Textbook of Lymphology, 2nd ed. Elsevier: Munich, Germany. 2006:434–47.

[16] Tran NT, Meissner MH. The epidemiology, pathophysiology, and natural history of chronic venous disease. Seminars in Vascular Surgery. 2002;15(1):5–12.

[17] Nicolaides A. Investigation of chronic venous insufficiency a consensus statement. Circulation. 2000;102(20):e126–e63.

[18] Welkie JF, Comerota AJ, Katz ML, Aldridge SC, Kerr RP, White JV. Hemodynamic deterioration in chronic venous disease. Journal of Vascular Surgery. 1992;16(5):733–40.

[19] Pappas P, Durán W, Hobson R. Pathology and cellular physiology of chronic venous insufficiency. Handbook of Venous Disorders, 2nd ed. Arnold: New York. 2001:58–67.

[20] Criqui MH, Denenberg JO, Langer RD, Kaplan RM, Fronek A. Epidemiology of chronic peripheral venous disease. In: Bergan JJ, editor. The Vein Book. Elsevier: USA. 2007. pp 27–37.

[21] Zicot M. Venous diseases and pregnancy. Revue medicale de Liege. 1999;54(5):424–8.

[22] Stvrtinová V, Kolesar J, Wimmer G. Prevalence of varicose veins of the lower limbs in the women working at a department store. International Angiology. 1990;10(1):2–5.

[23] Preziosi P, Galan P, Aissa M, Hercberg S, Boccalon H. Prevalence of venous insufficiency in French adults of the SUVIMAX cohort. International Angiology. 1999;18(2):171.

[24] Townsend Jr CM, Beauchamp RD, Evers BM, Mattox KL. Sabiston Textbook of Surgery. Elsevier Health Sciences: Philadelphia. 2012.

[25] Gourgou S, Dedieu F, Sancho-Garnier H. Lower limb venous insufficiency and tobacco smoking: a case-control study. American Journal of Epidemiology. 2002;155(11):1007–15.

[26] Coughlin L, Gandy R, Rosser S, De Cossart L. Factors associated with varicose veins in pregnant women. Phlebology. 2001;16(4):167–9.

[27] Berliner E, Ozbilgin B, Zarin DA. A systematic review of pneumatic compression for treatment of chronic venous insufficiency and venous ulcers. Journal of Vascular Surgery. 2003;37(3):539-44.

[28] Criqui MH, Jamosmos M, Fronek A, Denenberg JO, Langer RD, Bergan J, et al. Chronic venous disease in an ethnically diverse population the San Diego population study. American Journal of Epidemiology. 2003;158(5):448–56.

[29] Evans C, Fowkes F, Ruckley C, Lee A. Prevalence of varicose veins and chronic venous insufficiency in men and women in the general population: Edinburgh Vein Study. Journal of Epidemiology and Community Health. 1999;53(3):149–53.

[30] Carpentier P, Priollet P. Epidemiology of chronic venous insufficiency. Presse Medicale (Paris, France: 1983). 1994;23(5):197–201.

[31] Eklöf B, Rutherford RB, Bergan JJ, Carpentier PH, Gloviczki P, Kistner RL, et al. Revision of the CEAP classification for chronic venous disorders: consensus statement. Journal of Vascular Surgery. 2004;40(6):1248–52.

[32] Padberg FT. CEAP classification for chronic venous disease. Disease-A-Month. 2005; 51(2):176–82.

[33] Rabe E, Pannier F. Clinical, aetiological, anatomical and pathological classification (CEAP): gold standard and limits. Phlebology. 2012;27(suppl 1):114–8.

[34] Lacroix P, Aboyans V, Preux P, Houles M, Laskar M. Epidemiology of venous insufficiency in an occupational population. International Angiology. 2003;22(2):172.

[35] Staffa R. Chronic venous insufficiency epidemiology. Prevalence. 2002;60(70):55–7.

[36] Neglén P, Thrasher TL, Raju S. Venous outflow obstruction: an underestimated contributor to chronic venous disease. Journal of Vascular Surgery. 2003;38(5):879—85.

[37] Araki CT, Back TL, Padberg FT, Thompson PN, Jamil Z, Lee BC, et al. The significance of calf muscle pump function in venous ulceration. Journal of Vascular Surgery. 1994;20(6):872–9.

[38] Vasquez MA, Rabe E, McLafferty RB, Shortell CK, Marston WA, Gillespie D, et al. Revision of the venous clinical severity score: venous outcomes consensus statement: special communication of the American Venous Forum Ad Hoc Outcomes Working Group. Journal of Vascular Surgery. 2010;52(5):1387–96.

[39] Labropoulos N, Leon M, Nicolaides AN, Giannoukas AD, Volteas N, Chan P. Superficial venous insufficiency: correlation of anatomic extent of reflux with clinical symptoms and signs. Journal of Vascular Surgery. 1994;20(6):953–8.

[40] Periferik TKDCD. Arter ve Ven Hastalıklari Tedavi Kılavuzu. Ankara: Öncü Basımevi. 2008:97–123.

[41] Weiss RA, Munavalli G, editors. Endovenous ablation of truncal veins. Seminars in Cutaneous Medicine and Surgery: WB Saunders: Philadelphia, USA. 2005.

[42] Mariani F. Compression. Consensus Document Based on Scientific Evidence and Clinical Experiences. Minerva Medica: Torino. 2009.

[43] Bakar Y. Mastektomi sonrası gelişen lenfödemde fizyoterapinin etkinliği Ankara: Hacettepe University: Ankara. 2005.

[44] Vaidyanathan S, Menon RR, Jacob P, John B. Chronic venous disorders of the lower limbs. A Surgical Approach: Springer; 2014.

[45] Aguilar-Ferrándiz ME, Castro-Sánchez AM, Matarán-Peñarrocha GA, García-Muro F, Serge T, Moreno-Lorenzo C. Effects of kinesio taping on venous symptoms, bioelectrical activity of the gastrocnemius muscle, range of ankle motion, and quality of life in postmenopausal women with chronic venous insufficiency: a randomized controlled trial. Archives of Physical Medicine and Rehabilitation. 2013;94(12):2315–28.

[46] dos Santos Crisóstomo RS, Candeias MS, Ribeiro AMM, Martins CdLB, Armada-da-Silva PA. Manual lymphatic drainage in chronic venous disease: a duplex ultrasound study. Phlebology. 2014;29(10):667–676.

[47] Asmussen P, Strossenreuther R. Compression therapy. Foeldi's Textbook of Lymphology San Biotext: Francisco. 2006:563–627.

[48] Leduc O, Bourgeois P, Leduc A. Manual lymphatic drainage: scintigraphic demonstration of its efficacy on colloidal protein reabsorption. Progress in Lymphology. 1988;11:551–4.

[49] Tan I-C, Maus EA, Rasmussen JC, Marshall MV, Adams KE, Fife CE, et al. Assessment of lymphatic contractile function after manual lymphatic drainage using near-infrared fluorescence imaging. Archives of Physical Medicine and Rehabilitation. 2011;92(5):756–64.

[50] Steins A, Junger M. Physical therapy in patients with chronic venous insufficiency. Phlebologie-Stuttgart. 2000;29(2):48.

[51] Felty CL, Rooke TW. Compression therapy for chronic venous insufficiency. Seminars in vascular surgery: Elsevier. 2005;18(1):36–40.

[52] Földi E. The treatment of lymphedema. Cancer. 1998;83(S12B):2833–4.

[53] Ochałek K, Grądalski T. The use of manual lymph drainage in vascular diseases. Acta Angiol. 2011;17(3):189–98.

[54] Bakar Y, Öztürk A, Calisal MA, Ertürk K, Daglar B. Complete decongestive physiotherapy for older people with chronic venous insufficiency. Topics in Geriatric Rehabilitation. 2010;26(2):164–70.

[55] Kärki A, Anttila H, Tasmuth T, Rautakorpi U-M. Lymphoedema therapy in breast cancer patients–a systematic review on effectiveness and a survey of current practices and costs in Finland. Acta Oncologica. 2009;48(6):850–9.

[56] Szewczyk T. The importance of massage in edema of lower limbs in patients with chronic venous insufficiency. Valetudinaria Postępy Medycyny Klinicznej i Wojskowej. 2002;7:50–3.

[57] Partsch B, Partsch H. Calf compression pressure required to achieve venous closure from supine to standing positions. Journal of Vascular Surgery. 2005;42(4):734–8.

[58] Molski P, Kruczyński J, Molski A, Molski S. Manual lymphatic drainage improves the quality of life in patients with chronic venous disease: a randomized controlled trial. Archives of Medical Sciences. 2013;9(3):452–8.

[59] Szolnoky G, Dobozy A, Kemény L. Towards an effective management of chronic lymphedema. Clinics in Dermatology. 2014;32(5):685–91.

[60] Feldman J, Stout N, Wanchai A, Stewart B, Cormier J, Armer J. Intermittent pneumatic compression therapy: a systematic review. Lymphology. 2012;45(1):13.

[61] Belgrado J-P, Bourgeois P, Röh N, Moraine J. Intermittent pneumatic compression in the treatment of lymphedema: current state of knowledge. European Journal of Lymphology Related Probems. 2007;17(50):4–10.

[62] Kumar S, Walker MA. The effects of intermittent pneumatic compression on the arterial and venous system of the lower limb: a review. Journal of Tissue Viability. 2002;12(2):58–66.

[63] Partsch H. Indications for compression therapy in venous and lymphatic disease consensus based on experimental data and scientific evidence under the auspices of the IUP. International Angiology. 2008;27(3):193.

[64] Comerota AJ. Intermittent pneumatic compression: physiologic and clinical basis to improve management of venous leg ulcers. Journal of Vascular Surgery. 2011;53(4):1121–9.

[65] Brennan MJ, Miller LT. Overview of treatment options and review of the current role and use of compression garments, intermittent pumps, and exercise in the management of lymphedema. Cancer. 1998;83(S12B):2821–7.

[66] Werbel G, Shybut G. Acute compartment syndrome caused by a malfunctioning pneumatic-compression boot. A case report. Journal of Bone and Joint Surgery. American volume. 1986;68(9):1445–6.

[67] Strup S, Gudziak M, Mulholland S, Gomella L. The effect of intermittent pneumatic compression devices on intraoperative blood loss during radical prostatectomy and radical cystectomy. The Journal of Urology. 1993;150(4):1176–8.

[68] Arcelus JI, Caprini JA, Sehgal LR, Reyna JJ. Home use of impulse compression of the foot and compression stockings in the treatment of chronic venous insufficiency. Journal of Vascular Surgery. 2001;34(5):805–11.

[69] Güçük A, Peker Ö, Bircan Ç, Yiğit M, Şenocak Ö,Gülbahar S et al. The effectiveness of intermittent pneumatic compression ın patients with chronic venous insufficiency. Ege Fiziskel Tıp Rehabilitasyon Dergisi, 2001; 7(3–4): 117–122.

[70] van Uden CJ, van der Vleuten CJ, Kooloos JG, Haenen J, Wollersheim H. Gait and calf muscle endurance in patients with chronic venous insufficiency. Clinical Rehabilitation. 2005;19(3):339–44.

[71] Miller BF, Gruben KG, Morgan BJ. Circulatory responses to voluntary and electrically induced muscle contractions in humans. Physical Therapy. 2000;80(1):53–60.

[72] Kunimoto B, Cooling M, Gulliver W, Houghton P, Orsted H, Sibbald RG. Best practices for the prevention and treatment of venous leg ulcers. Ostomy Wound Management. 2001;47(2):34–51.

[73] Padberg FT, Johnston MV, Sisto SA. Structured exercise improves calf muscle pump function in chronic venous insufficiency: a randomized trial. Journal of Vascular Surgery. 2004;39(1):79–87.

[74] Kügler C, Strunk M, Rudofsky G. Venous pressure dynamics of the healthy human leg. Journal of Vascular Research. 2001;38(1):20–9.

[75] Davies J, Bull R, Farrelly I, Wakelin M. Improving the calf pump using home-based exercises for patients with chronic venous disease. Wounds UK. 2008;4(3):48–53.

[76] Kan YM, Delis KT. Hemodynamic effects of supervised calf muscle exercise in patients with venous leg ulceration: a prospective controlled study. Archives of Surgery. 2001;136(12):1364–9.

[77] Taheri SA, Heffner R, Williams J, Lazar L, Elias S. Muscle changes in venous insufficiency. Archives of Surgery. 1984;119(8):929–31.

[78] Back TL, Padberg FT, Araki CT, Thompson PN, Hobson RW. Limited range of motion is a significant factor in venous ulceration. Journal of Vascular Surgery. 1995;22(5):519–23.

[79] Yang D, Vandongen Y, Stacey M. Effect of exercise on calf muscle pump function in patients with chronic venous disease. British Journal of Surgery. 1999;86(3):338–41.

[80] Valentim da Silva RM, Cavalcanti RL, de França Rêgo LM, Leite Nunes PF, Meyer PF. Effects of Kinesio Taping® in treatment of Cellulite: randomized controlled blind trial. Manual Therapy, Posturology & Rehabilitation Journal. 2014;12:175.

[81] Murray H, Husk L. Effect of kinesio taping on proprioception in the ankle. The Journal of Orthopaedic and Sports Physical Therapy. 2001; 31(1): 689-26.

5

Influence of Auditory Pacing on the Control of Rhythmic Movement in Physical Therapy

Masanori Ito, Yuki Takahashi, Satoshi Fujiwara and Naoki Kado

Additional information is available at the end of the chapter

Abstract

The electromyographic reaction time data responses to various rhythm shifts are discussed in Section 2 of this chapter. The following four experimental designs were introduced: (1) subliminal rhythm shift with shortened interval, (2) subliminal rhythm shift with lengthened interval, (3) subliminal rhythm shift with random interval, and (4) differences in the rate of rhythm shift. We found that the periodic rhythmic stimulation is predicted to comprise some time duration. Furthermore, the reactive movements can be performed without delay under conditions with an interstimulus-onset interval shift of 7% of 1500 ms. When the physical therapist facilitates rhythmical reactive periodic movement using an external event such as a handclap, it will be desirable to keep the rhythm shift within 7% of the interstimulus-onset interval. The variabilities of the inter-tap interval in the continuation paradigm of sensorimotor synchronization are discussed in Section 3. The participants performed self-paced, synchronization-continuation, and syncopation-continuation tapping tasks. We found that the accuracy of the periodic movement with an interstimulus-onset interval of 1000 ms can be improved by using auditory pacing. However, the consistency of periodic movement is mainly dependent on innate skill; thus, improvement in consistency from pacing alone is unlikely.

Keywords: auditory, external pacing, rhythmic movement, reaction time, sensorimotor synchronization

1. Introduction

Producing rhythmic and periodic movement is one of the important aspects of movement control. In physical therapy, external events such as auditory stimuli and visual stimuli might be used as triggers for the facilitation of periodic movement. Rhythmic coordinated movement is impaired in patients with motor diseases such as Parkinson's or those who have experienced a stroke. It is possible that an auditory pacing event could be useful as physical therapy in treating movement disorders. In a physical therapy study, during a target-hitting task using flexion and extension of the elbow, variability of electromyogram patterns of the biceps brachii decreased with pacing using a regular auditory rhythm, compared with that during the no-pacing and irregular auditory rhythm conditions [1]. In clinical studies, it has been reported that an intervention using rhythmic auditory stimulation improved gait velocity, cadence, and stride length in patients with Parkinson's disease [2] and gait velocity, stride length, and electromyographic activity of the medial gastrocnemius in patients with hemiparetic stroke [3].

When performing a rhythmic movement using periodic auditory stimuli as a trigger, the subjects can select a variety of movement patterns (such as reaction, synchronization, and syncopation). In this chapter, the electromyographic reaction time (EMG-RT) data responses to various rhythm shifts [4–7] are discussed in Section 2, and the variabilities of intertap interval (ITI) in the continuation paradigm of sensorimotor synchronization [8] are discussed in Section 3. Furthermore, each section includes an explanation of the clinical consideration in physical therapy.

2. Influence of various rhythm shifts on reactive periodic movement

The EMG-RT is defined as the interval between the stimulation signal and the onset of voluntary electromyographic activity of a response, and reflects the time of the central process. The presentation of periodic stimuli creates predictions and expectations. During the reaction-time task, the EMG-RTs are shortened in the first three stimuli when applying the periodic stimuli. On the other hand, the different intervals inserted in periodic stimuli sequences causes a delay in EMG-RT [9]. Regarding the facilitation of reactive periodic movement during physical therapy, if the physical therapists provide periodic rhythm by handclap, it will be impossible to replicate the exact time interval without deviation in the absence of a metronome. The studies described in this section show the EMG-RT data responses to various rhythm shifts. Additionally, we clarify the relationship between the degree of stimulus interval deviation and the delay of EMG-RT in the reactive periodic movement.

2.1. Apparatus for recording the EMG-RT

The same apparatus was used for EMG-RT measurements in experiments 1–4, which are discussed in this section. The telemetry EMG measuring system (MQ8; KISSEICOMTEC, Matsumoto City, Japan) was loaded onto a PC (VersaPro VY20F/AG-W; NEC). The auditory stimulus system was set up using SoundTrigger2Plus (KISSEICOMTEC). Auditory stimuli were delivered via headphones. The presented auditory stimulus and EMG signals were recorded with a data acquisition system (VitalRecorder2; KISSEICOMTEC), and recorded signals were analyzed by an EMG signal analysis program (BIMUTAS-Video; KISSEICOMTEC). The surface electrodes (LecTrode NP; ADVANCE, Tokyo, Japan) were placed over the right tibialis anterior muscle.

2.2. EMG-RT measurements

2.2.1. Subliminal rhythm shift with shortened interval

The purpose of experiment 1 was to investigate the influence of a subliminal rhythm shift with a shortened interval on the control of reactive movement. Fourteen healthy subjects (10 men, 4 women; mean age, 25.4 years) participated in this experiment. The subjects were right-foot dominant and kicked the balled with their right foot. Subjects had no motor function abnormalities of the right ankle and no hearing abnormalities. The experiment was conducted in a quiet room. The subjects were seated with 90° of knee flexion. All subjects performed the reaction-time tasks, raising their right ankles in response to the auditory stimuli. Their eyes were closed to exclude the influence of vision during the tasks. The following three test conditions were applied: (1) periodic auditory stimuli with an interstimulus-onset interval (ISI) of 1500 ms and a shift in the last stimulus interval only to (2) 1425 ms (the interval shortened 5% of 1500 ms), and (3) 1200 ms (the interval shortened 20% of 1500 ms), respectively, in successive stimulus sequences with an ISI of 1500 ms. Each condition was composed of 6–10 stimuli. There were 15 trials performed during each condition for a total of 45 trials. EMG-RT values for the last stimulus were compared among the three conditions. One-way repeated measures analysis of variance (ANOVA) revealed a significant difference between the EMG-RT values under different conditions (see **Figure 1**). Tukey's posthoc test showed that the EMG-RT was

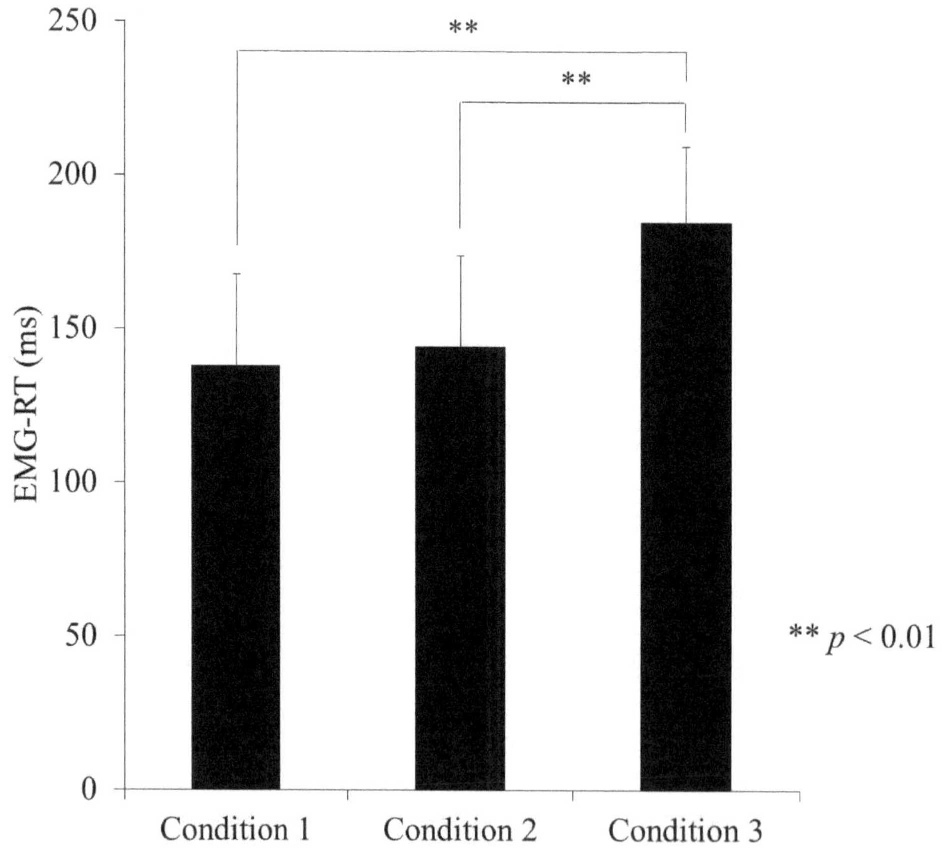

Figure 1. EMG-RT values of conditions 1–3.

significantly delayed under condition 3 (184.7 ± 24.6 ms, $p < 0.01$) compared with that under conditions 1 (138.0 ± 29.7 ms) and 2 (144.3 ± 29.4 ms). A comparison of conditions 1 and 2 revealed no significant differences.

2.2.2. *Subliminal rhythm shift with lengthened interval*

Experiment 2 aimed to investigate the influence of a subliminal rhythm shift with a lengthened interval on the control of reactive movement. Thirteen healthy individuals (10 men, 3 women; mean age, 27.4 years) were included in this study. All subjects were right-footed according to the Chapman's foot-preference inventory (mean score, 14.8) [10]. The subjects had no motor function abnormalities of the right ankle and no hearing abnormalities. All subjects performed the same reaction-time tasks as those in experiment 1. The following three test conditions were applied: (1) periodic auditory stimuli with an ISI of 1500 ms, and a shift in the last stimulus interval only to (2) 1575 ms (the interval lengthened 5% of 1500 ms), and (3) 1800 ms (the interval lengthened 20% of the 1500 ms), respectively, in successive stimuli sequences at an ISI of 1500 ms. Each condition was composed of 6–10 stimuli. There were 15 trials performed during each condition for a total of 45 trials. EMG-RT values for the last stimulus were compared among the three conditions. One-way repeated measures ANOVA revealed a significant difference between the EMG-RT values under different conditions (see **Figure 2**). Tukey's posthoc test showed that the EMG-RT was significantly delayed under

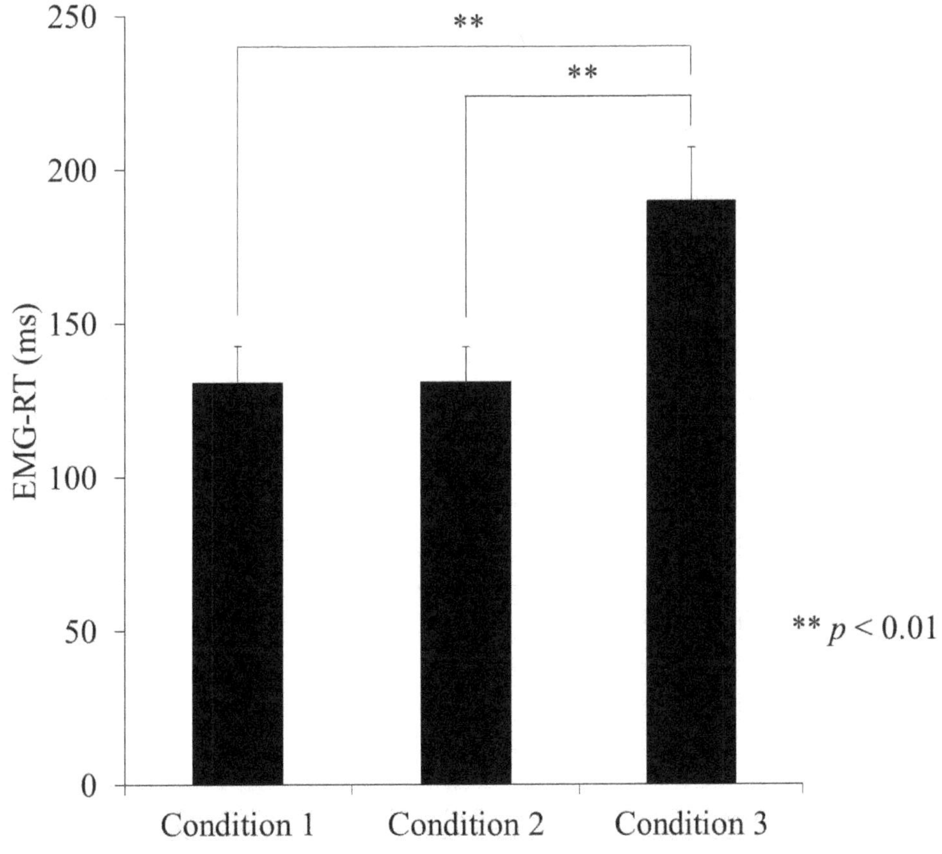

Figure 2. EMG-RT values of conditions 1–3.

condition 3 (189.8 ± 17.3 ms, $p < 0.01$) compared with that under conditions 1 (130.9 ± 11.8 ms) and 2 (131.1 ± 11.2 ms). A comparison of conditions 1 and 2 revealed no significant differences.

2.2.3. Subliminal rhythm shift with random interval

Experiment 3 included 14 healthy subjects (11 men, 3 women; mean age, 28.5 years) who performed the same reaction-time tasks as those in experiments 1 and 2. All subjects were right-footed according to the Chapman's foot-preference inventory (mean score, 14.6) [10]. EMG-RT was measured under the following three test conditions: (1) periodic auditory stimuli with an ISI of 1500 ms, (2) a random ISI shift in the range of 1463–1537 ms (range of ±5% of the 1500 ms), and (3) a random ISI shift in the range of 1350–1650 ms (range of ±20% of 1500 ms). In condition 3, the time differences between consecutive ISIs were set longer than 75 ms and 10 auditory stimuli were provided per trial. There were 10 trials performed during each condition for a total of 30 trials. EMG-RT values corresponding to the 1st–10th stimuli were compared within each condition using one-way repeated measures ANOVA. When a significant difference was recognized, paired comparisons were performed using Tukey's posthoc test. The EMG-RT values for conditions 1–3 are shown in **Table 1**. In conditions 1 and 2, EMG-RT value responses to the 2nd–10th stimuli were significantly shortened compared with the response to the 1st stimulus ($p < 0.01$), and the responses to the 3rd–10th stimuli were significantly shortened compared with the response to the 2nd stimulus ($p < 0.01$). In condition 3, EMG-RT value responses to the 2nd–10th stimuli were significantly shortened compared with the response to the 1st stimulus ($p < 0.01$), and the responses to the 3rd stimulus was significantly shortened compared with the response to the 2nd stimulus ($p < 0.01$). On the other hand, EMG-RT value responses to the 7th–10th stimuli were significantly delayed compared with the response to the 3rd stimulus ($p < 0.01$).

2.2.4. Differences in rate of rhythm shift

Experiment 4 aimed to investigate the influence of differences in the rate of rhythm shift on the control of reactive movement. Ten healthy individuals (8 men, 2 women; mean age, 25.5 years) performed the same reaction-time tasks as those in the previous EMG-RT measurements. All subjects were right-footed according to the Chapman's foot-preference inventory (mean score,

	Stimulus number									
	1st	**2nd**	**3rd**	**4th**	**5th**	**6th**	**7th**	**8th**	**9th**	**10th**
Condition 1	196.7 (19.4)	158.3 (17.5)	134.2 (15.5)	132.4 (14.2)	132.7 (13.0)	133.8 (14.6)	134.9 (13.7)	134.5 (13.2)	136.7 (15.8)	136.2 (14.0)
Condition 2	198.6 (19.6)	159.9 (21.0)	133.7 (12.9)	133.4 (13.1)	134.3 (13.5)	134.8 (13.3)	136.6 (12.8)	137.1 (13.7)	137.6 (13.6)	138.7 (11.9)
Condition 3	199.5 (15.0)	159.3 (15.3)	138.8 (15.3)	149.1 (19.0)	152.1 (14.4)	153.8 (14.5)	159.6 (12.7)	160.0 (13.0)	161.0 (10.8)	165.0 (11.5)

Note. Values are mean (SD, standard deviation).

Table 1. EMG-RT values for conditions 1–3 (unit: ms).

13.8) [10]. The following 21 test conditions were applied: periodic auditory stimuli with an ISI of 1500 ms, and only the last stimulus interval shifted to 1485, 1470, 1455, 1440, 1425, 1410, 1395, 1380, 1365, 1350, 1335, 1320, 1305, 1290, 1275, 1260, 1245, 1230, 1215, and 1200 ms (intervals shortened from 1 to 20% of 1500 ms), in successive stimuli sequences at an ISI of 1500 ms. Each condition was composed of 6–10 stimuli. There were 10 trials performed during each condition for a total of 210 trials; each subject performed the 210 trials over a period of 5 days (42 trials per day). EMG-RT values for the last stimulus were compared among the 21 conditions. EMG-RT value responses to stimuli with an ISI of 1500 ms (no rhythm shift) were 142.4 ± 8.9 ms. The EMG-RT values for 20 test conditions with rhythm shift are shown in **Table 2.** The EMG-RT values of shifts in ISI from 8 to 20% of the 1500 ms were significantly delayed compared with those during the periodic auditory stimuli with an ISI of 1500 ms with shifts in ISI from 1 to 7% of 1500 ms ($p < 0.01$). The EMG-RT values of shifts in ISI from 15 to 20% of 1500 ms were significantly delayed compared with shifts in ISI from 8 to 11% of 1500 ms ($p < 0.01$).

2.3. Practical considerations for the use of reactive periodic movement in physical therapy

Small changes below 5% of the base interval are considered to be below the threshold of conscious recognition [11]. For a base interval of 1500 ms, our three experiments revealed that the reactive movements can be performed without delay under conditions with an ISI shift below the threshold of conscious recognition. The periodic rhythmic stimulation is predicted to comprise some time duration. The prediction system for stimuli plays the same role as in the case of constant rhythm in such an ISI shift, and the readiness for movement will be maintained in the central nervous system. On the other hand, changes of 20% of the base interval are considered to be above the threshold of conscious recognition [11]. Our data showed that EMG-RTs were delayed during the 20% ISI shift. The prediction system for the stimulus loses its ability, and the central nervous system will need to provide new motor commands. Furthermore, experiment 4 revealed that the periodic rhythmic stimulation with the 1500-ms interval is predicted to comprise an approximately 100 ms duration. The reactive movements can be performed without delay with an ISI shift of 7% of 1500 ms. Finger tapping produces a series of intervals with substantial variability, even when they are intended to be regular; the typical SD is 3–6% of an ISI within a range of 200–2000 ms [12]. When the physical therapist facilitates rhythmical reactive periodic movement using a handclap, it will be desirable to keep the rhythm shift in a range within 7% of the ISI.

Rate of rhythm shift									
1%	**2%**	**3%**	**4%**	**5%**	**6%**	**7%**	**8%**	**9%**	**10%**
141.6 (8.6)	141.9 (8.6)	143.3 (5.7)	146.9 (8.9)	145.4 (8.6)	142.9 (7.2)	147.3 (8.0)	164.2 (10.0)	166.5 (7.5)	165.0 (4.8)
11%	**12%**	**13%**	**14%**	**15%**	**16%**	**17%**	**18%**	**19%**	**20%**
164.7 (9.6)	174.0 (12.0)	175.2 (10.7)	174.8 (11.8)	181.3 (8.5)	182.7 (12.5)	186.9 (7.3)	187.0 (9.7)	186.8 (8.3)	189.3 (14.4)

Note. Values are mean (SD).

Table 2. EMG-RT values for 20 test conditions with rhythm shift (unit: ms).

3. External pacing on the control of periodic movement

3.1. Influence of pacing with auditory stimuli on movement continuation

The purpose of this study was to determine if the pacing of external events could be used to control rhythmic movement by comparing the variability of periodic tapping using the self-paced, synchronization-continuation, and syncopation-continuation paradigms.

Eighteen healthy subjects (8 men, 10 women; mean age, 23.9 years) participated in this study. All subjects were strongly right-handed according to the Edinburgh Handedness Inventory (mean laterality quotient, 91.2) [13]. The subjects had no motor function abnormalities of the right index finger and no hearing abnormalities. Regarding the apparatus, the MQ8, VitalRecorder2, and BIMUTAS-Video introduced in the previous section were also used in this study. The auditory stimulus system was set up using Viking Quest (Nicolet Biomedical, Wisconsin, USA).

The experiment was conducted in a quiet room. The subjects were seated with eyes closed and the right forearm was placed in a pronated position on a desk in front of them. They were required to tap with the right index finger during the following three tasks: task 1, self-paced tapping with no auditory stimuli with the subjects performing 15 successive taps for the directed interval; task 2, synchronization-continuation tapping, which incorporated the subjects tapping in synchrony with 15 periodic auditory stimuli (pacing phase), and then continuing to perform 15 taps at the same rate without the auditory stimuli (continuation phase); task 3, syncopation-continuation tapping, which involved the subjects tapping in synchrony with the midpoint of each stimulus of 15 periodic auditory stimuli (pacing phase), and then continuing to perform 15 taps at the same rate without the auditory stimuli (continuation phase). The time difference between the onset of two successive stimuli was defined as the ISI, and a total of three different ISIs were used in the pacing phase of tasks 2 and 3: 1000, 2000, and 5000 ms. These were also the directed intervals used in task 1. Each task was repeated three times and a total of nine trials were performed at random by each subject. The execution of each task in each subject was carried out over 3 days. Task 1 was performed on day 1, and then tasks 2 and 3 were performed at random. The parameters evaluating the tapping were the mean and coefficient of variation (CV) of the ITI. Synchronization error (SE) in the pacing phase of task 2 was defined as the time difference between the taps and stimulus onset. SE in the pacing phase of task 3 was defined as the time difference between the taps and midpoint of successive stimuli. In all tasks, the latter 10 ITIs in each sequence were used for analysis. The paired *t*-test was used to compare the pacing phases of tasks 2 and 3. One-way repeated measures ANOVA was used to compare task 1 and the continuation phases of tasks 2 and 3. When a significant difference was recognized, paired comparisons were performed using Tukey's posthoc test. In the pacing phases of tasks 2 and 3, the distribution of SE was also considered within these comparisons.

The mean and CV values of the ITI for the pacing phases of tasks 2 and 3 are shown in **Table 3**. There were no significant differences according to the paired *t*-test. Distributions of SEs for the pacing phases of tasks 2 and 3 are shown in **Figures 3** and **4**. A positive asynchrony for any ISI was observed in task 3 compared with that during task 2. In addition, as the duration of ISI increased, the distribution became less peaked. The mean and CV values

	Task 2	Task 3
Mean (ms)		
1000 ms	996.3 ± 3.7	997.3 ± 4.4
2000 ms	1999.2 ± 10.9	1994.1 ± 15.6
5000 ms	5003.4 ± 19.9	5004.1 ± 49.0
CV (%)		
1000 ms	3.1 ± 0.9	3.0 ± 1.3
2000 ms	3.8 ± 1.4	4.2 ± 2.5
5000 ms	4.4 ± 2.0	4.4 ± 2.4

Note. Values are mean ± SD.

Table 3. Mean and CV values in the pacing phases of tasks 2 and 3.

of the ITI for task 1 and the continuation phases of tasks 2 and 3 are shown in **Table 4**. For the ISI of 1000 ms, one-way ANOVA revealed a significant difference between the mean ITIs for different tasks. Posthoc analyses showed that the mean ITI was significantly smaller in tasks 2 and 3 when compared to that in task 1. For the ISI of 2000 ms, the CV was significantly larger for task 3 than for task 1. For the ISI of 5000 ms, the mean ITI was significantly larger for tasks 2 and 3 than for task 1, and the CV was significantly larger for tasks 2 and 3 than for task 1. There were no significant differences among other comparisons.

In the pacing phase, there was no difference in the accuracy or consistency of tapping between the synchronization and syncopation patterns. On the other hand, the distribution of SE showed different characteristics between the two paradigms. The SE distribution of the synchronization paradigm for the ISIs 1000 and 2000 ms displayed similar tendencies to a previous study in which SE almost always indicated negative asynchrony with a small spread in SE distribution for ISIs from 450 to 1500 ms, and anticipatory tapping with a large negative SE and reactive tapping were mixed in SE distribution for ISIs from 1800 to 3600 ms [14]. In both paradigms, positive asynchrony representing reactive tapping was seen. In the synchronization tapping task, anticipatory tapping and reactive tapping were identified when the standard value of SE was set at 100 ms [14]. When we adopted this criterion, the SE data for task 2 identified reactive tapping (0, 13, and 52 of 180 trials for ISIs 1000, 2000 and 5000 ms, respectively). The distribution of SE in syncopation tapping using isochronous auditory stimuli has not been reported in previous studies. Although the SE distributions of the pacing phase of synchronization and syncopation were different, there was no difference in the accuracy and consistency of tapping between these patterns. Rhythmic synchronization tasks require two timing demands: rhythm production at the same frequency as an external stimulus and motor responses that coincide in time with the stimulus. In the pacing phase of this study, the rhythmicity of periodic movement might have been mainly controlled by temporal information from the auditory stimulus rather than the error between auditory stimuli and tapping.

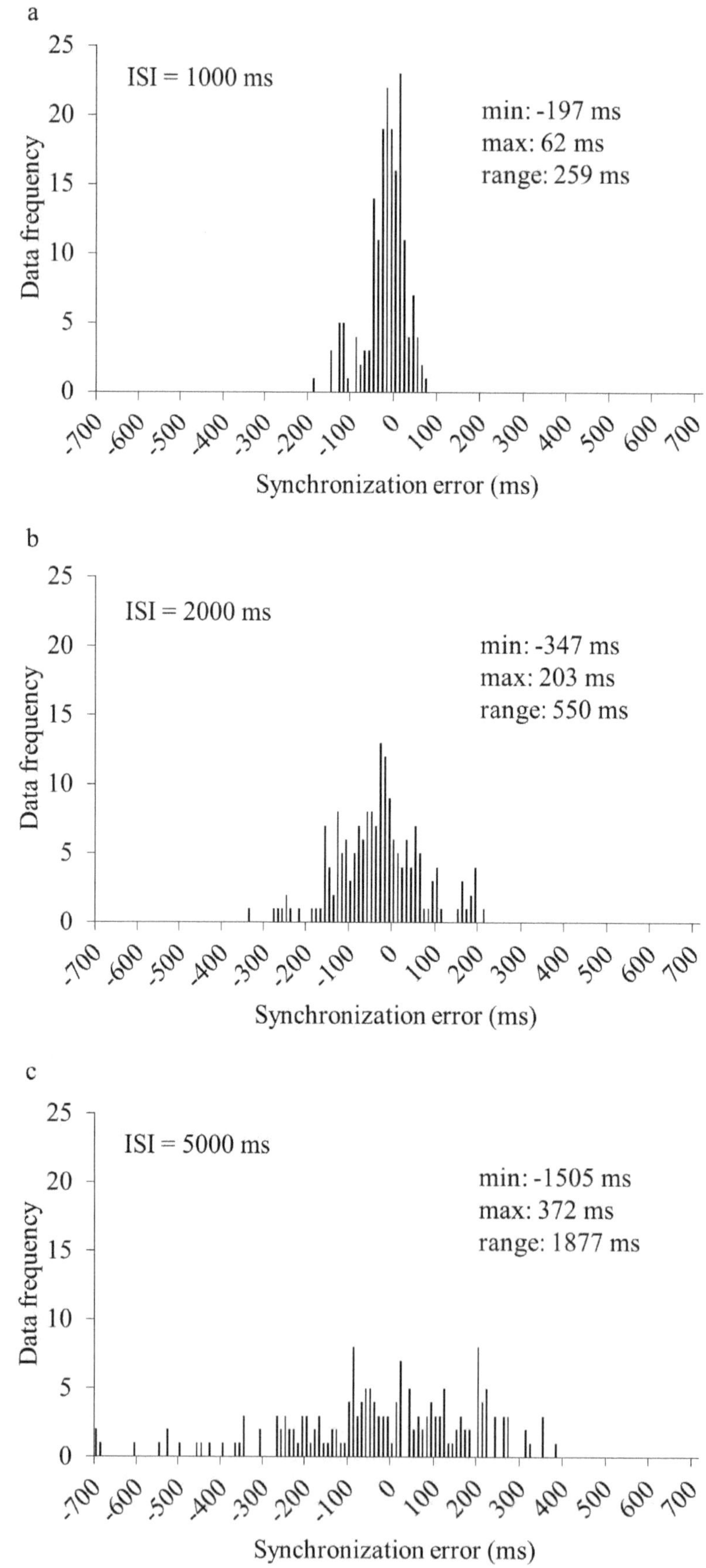

Figure 3. Distribution of SE for the ISI of (a) 1000, (b) 2000, and (c) 5000 ms in the pacing phase of task 2.

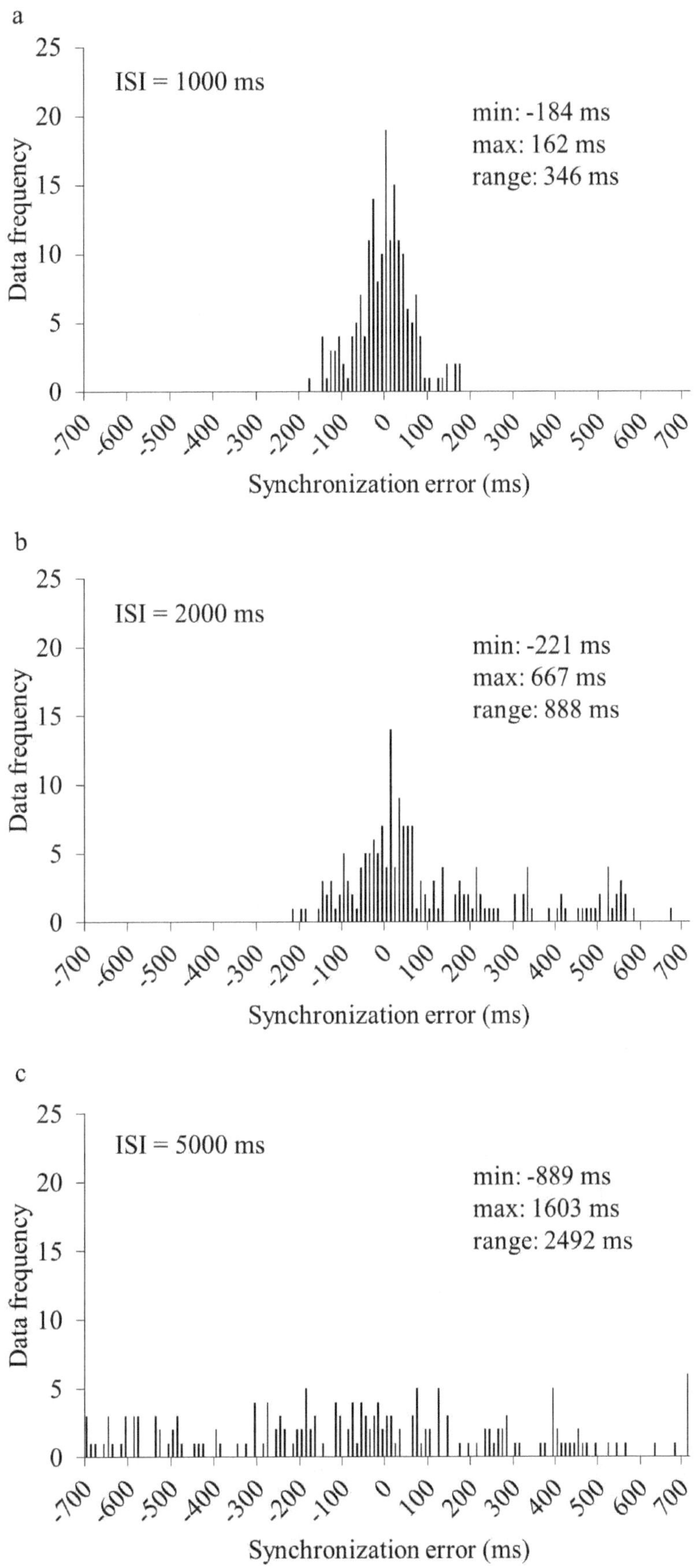

Figure 4. Distribution of SE for the ISI of (a) 1000, (b) 2000, and (c) 5000 ms in the pacing phase of task 3.

	Task 1	Task 2	Task 3
Mean (ms)			
1000 ms	1137.0 ± 202.9	1000.7 ± 51.7**	1022.8 ± 77.8*
2000 ms	1847.9 ± 368.8	1982.5 ± 187.2	2077.6 ± 325.5
5000 ms	4177.8 ± 1050.8	5202.6 ± 381.8**	5342.8 ± 511.4**
CV (%)			
1000 ms	4.0 ± 1.2	3.4 ± 0.9	4.0 ± 1.7
2000 ms	3.6 ± 1.1	4.1 ± 1.9	4.9 ± 1.5*
5000 ms	3.5 ± 2.0	5.4 ± 1.7*	5.9 ± 2.7**

Note: Values are mean ± SD.
*$p < 0.05$ compared with task 1.
** $p < 0.01$ compared with task 1.

Table 4. Mean and CV values in task 1 and the continuation phases of tasks 2 and 3.

For the ISI of 1000 ms, a comparison of task 1 with the continuation phase of tasks 2 and 3 showed that accuracy improved following a pacing phase, which suggests a close relationship between the length of the stimulus interval and attentional resources. A study using synchronization tapping in parallel with word-memory task demonstrated that a reduction in attentional resources caused by the execution of a secondary task did not have a significant effect on automatic anticipation in the 450–1500 ms ISI range [14]. However, in the ISI range of 1800–3600 ms, anticipatory tapping was substantially affected by tasks that decreased attentional resources. These results suggest that a timing control mechanism independent of attentional resources, the so-called "automatic movement," exists in the case of an ISI below 1800 ms, and that tapping was controlled in a feed-forward rather than feed-back manner. The results of previous studies suggest that the mechanism for anticipatory timing control is different and has an ISI threshold of 1800 ms. In addition, it was shown that prediction of the next stimulus becomes more difficult with longer ISIs. The accuracy of tapping in the continuation phase was improved by pacing at an ISI of 1000 ms. This is most likely because the interval was shorter than 1800 ms.

For the ISI of 2000 ms, a comparison of task 1 with the continuation phase of tasks 2 and 3 showed that the CV was significantly high under self-paced conditions, but only for the syncopation component. The ITI series of task 3 for an ISI of 2000 ms indicates that several subjects drift away from the 2000-ms interval during the continuation phase, although the mean ITI for the 18 subjects was 2077.6 ms. During additional analysis, the autocorrelation functions (ACF) were used for analysis of the ITI time series data. Regarding the ACF for the time series data (10 pacing phase ITIs and 10 continuation phase ITIs), the criteria for data selection of ITI drift were set as lag 1 > 0.4. Based on results of the ACF, the 18 subjects were divided evenly into two groups (the ITI drift group and ITI nondrift group). The mean ACF for the ITI series of both groups are shown in **Figure 5**. For the ITI drift group, a positive peak appears in the lag 1 autocorrelation and a negative peak appears in the lag 10 autocorrelation.

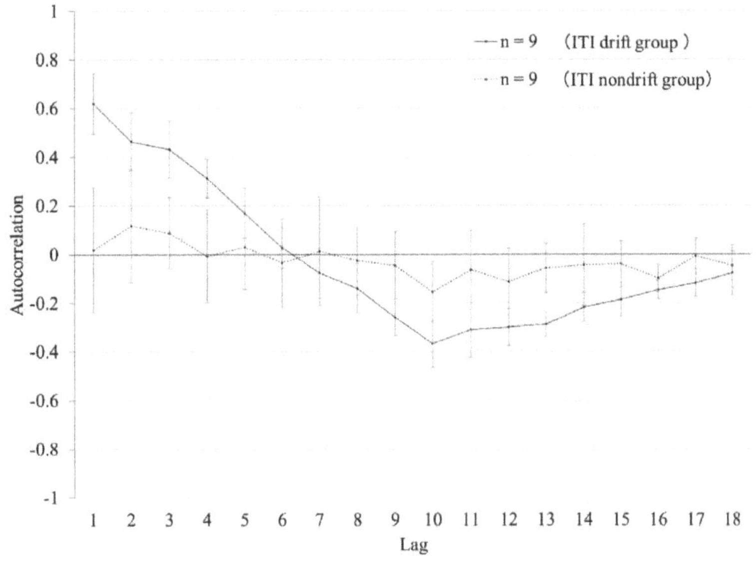

Figure 5. Mean autocorrelation functions for the ITI series in ITI drift and nondrift groups.

In a comparison of both groups, an unpaired *t*-test revealed no significant differences in the pacing (syncopation) phase. In the continuation phase, the CV of the ITI drift group (5.8 ± 1.1%) was significantly higher than that of the ITI nondrift group (3.9 ± 1.4%) (**Figure 6**).

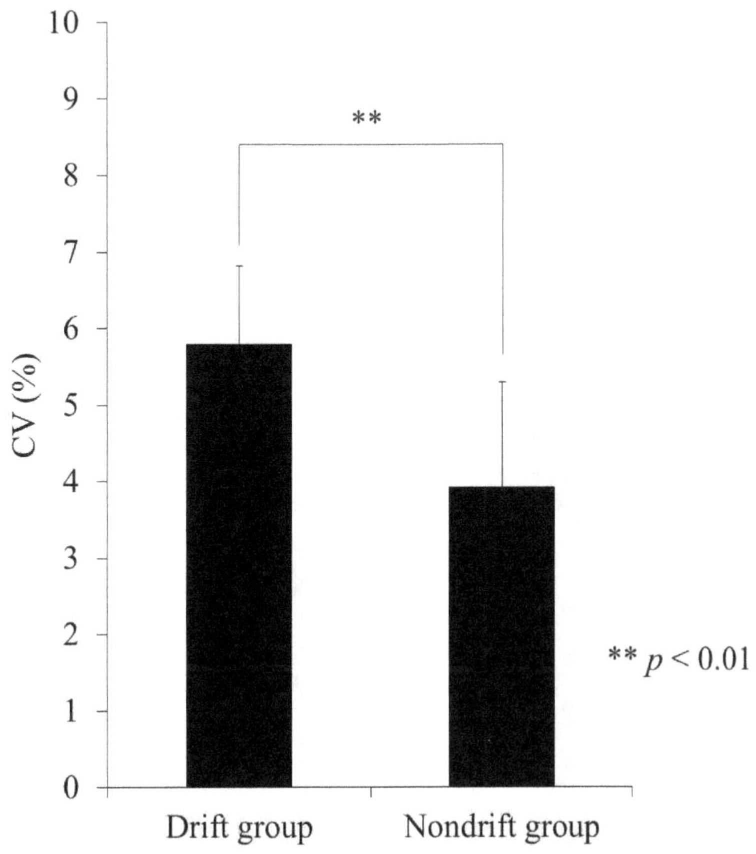

Figure 6. CV values for continuation phase of task 3 in ITI drift and nondrift groups.

We observed a large variation in the ITI during the continuation phase in subjects with ITI drift. The interval of 2000 ms was similar to the 1800-ms interval reported in a previous study [14], and the difficulty of the periodic movement with the 2000-ms interval was different for each individual.

A strategy used to perform syncopation tapping with a 2000-ms interval involves a stimulus and tap repeated at intervals of 1000 ms. The accurate estimation of the 1000 ms interval is required to execute this strategy. In comparing the self-paced tapping (1000 ms) in both groups, an unpaired *t*-test revealed that the CV of the ITI drift group (4.5 ± 0.9%) was significantly higher than that of the ITI nondrift group (3.3 ± 1.1%) (**Figure 7**).

Additional analysis demonstrated that the correlation coefficient was 0.42 for the mean ITI between task 1 (target duration: 1000 ms) and the continuation phase of task 3 (target duration: 2000 ms) (**Figure 8**). The area surrounded by gray in **Figure 8** shows that the ITIs for the continuation phase of task 3 are about twice the value of the ITIs for task 1.

In the continuation phase following the syncopation tapping, the subjects had to estimate the 1000 ms interval to determine the time between the lack of stimulus and their tap. However,

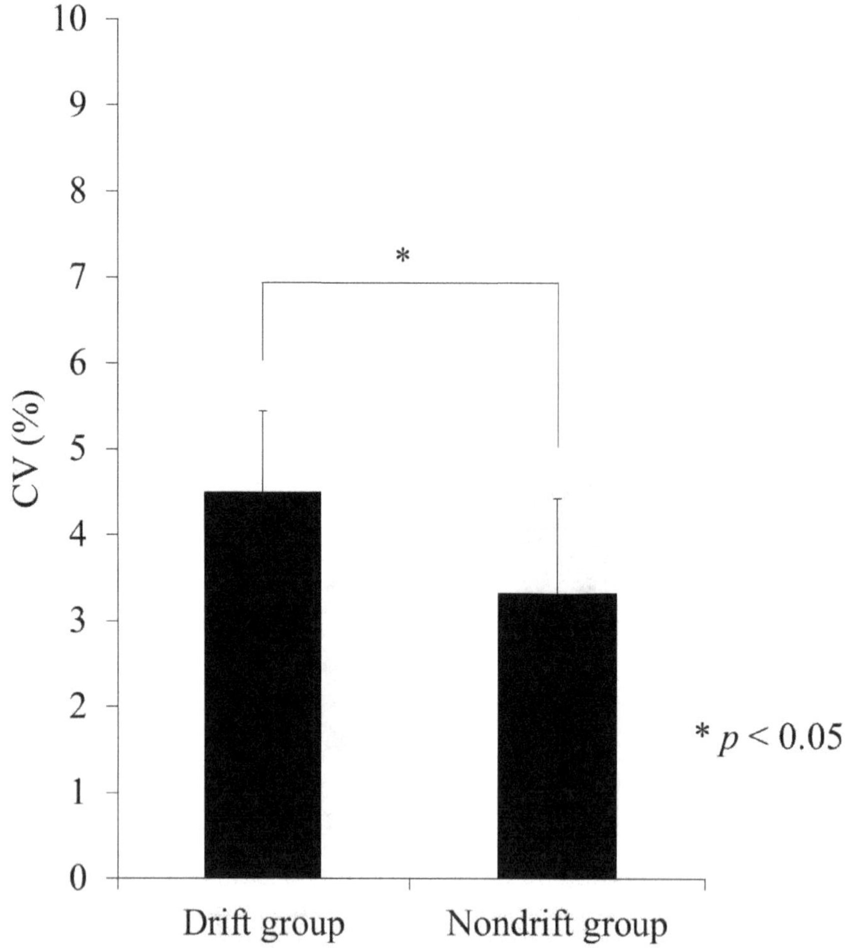

Figure 7. CV values for task 1 (1000 ms) in ITI drift and nondrift groups.

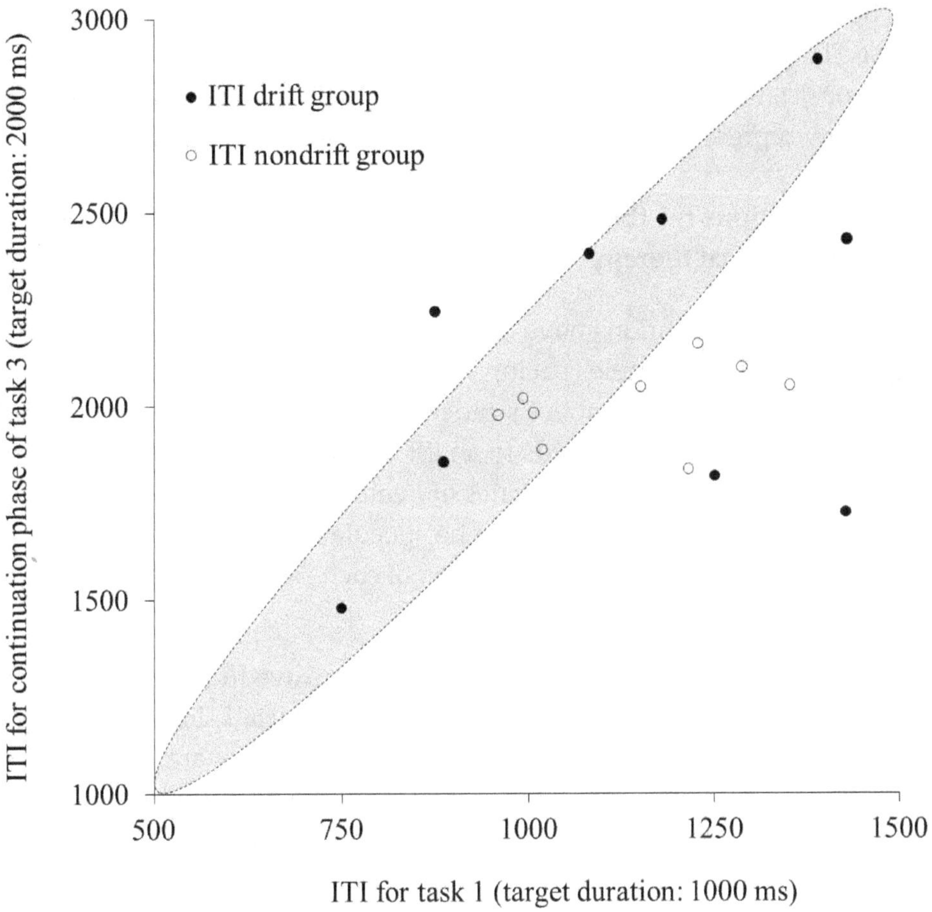

Figure 8. Correlation for the mean ITI between task 1 (target duration: 1000 ms) and the continuation phase of task 3 (target duration: 2000 ms).

since deviations from the target duration were large during the self-paced tapping for the 1000-ms interval (i.e., the ability to estimate a 1000 ms interval was poor), accurate movement in the continuation phase would be more difficult. If the syncopation tapping of the interval for 2000 ms is adopted as the pacing interval, the subjects should be able to accurately estimate the halfway point of the time interval.

For ISI > 5000 ms, estimation of temporal duration was shown to involve memory [15], which concurs with the finding in our study that reactive tapping markedly increased with an ISI of 5000 ms. Reactive tapping is one when the movement is performed after identification of a stimulus, and indicates that the prediction of the next stimulus input was difficult. Therefore, for an ISI of 5000 ms, negative asynchrony and positive asynchrony were intermingled and the SE distribution was broad. Regarding the syncopation pattern, positive asynchrony had a larger spread because participants were not able to react to the stimulus since there was no stimulus corresponding to the tap. These findings showed the 5000 ms task is performed in a nonrhythmical manner and relies on memory more than timing. True rhythm should refer only to events within the time scale of short-term memory [11]. Intervals of 5000 ms are likely too long for the facilitation of movement using pacing, as movement under both the synchronization and syncopation conditions will be controlled by memory; thus, variability in the periodic movement will be large. Even though the ITI for the self-paced condition deviated considerably from the actual 5000-ms interval, the consistency of the tapping was maintained. Despite individual differences, we believe the variability represented the maximum performance for finger tapping.

3.2. Practical considerations for the use of continuation paradigm of sensorimotor synchronization in physical therapy

Investigations of clinical applications have demonstrated that pacing is effective when the ISI is shorter than 1000 ms; for example, pacing during the time when the interval of auditory stimulus was set up based on each patient's cadence. The average cadence of healthy subjects was 110 steps/min [16], which corresponds to an ISI of about 545 ms. During the sensorimotor synchronization task, the preferred tempo rates of healthy subjects were reported to be 767 ms [17]. Based on the findings of this study, it can be speculated that the pacing of periodic auditory stimuli might function in refining the precision of each individual's internal timing mechanism, particularly at an ISI of 1000 ms.

On the other hand, the consistency of tapping did not improve in a continuation phase when compared with that during self-paced tapping in any of the trials. Finger tapping produces a series of intervals whose variability is substantial, even when they are intended to be regular, and the typical standard deviation corresponds to 3–6% of the ISI within a range of 200–2000 ms [12]. The values of CV in task 1 of this study were 4.0, 3.6, and 3.5% for intervals of 1000, 2000, and 5000 ms, respectively. Although there were individual differences, this variability probably represented the innate maximum performance for finger tapping in each interval. When periodic movement was produced as they were in task 1, it indicates innate skill, which produces the consistent rhythm, even if error exists between the directed interval and ITI. Although the auditory rhythm was provided as a trigger in the pacing phase, movement in the subsequent continuation phase would be dependent on innate skill.

In conclusion, in physical therapy, the accuracy of periodic movement with an ISI of 1000 ms can be improved using auditory pacing. In addition, the consistency of periodic movement is mainly dependent on each individual's innate skill, and thus improvement in consistency based on pacing is unlikely. The limitation of this study was that the periodic movement of intervals around 1000 ms was not examined in detail. In the future, it is expected that the periodic movement of short intervals will be evaluated to examine not only the instant effect of pacing but also the training effect on longitudinal intervention.

Author details

Masanori Ito*, Yuki Takahashi, Satoshi Fujiwara and Naoki Kado

*Address all correspondence to: itou@sumire-academy.ac.jp

Department of Physical Therapy, Kobe College of Rehabilitation and Welfare, Kobe-shi, Hyogo, Japan

References

[1] Safranek MG, Koshland GF, Raymond G. Effect of auditory rhythm on muscle activity. Physical Therapy. 1982;**62**(2):161–168.

[2] McIntosh GC, Brown SH, Rice RR, Thaut MH. Rhythmic auditory-motor facilitation of gait patterns in patients with Parkinson's disease. Journal of Neurology, Neurosurgery, and Psychiatry. 1997;**62**(1):22–26. DOI: 10.1136/jnnp.62.1.22

[3] Thaut MH, McIntosh GC, Rice RR. Rhythmic facilitation of gait training in hemiparetic stroke rehabilitation. Journal of Neurological Sciences. 1997;**151**(2):207–212. DOI: 10.1016/S0022-510X(97)00146-9

[4] Takahashi Y, Fujiwara S, Ito M, Kado N, Suzuki T. Influence of subliminal rhythm shift on reactive periodic movement. Rigakuryoho Kagaku. 2013;**28**(2):249–252. DOI: 10.1589/rika.28.249

[5] Takahashi Y, Fujiwara S, Ito M, Kado N, Suzuki T. Influence of subliminal rhythm shift with a lengthened interval on reactive periodic movement. The Journal of Japanese Physical Therapy Association. 2014;**41**(5):306–311.

[6] Takahashi Y. The influence of auditory stimulation rhythm shift prediction on electromyographic reaction time [thesis]. Osaka: Graduate School of Kansai University of Health Sciences; 2013. 193 p.

[7] Takahashi Y, Fujiwara S, Ito M, Kado N, Suzuki T. Difference in rate of rhythm shift of auditory stimulation on rhythmical reactive periodic movement. Journal of Kansai Physical Therapy. 2014;**14**:49–58. DOI: 10.11354/jkpt.14.49

[8] Ito M, Kado N, Suzuki T, Ando H. Influence of pacing by periodic auditory stimuli on movement continuation: comparison with self-regulated periodic movement. Journal of Physical Therapy Science. 2013;**25**(9):1141–1146. DOI: 10.1589/jpts.25.1141

[9] Fujiwara S, Ito M, Kado N, Suzuki T, Shimada T. Influence of varying the interstimulus interval on electromyographic reaction time during exercise using a rhythmic auditory stimulus – effect of increasing the stimulus number and changing the interstimulus interval. Journal of Kansai Physical Therapy. 2010;**10**:71–76. DOI: 10.11354/jkpt.10.71

[10] Chapman JP, Chapman LJ, Allen JJ. The measurement of foot preference. Neuropsychologia. 1987;**25**(3):579–584.

[11] Thaut MH. Rhythm, music, and the brain: scientific foundations and clinical applications. 1st ed. New York: Routledge; 2008. 247 p.

[12] Madison G. Variability in isochronous tapping: higher order dependencies as a function of intertap interval. Journal of Experimental Psychology: Human Perception and Performance. 2001;**27**(2):411–422. DOI: 10.1037//0096-1523.27.2.411

[13] Oldfield RC. The assessment and analysis of handedness: the Edinburgh inventory. Neuropsychologia. 1971;**9**(1):97–113. DOI: 10.1016/0028-3932(71)90067-4

[14] Miyake Y, Onishi Y, Pöppel E. Two types of anticipation in synchronization tapping. Acta Neurobiologiae Experimentalis (Wars). 2004;**64**(3):415–426.

[15] Fraisse P. Perception and estimation of time. Annual Review of Psychology. 1984;**35**:1–36. DOI: 10.1146/annurev.ps.35.020184.000245

[16] Neumann DA. Kinesiology of the musculoskeletal system: foundations for physical rehabilitation. 1st ed. St. Louis: Mosby; 2002. 597 p.

[17] Thaut MH, Kenyon GP. Rapid motor adaptations to subliminal frequency shifts during syncopated rhythmic sensorimotor synchronization. Human Movement Science. 2003;**22**(3):321–338. DOI: 10.1016/S0167-9457(03)00048-4

6

Comprehensive Physical Function Assessment in Elderly People

Tadashi Ito

Additional information is available at the end of the chapter

Abstract

In elderly people with mobility limitations, abnormalities in posture and gait contribute to the greater decline of physical motor function. The aim of the review article was to determine the comprehensive physical motor function assessment. Muscle function was assessed with the grip strength. Gait function was assessed with walking time tests conducted at a normal pace. Balance function was assessed with one-legged standing time. The 6-min walking distance test (6MD) was performed in a 10-m, straight corridor. Walking efficiency during the 6MD trials was measured using the Cosmed K4b2 (Rome, Italy), an indirect calorimetry system specifically designed to measure energy expenditure in nonlaboratory settings. The center of pressure was recorded using a balance board (Wii; Nintendo Co., Ltd., Kyoto, Japan). A vibratory stimulus was applied alternately to two muscles by fixing two vibrators from the vibration device onto the participant's gastrocnemius and lumbar multifidus muscle. These findings show that an assessment affecting postural control under proprioceptive stimulation might be a good indicator of elderly people. Also, the objective assessment of walking efficiency might be important for identifying the risk of external activity limitation or functional limitations among the late elderly.

Keywords: elderly people, physical function assessment, walking efficiency, proprioceptive system

1. Introduction

The ability to walk safely and postural control stabilization are vital for elderly people to decrease their risk of falling and to maintain their independence. A function of walking that accompanies aging is a higher energy cost of movement, often referred to as a lower economy of walking [1, 2]. In addition, a defect or slowing of this mechanism has been suggested to explain the difficulties experienced by older persons when trying to control their posture [3, 4]. Moreover, both muscle strength and lower postural stability decline with aging [5, 6]. Therefore, aging is characterized by changes in the neuromuscular system that decreases muscle strength, balance, and proprioception.

Meanwhile, this progressive decline in physical capacities reduces the ability of elderly people to perform complex motor tasks and is associated with impaired mobility and a reduction in the ability [7]. Assessment of motor function contributes to the identification of factors that generate impairments to the performance of daily activities and an increase in the risk of falls for elderly people. Moreover, assessment of motor function by physical therapist provides important information about age-related progressive reduction in muscle strength, ability to walk, and postural control.

This chapter provides an overview of the assessment method on motor function in elderly people.

2. The relationship between walking efficiency and life-space assessment in elderly people

2.1. Life-space assessment

The increased metabolic cost of walking can detract from the activity and quality of life of elderly people as a decline in physical activity rapidly degrades physical and psychological functions [8, 9]. Life space has been reported to have good construct and criterion validity for measuring the severity of mobility limitations, and achieving efficient walking plays a crucial role in the extension of life space. Life-space assessment (LSA) is a tool that measures mobility and reflects participation in society based on the distance through which a person reports moving during the 4 weeks prior to the assessment [10, 11]. Life space, a relatively understudied concept in gerontology, can be defined as the size of the spatial area a person intentionally moves through in daily life, as well as the frequency of travel within a specific time frame [10]. Also, a reduced frequency of going outdoors could represent reduced life space, which has been hypothesized to be a risk factor in future physical disability. Murata et al. reported that life space was related not only to age or health status but also to environmental or psychosocial factors [12]. Shimada et al.'s reports confirm that LSA was more strongly associated with gait speed than the other gait variables [13] and also show that these declines in physical performances were apparent at age 80 years and over in women and at age 90 years and over in men [13].

LSA may reflect the physical activity status indirectly in elderly people because the LSA score is associated with physical performance, Activities of Daily Living (ADL), and sociodemographic factors [11].

Life-space mobility was measured using a Japanese translation of the LSA [14]. The LSA provided a score based on the distance a person reported moving during the 4 weeks before the assessment [10, 13].

The LSA scores range from 0 ("completely room-bound") to 120 ("travel out of town every day without assistance") [13].

2.2. Walking efficiency in elderly people

It may be that the decline in walking efficiency is a common result of the decrease of many bodily functions that capture the overall impact of life space and is an important indicator of life space. However, the mechanism by which older people's life space and walking efficiency decline is not well investigated and remains poorly understood. Also, the specific mechanisms that explain the difference between the decline in walking efficiency and life space in early elderly and late elderly are not yet clear. Additionally, little is known about the relationship between the walking efficiency decline and confined life space to influence on aging.

In older adults with mobility limitations, abnormalities in posture and gait contribute to the greater energy cost of inefficient gait, with adjustments for age and gait speed [15]. Limitations in life space, as measured by the University of Alabama at Birmingham (UAB) life-space assessment, reflect lifestyle as well as walking efficiency and may be a valuable measure of functional decrease for community-dwelling elderly people, especially since life space specifically relates to mobility and a person's participation in society.

2.2.1. Walking efficiency assessment

Walking efficiency during the 6MD trials was measured using the Cosmed K4b2 (Rome, Italy), an indirect calorimetry system specifically designed to measure energy expenditure in nonlaboratory settings (**Figure 1**).

In brief, it uses a breath-by-breath measurement of gas exchange through a rubberized facemask and a turbine for gas collection, secured by a head harness. A flexible facemask that the participants keep in place by a head harness covers the participants' mouth and nose. Flexible facemask is attached to a digital turbine flowmeter to measure the volume of expired air and inspired. Sampling line from the turbine to analyzer unit system delivers expired air for the measurement (O_2, CO_2 content). Before test, the K4b2 was calibrated according to the manufacturer's guidelines. After warming up the unit for 60 min, the CO_2 and O_2 analyzers were calibrated against room air as well as a reference gas of known composition (4.94% CO_2, 16.07% O_2). Before walking efficiency assessment, each participant was required to sit quietly for 10 min as a rest period. The speed and distance of the 6-min walking distance test (6MD) was recorded using standardized procedures.

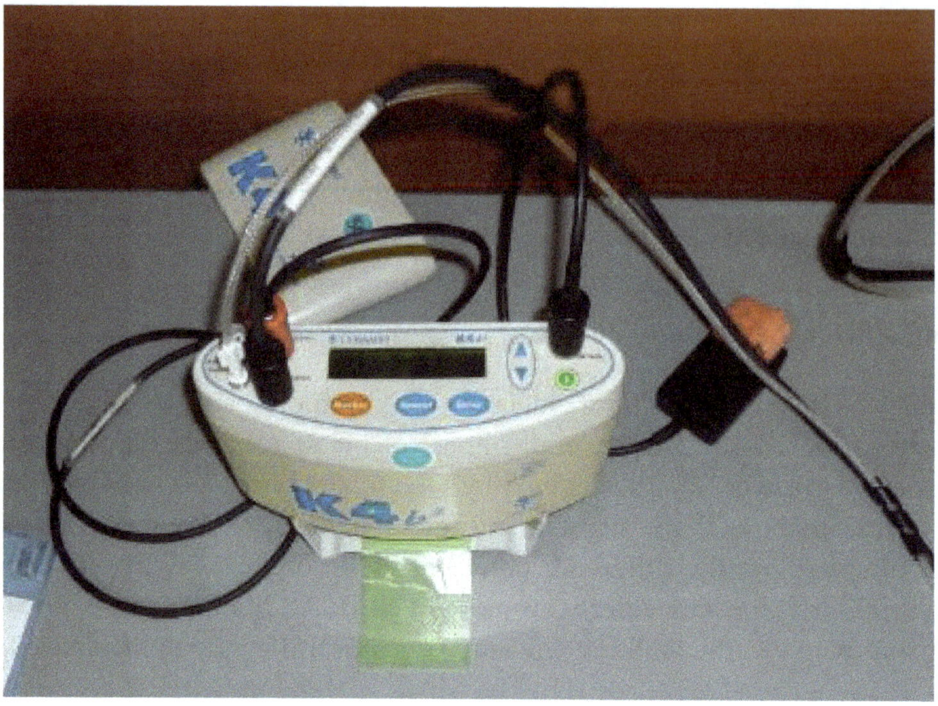

Figure 1. Expiration gas analyser.

Walking efficiency was calculated based on net efficiency as follows: Walking efficiency = (walking VO_2 ml/kg - resting VO_2 ml/kg)/6MD average walking speed (m/s) (**Figure 2**) [16]. The Cosmed K4b2 system uses the increased VO_2/kg ratio after noise processing to predict walking efficiency from O_2 consumption.

Breath-by-breath values from the Excel spreadsheet were calculated from the increased ratio over 1-breath intervals. Outliers from the increased ratio were calculated from exploratory data analysis of participants. We defined outliers (noise) as values beyond an increased ratio of 100%. Data that were more than 100% of the increased ratio were removed, and a below-100% value was calculated from the remaining test data. This method contributes to noise processing of the VO_2/kg signal. For each subject, walking efficiency was calculated by recording the noise-processed VO_2/kg values.

2.3. Relationship between walking efficiency and life-space assessment

Ito et al. reported the significant relationship between walking efficiency and LSA in late elderly [16]. Moreover, the data from this study suggest that as walking efficiency declines with age, life space increasingly declines (**Figure 3**). This suggests that the age-related decline of walking efficiency is caused by physiological changes of the late elderly. Other studies have suggested that as aerobic capacity declines with age, walking at a habitual speed becomes an increasingly more intense and therefore difficult activity, resulting in a slowing of walking speed in an effort to reduce fatigue [17]. Also, the previous study has shown that the walking energy cost for a comparable speed is generally higher for healthy

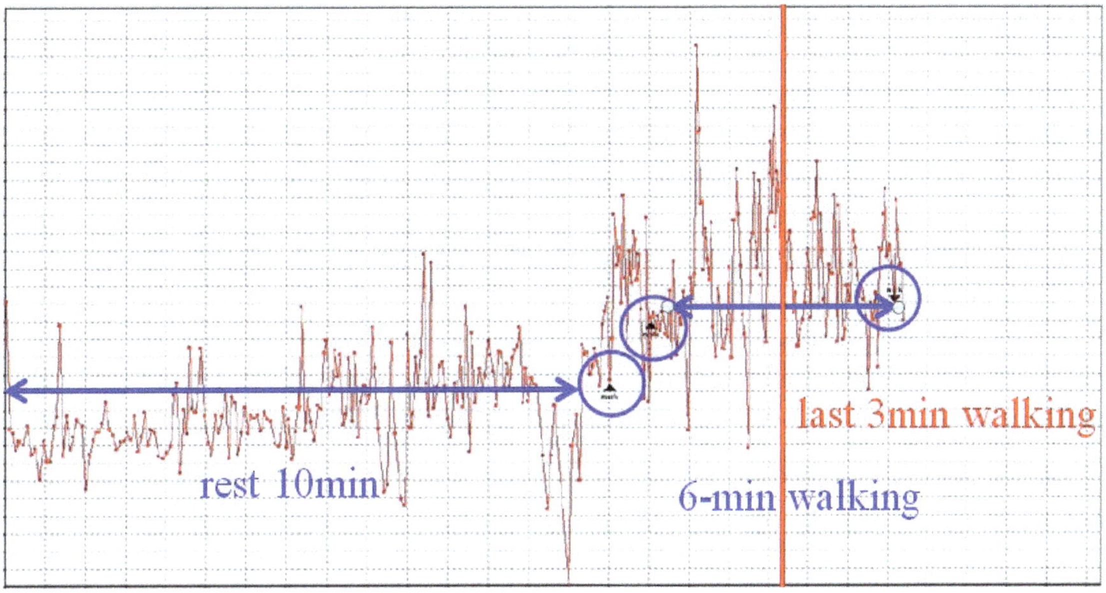

Figure 2. Walking efficiency = (walking VO_2 ml/kg - resting VO_2 ml/kg)/6MD average walking speed (m/s). Horizontal axis of blue shows the meaning of 10 min of the rest period and 6-min walking trial. Vertical axis of red shows the meaning of last 3 min of the 6-min walking trial. Following the transfer of data from the instrument, an Excel spreadsheet was used to calculate steady-state VO_2/kg and mean counts per minute during the last 3 min of the 6MD trial and 10 min of the rest period.

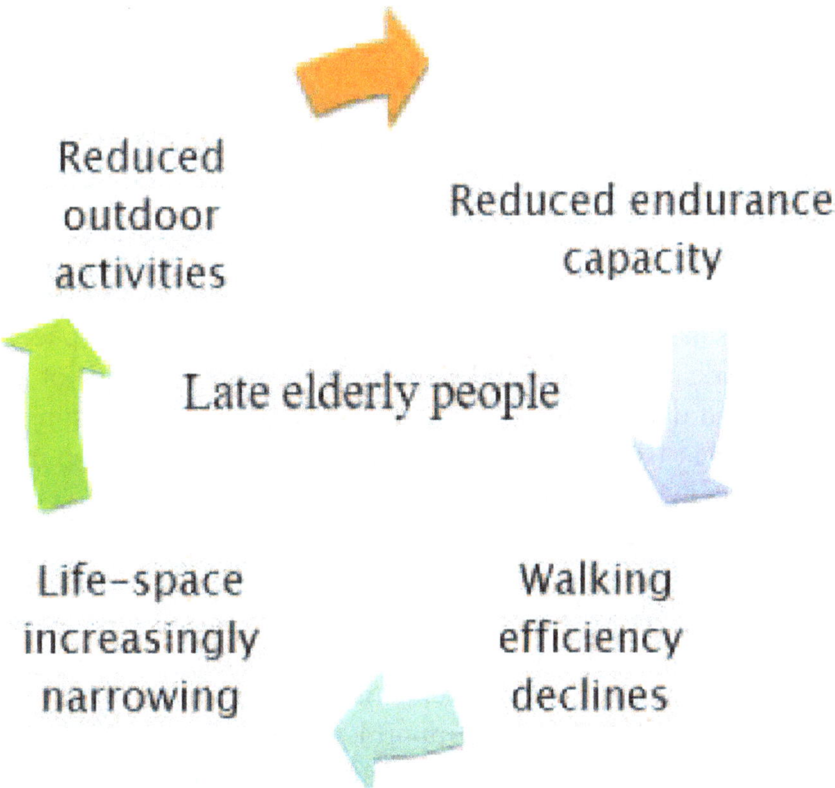

Figure 3. Schematic diagram of the incidence of walking efficiency decline in late elderly people.

elderly people, particularly those above 65 years, compared with younger people [18, 19]. Mechanisms related to the initiation and stepping patterns of gait, such as hip extension, step width, and cadence, have previously been reported to be related to the energy cost of walking in older adults with slow and variable gait [15]. Abe et al. reported that women of advanced age (75 years or older) have diminished pulmonary function, physical function, and mobility, and that diminished pulmonary function is associated with declining physical function [20]. Malatesta et al. reported that healthy octogenarians exhibited higher walking cost and greater stride time variability [21] and also reported that these declines in physical performances were apparent at age 80 years and over in women and at age 90 years and over in men [13]. Shimada reported that increased VO_2 in older adults manifests as walking becomes inefficient and reduced endurance capacity occurs [22].

This suggests that going activity to extension of LSA may better impact walking efficiency than efforts to improve gait speed and muscle strength.

3. Physical function assessments in elderly people

3.1. Performance assessment

The assessment measures are taken by well-trained staff who had nursing, physiotherapy, occupational therapy, or similar qualifications.

3.1.1. Grip strength assessment

Muscle function is assessed by the grip strength (GS) (**Figure 4**). GS is measured in kilograms in the participant's dominant hand using a Smedley-type handheld dynamometer (GRIP-D; Takei Ltd, Niigata, Japan).

3.1.2. Five-meter walk test

Five-meter walk test is assessed with walking conducted at a normal pace (usual walking speed; UWS). Two marks are used to indicate the path (start and end) of a 5-m walk path space. UWS is measured using a stopwatch system. Examiner tells the subjects to walk on a straight and flat surface at UWS. Moreover, examiner tells the subjects to maintain gait past the end of the walk path for a further 2.5 m.

3.1.3. One-legged standing time test

Balance function is assessed with one-legged standing time (**Figure 5**). One-legged standing time is used to measure how long a subject remains standing on one leg (eyes open). Subjects are allowed to decide which leg to use as support leg. Next, examiner tells the subjects to lift the converse foot from flat floor. Moreover, examiner tells the subjects to confirm sure not to press the lifted leg against support leg. The test ended when lifted leg touched the support leg, the lifted leg touched the floor, or after 60 s of successful balance.

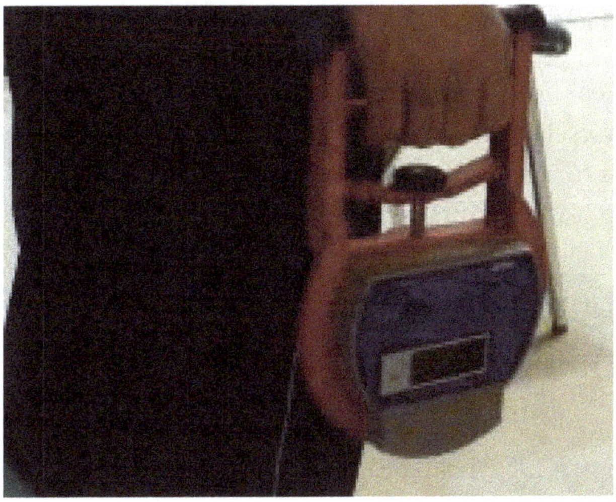

Figure 4. Grip strength assessment.

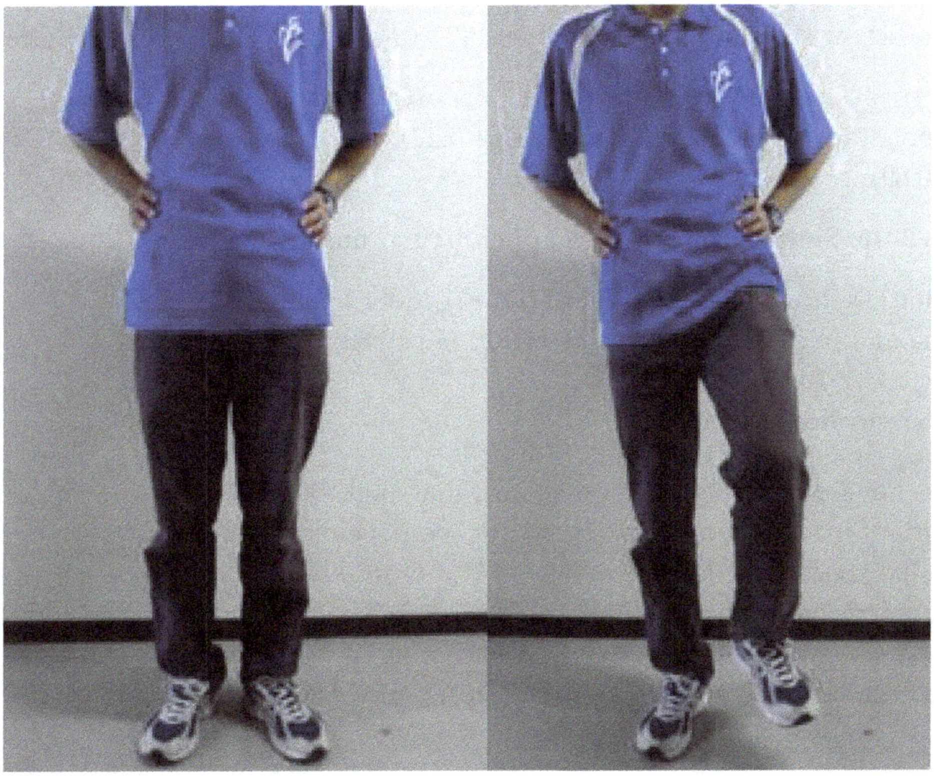

Figure 5. One-legged standing time test.

3.1.4. The 6-min walking distance test

6MD is performed in a 10-m, straight corridor. In the 6MD, participants are instructed to walk as quickly as possible to cover the longest distance possible within 6 min. This test measures the distance that a participant could quickly walk on a flat, hard surface in a period of 6 min.

3.1.5. Appendicular skeletal muscle mass assessment

In the elderly, muscle weakness is associated with the muscle atrophy aging (sarcopenia) progressive loss. Skeletal muscle mass loss may also have the potential to impact quality of life and ultimately the need for long-term care in elderly people [23]. Several studies developed equations for estimating skeletal muscle mass [24–26].

3.1.6. Prediction models

Sanada K, et al., 2010: Prediction models of sarcopenia [24]

Men: appendicular skeletal muscle mass = 0.326 × body mass index (BMI) − 0.047 × waist circumference - 0.011 × Age + 5.135 ($R^2 = 0.68$).

Women: appendicular skeletal muscle mass = 0.156 × BMI + 0.044 × hand grip strength − 0.010 × waist circumference + 2.747 ($R^2 = 0.57$).

Yoshida D, et al., 2014: Bioelectrical impedance analysis [25]

Men: appendicular skeletal muscle mass = 0.197 × (impedance index) + 0.179 × (weight) 0.019 ($R^2 = 0.87$).

Women: appendicular skeletal muscle mass = 0.221 × (impedance index) + 0.117 × (weight) + 0.881 ($R^2 = 0.89$).

Ito T, et al., 2016: Simple estimation of appendicular muscle mass [26]

Appendicular skeletal muscle mass = 5.051 × (gender: men = 1, women = 0) + 0.364 × (BMI) + 0.168 × (maximum calf circumference) − 0.815 ($R^2 = 0.80$).

3.2. Reduced physical activity

Past studies have provided the first evidence that slightly constricted life space may serve as an important marker and/or risk factor for the development of frailty, whereas severely constricted life space may indicate a high risk of mortality [27]. Webber et al. reported how mobility impairments can lead to limitations in accessing different life spaces and stressed the associations among determinants that influence mobility [28]. Previous study reported falls and reduced life space closely related to physical performance [29, 30].

4. Assessment of relative proprioceptive weighting ratio in elderly people with lumbar spondylosis

4.1. Sensory proprioceptive inputs in postural control

In daily life, an upright postural control task is essential for the activities of elderly people. After processing of the sensory inputs, individuals must integrate the respective contributions of the various sources of sensory information for regulating posture. Hay et al. reported that older persons have difficulties in taking advantage of sensory redundancy in postural control [31]. In addition, a defect or slowing of this mechanism has been suggested to explain the difficulties experienced by older persons when trying to control their posture [32, 33]. Proprioceptive input from the muscles of the legs and trunk plays an important role in maintaining postural stability [34]. Previous studies have reported that proprioception and vibration sensation in the lower limbs decrease during normal aging [3, 4] and also reported that postural instability has been observed in elderly people [35]. Therefore, a vibratory stimulus that matches the response frequency of the receptors present in skeletal muscle may influence body sway (**Figure 6**).

Previous studies have reported that patients with recurrent low back pain (LBP) have impaired motor control [36] and altered lumbosacral proprioceptive acuity [37, 38]. LBP is a widespread pathological condition that is often related to impaired or degenerated trunk mobility, which becomes evident during common activities [39, 40]. Taimela et al. reported that lumbar muscle fatigue impaired lumbar positional sense in both patients with LBP and healthy subjects [41]. These impairments lead to pain and declines in postural strategy, muscle function, and proprioception [42, 43].

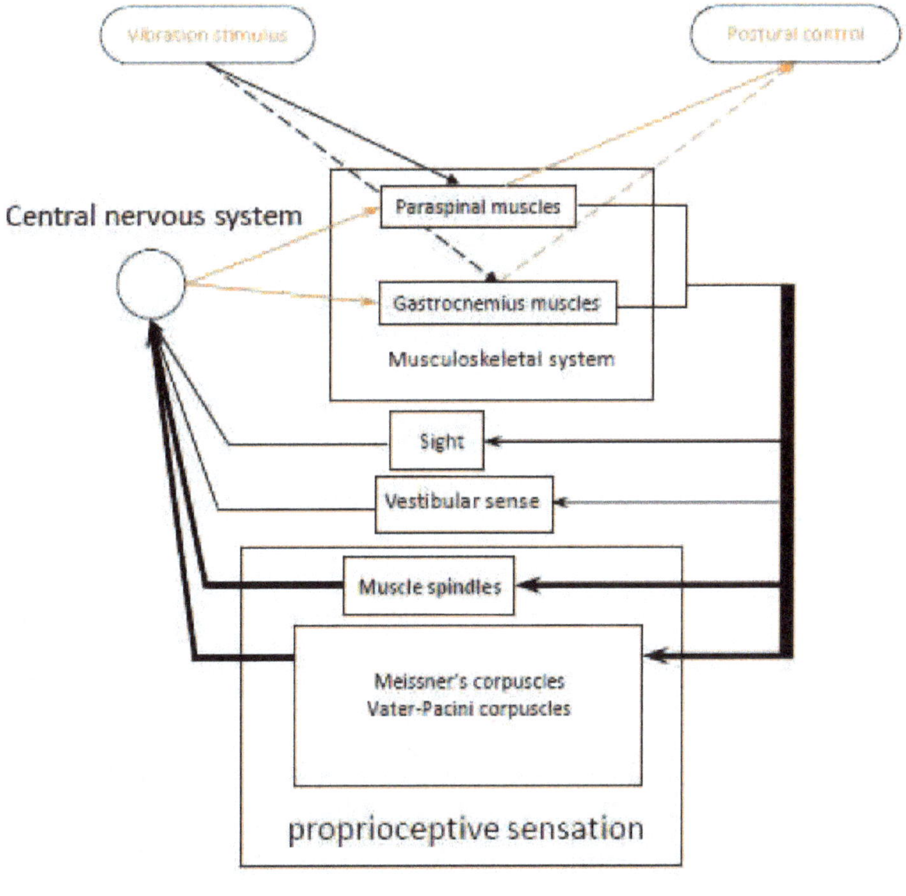

Figure 6. The representative receptor and response frequencies are 30 Hz in Meissner's corpuscles, 60 Hz in muscle spindles, and 240 Hz in Vater-Pacini corpuscles.

Muscle vibration, known to be a strong stimulus for muscle spindles and Vater-Pacini corpuscles, has been used to assess the role of proprioception [44, 45]. Both of these studies suggest that pain is a possible cause of decreased variability in postural strategy. These impairments lead to pain and declines in postural strategy, muscle function, and proprioception.

4.2. Assessment of relative proprioceptive weighting ratio

The center of pressure (COP) was recorded using a balance board (Wii; Nintendo Co., Ltd., Kyoto, Japan) (**Figure 7**) [46–48]. A vibratory stimulus is applied alternately to each muscle by fixing vibrators from the vibration device onto the subjects' lumbar multifidus (LM) muscle and gastrocnemius (GS). The device consists of an amplifier, laptop computer, and four vibrators (**Figure 8**). This mechanical vibration test has been used to analyze the role of proprioception in the postural control strategy [49–53].

The subjects stood barefoot on the Wii Balance Board with their feet together and their eyes closed. They were instructed to remain still and relax in the standing posture with their arms hanging loosely at their sides (**Figure 9**).

To provide information regarding relative proprioceptive sensation dominance, the relative proprioceptive weighting (RPW) ratio was calculated using following computation expression.

$$RPW = (Abs\ GS)/(Abs\ LM + Abs\ GS) \times 100[\%]$$

RPW of near to 0 conform to 100 [%] dependence on trunk strategy, whereas RPW of near to 100 conform to 100 [%] dependence on lower limb strategy [54–56].

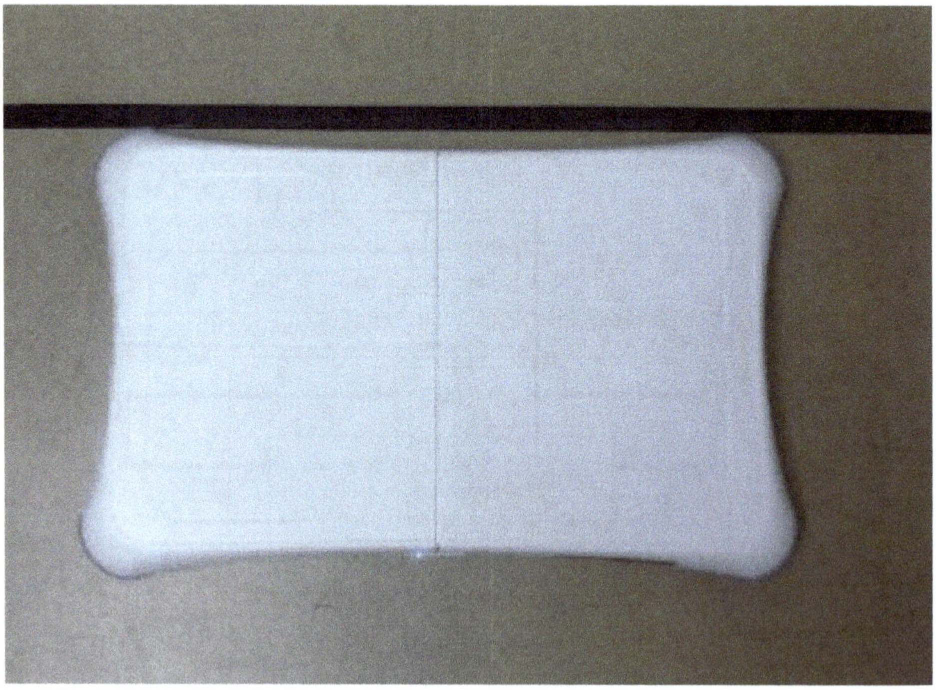

Figure 7. Recently, the Wii Balance Board has been much used in the field of medical research, and it has been reported that results from the Wii Balance Board correlate closely with those of commercially available force plates.

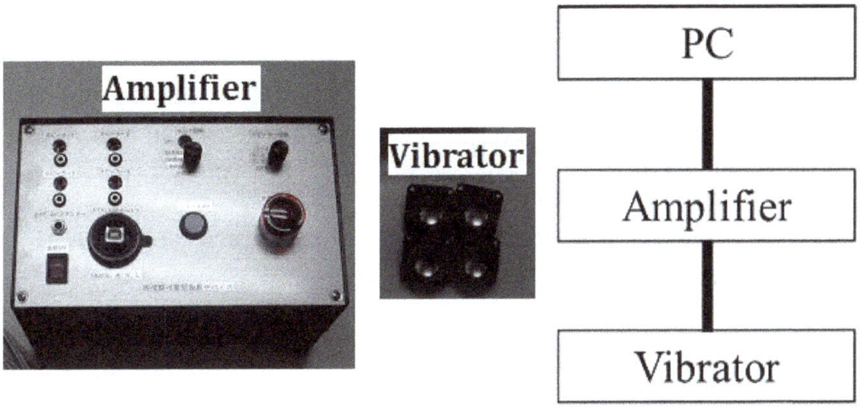

Figure 8. Photograph and block diagram of variable-frequency vibratory stimulation device.

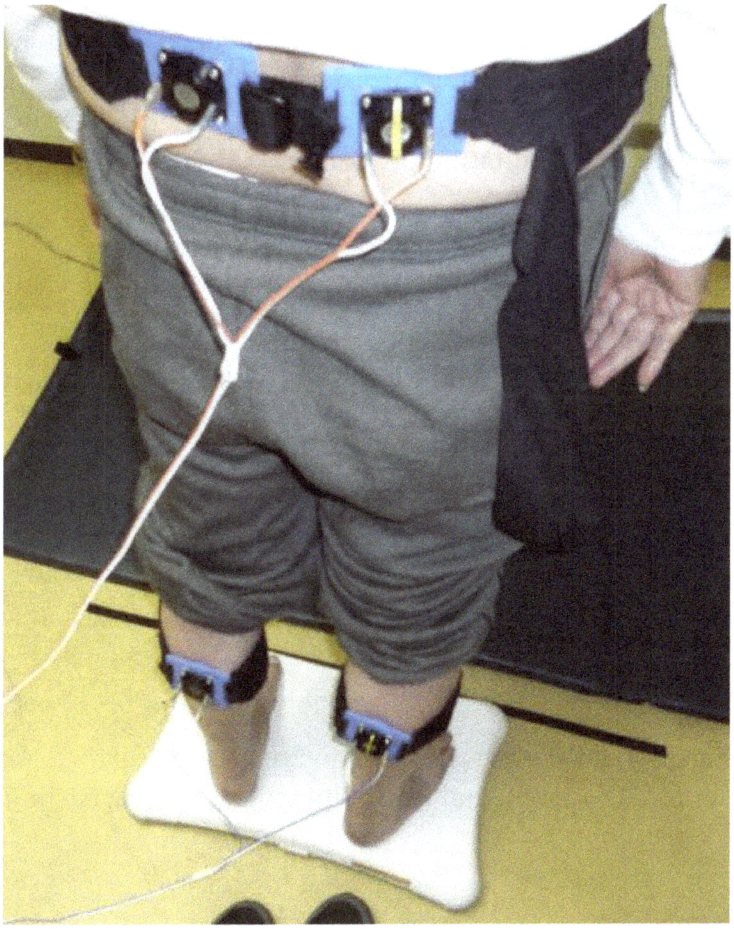

Figure 9. Experimental setup: paraspinal muscles and gastrocnemius muscles in vibration trial.

4.3. Proprioceptive input decline from the muscles of the legs or trunk

Recent studies in which a vibratory stimulation of 60 Hz was used have suggested that people with LBP adopt a lower leg-derived postural control strategy [57]. A possible explanation is that these participants were exploiting this strategy to its maximum effect during vibratory stimulation of 60 Hz. Also, according to other study, the impairment of back muscle strength leads to the motor function and sensory deficit that affects balance performance [58]. Moreover, according to another study, the lower leg's response to balance control under 30 Hz proprioceptive stimulation might be a good indicator of declining gait function [59].

These differences may result from differences between the measurement conditions and physical status of the participants.

5. Conclusions

Comprehensive physical function assessment has been proved useful for understanding the ability of elderly people. Walking efficiency is closely correlated with life space, and it can be used for comparing physical function. Performance assessment, such as the grip strength, skeletal muscle mass, and postural control stabilization, may help slow the events that ultimately can lead to motor function disorder and disability. This chapter suggests that comprehensive physical function assessment is a useful method to evaluate the physical function and therefore aids rehabilitation programs.

Acknowledgements

We also thank Yoshihito Sakai, Yoshifumi Morita, Noritaka Sato, and Kazunori Yamazaki for their help in this chapter.

Author details

Tadashi Ito

Address all correspondence to: sanjigen@mikawa-aoitori.jp

Three-dimensional motion analysis room, Aichi Prefecture Mikawa Aoitori Medical and Rehabilitation Center for Developmental Disabilities, Okazaki-shi, Aichi, Japan

References

[1] Wert DM, Brach JS, Perera S, et al. The association between energy cost of walking and physical function in older adults. Arch Gerontol Geriatr. 2013;**57**(2):198–203.

[2] Schrack JA, Simonsick EM, Ferrucci L. The relationship of the energetic cost of slow walking and peak energy expenditure to gait speed in mid-to-late life. Am J Phys Med Rehabil. 2013;**92**(1):28–35.

[3] Skinner HB, Barrack RL, Cook SD. Age-related decline in proprioception. Clin Orthop Relat Res. 1984;**184**:208–11.

[4] Steinberg FU, Graber AL. The effect of age and peripheral circulation on the perception of vibration. Arch Phys Med Rehabil. 1963;**44**:645–50.

[5] Thelen DG, Schultz AB, Alexander NB, et al. Effects of age on rapid ankle torque development. J Gerontol A Biol Sci Med Sci. 1996;**51**(5):M226–32.

[6] Woodhull-McNeal AP. Changes in posture and balance with age. Aging (Milano). 1992;**4**(3):219–25.

[7] Meuleman JR, Brechue WF, Kubilis PS, et al. Exercise training in the debilitated aged: strength and functional outcomes. Arch Phys Med Rehabil. 2000;**81**(3):312–18.

[8] Bäckmand H, Kaprio J, Kujala UM, et al. Physical and psychological functioning of daily living in relation to physical activity. A longitudinal study among former elite male athletes and controls. Aging Clin Exp Res. 2006;**18**(1):40–9.

[9] Young DR, Masaki KH, Curb JD. Associations of physical activity with performance-based and self-reported physical functioning in older men: the Honolulu Heart Program. J Am Geriatr Soc. 1995;**43**(8):845–54.

[10] Baker PS, Bodner EV, Allman RM. Measuring life-space mobility in community-dwelling older adults. J Am Geriatr Soc. 2003;**51**(11):1610–4.

[11] Peel C, Sawyer Baker P, Roth DL, et al. Assessing mobility in older adults: The UAB Study of Aging Life-Space Assessment. Phys Ther. 2005;**85**(10):1008–19.

[12] Murata C, Kondo T, Tamakoshi K, et al. Factors associated with life space among community-living rural elders in Japan. Public Health Nurs. 2006;**23**(4):324–31.

[13] Shimada H, Kim H, Yoshida H, et al. Relationship between age-associated changes of gait and falls and life-space in elderly people. J Phys Ther Sci. 2010;**22**(4):419–24.

[14] Shimada H, Sawyer P, Harada K, et al. Predictive validity of the classification schema for functional mobility tests in instrumental activities of daily living decline among older adults. Arch Phys Med Rehabil. 2010;**91**(2):241–6.

[15] Wert DM, Brach J, Perera S, et al. Gait biomechanics, spatial and temporal characteristics, and the energy cost of walking in older adults with impaired mobility. Phys Ther. 2010;**90**(7):988–85.

[16] Ito T, Shimada H, Yoshida D, et al. The relationship between walking efficiency and Life-space assessment in elderly people. In: The 49nd Congress of Japanese Society of Physical Therapy; May 31; Kanagawa Japan. Rigakuryohogaku: Japanese Physical Therapy Association; 2014. p. 1246.

[17] Fiser WM, Hays NP, Rogers SC, et al. Energetics of walking in elderly people: factors related to gait speed. J Gerontol A Biol Sci Med Sci. 2010;**65**(12):1332–7.

[18] Waters RL, Hislop HJ, Perry J, et al. Comparative cost of walking in young and old adults. J Orthop Res. 1983;**1**(1):73–6.

[19] McCann DJ, Adams WC. A dimensional paradigm for identifying the size-independent cost of walking. Med Sci Sports Exerc. 2002;**34**(6):1009–17.

[20] Abe T, Suzuki T, Yoshida H, et al. The relationship between pulmonary function and physical function and mobility in community-dwelling elderly women aged 75 years or older. J Phys Ther Sci. 2011;**23**(3):443–9.

[21] Malatesta D, Simar D, Dauvilliers Y, et al. Energy cost of walking and gait instability in healthy 65- and 80-yr-olds. J Appl Physiol. 2003;**95**(6):2248–56.

[22] Shimada H, Sturnieks D, Endo Y, et al. Relationship between whole body oxygen consumption and skeletal muscle glucose metabolism during walking in older adults: FDG PET study. Aging Clin Exp Res. 2011;**23**(3):175–82.

[23] Janssen I, Heymsfield SB, Ross R. Low relative skeletal muscle mass (sarcopenia) in older persons is associated with functional impairment and physical disability. J Am Geriatr Soc. 2002;**50**(5):889–96.

[24] Sanada K, Miyachi M, Yamamoto K, et al. Prediction models of sarcopenia in Japanese adult men and women. Tairyoku Kagaku. 2010;**59**(3):291–301.

[25] Yoshida D, Shimada H, Park H, et al. Development of an equation for estimating appendicular skeletal muscle mass in Japanese older adults using bioelectrical impedance analysis. Geriatr Gerontol Int. 2014;**14**(4):851–7.

[26] Ito T, Sakai Y, Morita Y, et al. Simple estimation of appendicular muscle mass using the maximum calf circumference of elderly inpatients. Rigakuryoho Kagaku. 2016;**31**(4): 511–5.

[27] Xue QL, Fried LP, Glass TA, et al. Life-space constriction, development of frailty, and the competing risk of mortality: the Women's Health And Aging Study I. Am J Epidemiol. 2008;**167**(2):240–8.

[28] Webber SC, Porter MM, Menec VH. Mobility in older adults: a comprehensive framework. Gerontologist. 2010;**50**(4):443–50.

[29] Imms FJ, Edholm OG. Studies of gait and mobility in the elderly. Age Ageing. 1981;**10**(3): 147–56.

[30] Bootsma-van der Wiel A, Gussekloo J, De Craen AJ, et al. Common chronic diseases and general impairments as determinants of walking disability in the oldest-old population. J Am Geriatr Soc. 2002;**50**(8):1405–10.

[31] Hay L, Bard C, Fleury M, et al. Availability of visual and proprioceptive afferent messages and postural control in elderly adults. Exp Brain Res. 1996;**108**(1):129–39.

[32] Shumway-Cook A, Woollacott M. Attentional demands and postural control: the effect of sensory context. J Gerontol A Biol Sci Med Sci. 2000;**55**(1):M10–6.

[33] Teasdale N, Stelmach GE, Breunig A, et al. Age differences in visual sensory integration. Exp Brain Res. 1991;**85**(3):691–6.

[34] Bloem BR, Allum JH, Carpenter MG, et al. Is lower leg proprioception essential for triggering human automatic postural responses?. Exp Brain Res. 2000;**130**(3):375–91.

[35] Pyykkö I, Jäntti P, Aalto H. Postural control in elderly subjects. Age Ageing. 1990;**19**(3): 215–21.

[36] Hodges PW, Richardson CA. Inefficient muscular stabilization of the lumbar spine associated with low back pain. A motor control evaluation of transversus abdominis. Spine (Phila Pa 1976). 1996;**21**(22):2640–50.

[37] Brumagne S, Cordo P, Lysens R, et al. The role of paraspinal muscle spindles in lumbosacral position sense in individuals with and without low back pain. Spine (Phila Pa 1976). 2000;**25**(8):989–94.

[38] Newcomer KL, Laskowski ER, Yu B, et al. Differences in repositioning error among patients with low back pain compared with control subjects. Spine (Phila Pa 1976). 2000;**25**(19):2488–93.

[39] Luoto S, Aalto H, Taimela S, et al. One-footed and externally disturbed two-footed postural control in patients with chronic low back pain and healthy control subjects. A controlled study with follow-up. Spine (Phila Pa 1976). 1998;**23**(19):2081–9; discussion 2089-90.

[40] Radebold A, Cholewicki J, Polzhofer GK, et al. Impaired postural control of the lumbar spine is associated with delayed muscle response times in patients with chronic idiopathic low back pain. Spine (Phila Pa 1976). 2001;**26**(7):724–30.

[41] Taimela S, Kankaanpää M, Luoto S. The effect of lumbar fatigue on the ability to sense a change in lumbar position. A controlled study. Spine (Phila Pa 1976). 1999;**24**(13):1322–7.

[42] Moseley GL, Hodges PW. Are the changes in postural control associated with low back pain caused by pain interference?. Clin J Pain. 2005;**21**(4):323–9.

[43] Brumagne S, Lysens R, Swinnen S, et al. Effect of paraspinal muscle vibration on position sense of the lumbosacral spine. Spine (Phila Pa 1976). 1999;**24**(13):1328–31.

[44] Roll JP, Vedel JP. Kinaesthetic role of muscle afferents in man, studied by tendon vibration and microneurography. Exp Brain Res. 1982;**47**(2):177–90.

[45] Frost LR, Bijman M, Strzalkowski ND, et al. Deficits in foot skin sensation are related to alterations in balance control in chronic low back patients experiencing clinical signs of lumbar nerve root impingement. Gait Posture. 2015;**41**(4):923–8.

[46] Clark RA, Bryant AL, Pua Y, et al. Validity and reliability of the Nintendo Wii Balance Board for assessment of standing balance. Gait Posture. 2010;**31**(3):307–10.

[47] Young W, Ferguson S, Brault S, et al. Assessing and training standing balance in older adults: a novel approach using the 'Nintendo Wii' Balance Board. Gait Posture. 2011;**33**(2):303–5.

[48] Holmes JD, Jenkins ME, Johnson AM, et al. Validity of the Nintendo Wii® balance board for the assessment of standing balance in Parkinson's disease. Clin Rehabil. 2013;**27**(4): 361–6.

[49] Capicíková N, Rocchi L, Hlavacka F, et al. Human postural response to lower leg muscle vibration of different duration. Physiol Res. 2006;**55**(Suppl 1):S129–34.

[50] Barbieri G, Gissot AS, Fouque F, et al. Does proprioception contribute to the sense of verticality?. Exp Brain Res. 2008;**185**(4):545–52.

[51] Thompson C, Bélanger M, Fung J. Effects of bilateral Achilles tendon vibration on postural orientation and balance during standing. Clin Neurophysiol. 2007;**118**(11):2456–67.

[52] Ivanenko YP, Solopova IA, Levik YS. The direction of postural instability affects postural reactions to ankle muscle vibration in humans. Neurosci Lett. 2000;**292**(2):103–6.

[53] Ceyte H, Cian C, Zory R, et al. Effect of Achilles tendon vibration on postural orientation. Neurosci Lett. 2007;**416**(1):71–5.

[54] Brumagne S, Janssens L, Janssens E, et al. Altered postural control in anticipation of postural instability in persons with recurrent low back pain. Gait Posture. 2008;**28**(4):657–62.

[55] Janssens L, Brumagne S, Polspoel K, et al. The effect of inspiratory muscles fatigue on postural control in people with and without recurrent low back pain. Spine (Phila Pa 1976). 2010;**35**(10):1088–94.

[56] Janssens L, Brumagne S, McConnell AK, et al. Proprioceptive changes impair balance control in individuals with chronic obstructive pulmonary disease. PLoS One. 2013;**8**(3): e57949.

[57] Brumagne S, Janssens L, Knapen S, et al. Persons with recurrent low back pain exhibit a rigid postural control strategy. Eur Spine J. 2008;**17**(9):1177–84.

[58] Ito T, Sakai Y, Nakamura E, et al. Relationship between paraspinal muscle cross-sectional area and relative proprioceptive weighting ratio of older persons with lumbar spondylosis. J Phys Ther Sci. 2015;**27**(7):2247–51.

[59] Ito T, Sakai Y, Kubo A, et al. The relationship between physical function and postural sway during local vibratory stimulation of middle-aged people in the standing position. J Phys Ther Sci. 2014;**26**(10):1627–30.

7

Physiotherapy and Mental Health

Michel Probst

Additional information is available at the end of the chapter

Abstract

Physiotherapy in mental health care and psychiatry is a recognized specialty within physiotherapy. It offers a rich variety of observational and evaluation tools as well as a range of interventions that are related to the patient's physical and mental health problems based on evidence-based literature and a 50-year history. Physiotherapy in mental health care addresses human movement, function, physical activity and exercise in individual and group therapeutic settings. Additionally, it connects the physical and mental health needs of humans. This chapter offers general reflections on mental health, the scope of physiotherapy in mental health care and physiotherapy research. Physiotherapy in mental health care and psychiatry can offer added and beneficial value to the treatment of people with mental health problems.

Keywords: psychomotor therapy, exercise, physical activity, body awareness, psychosomatic physiotherapy

1. Introduction

Mental health is a topic of growing interest in society. Various mental health organizations are engaged in the prevention, treatment and rehabilitation of persons with mental health problems and disorders. Unfortunately, physiotherapy is not always considered to be a significant profession within mental health because the role and the added value it offers can remain unclear among patients and other health care providers. However, physiotherapy is a recognized conventional profession within health care and can offer an extensive range of physical approaches (physical activity, exercise, movement, relaxation techniques and body and movement awareness). These approaches are aimed at symptom relief, the enhancement of self-confidence and the improvement of quality of life. Additionally, they are relevant to rehabilitation programmes in mental health care.

The goal of this chapter is to present an overview of why physiotherapy in mental health is necessary and what it can offer to fulfil requests for help and to increase the quality of life of persons with mental health problems. It describes physiotherapy methods and their applications in the fields of mental health and psychiatry.

2. Mental health

Mental health refers to cognitive and/or emotional well-being. More concretely, it refers to how a person thinks, feels and behaves. Mental health can affect daily life, relationships, the ability to enjoy life and even physical health. Mental health involves finding a balance between life activities and efforts to achieve resilience. According to the World Health Organization (WHO) [1], mental health is 'a state of well-being in which the individual realizes his or her own abilities, can cope with the normal stresses of life, can work productively and fruitfully, and is able to make a contribution to his or her community'. More concrete mental health includes different components of life; for example, in terms of relationships, having a good relationship with family and having supportive friends, with the ability to talk about feelings. For leisure time it is about having hobbies, doing exercises on regular basis and having regular holidays. Furthermore, it is important to follow a healthy lifestyle that includes, having healthy eating habits, not smoking or drinking and not taking no-prescribed drugs and at least being able to achieve some goals in life [2]. Mental health is not merely the absence of a mental disorder. It exists on a continuum to include flourishing mental health, very good mental health, mean mental health, decreased mental health, mental health problems and mental health disorders [3].

3. Mental health problems and disorders

It is important to distinguish between mental health problems and mental health disorders. A mental health problem is a negative mental experience that is part of everyday life and interferes with emotional and/or social abilities. These problems are less severe than those associated with a mental health disorder. As previously mentioned, persons with mental disorders have a growing imbalance in their abilities. A mental disorder is defined as a syndrome characterized by a clinically significant disturbance in an individual's cognition, emotion regulation or behaviour [see **Box 1**]. It reflects a common or severe dysfunction in the psychological, biological or developmental process underlying mental functioning [4, 5].

One out of four persons might face a mental health disorder at a certain point in their life. Depression, anxiety, post-traumatic stress disorder and other problems can be triggered by personal and lifestyle pressures such as bereavement, relationship breakdown or job loss. Drug or alcohol dependency, illness or long-term physical disability can cause depression. This mental health disorder is the fourth most significant cause of disability worldwide.

Common mental health disorders

Common disorders refer to obsessive-compulsive and related disorders, trauma and stressor-related disorders, dissociative disorders, somatic symptom and related disorders, eating disorders, disruptive, impulse-control and conduct disorders, substance-related and addictive disorders and neurocognitive disorders

Severe mental health disorders: Severe mental disorders include schizophrenia, bipolar disorders, mood disorders.

For the diagnostic criteria see:

World Health Organization: International classification [5]

American Psychiatric Association: diagnostic [4]

Box 1: Common and severe mental health disorders

Mental health problems/disorders often begin with the thoughts and beliefs related to a (physical or mental) problem. These thoughts and beliefs are the source of emotions and feelings that act as a driver of actions/behaviours. Behaviours are a choice and have consequences at some point.

4. Mental health and physiotherapy

The importance of the implementation of physiotherapy in both common and severe mental health disorders and psychiatry is underestimated, even if there is a tradition of more than 50 years in some countries (Belgium, Scandinavia, etc.), even if the attention to 'the moving body' increases in society and even if the moving body is an important issue that is integral to psychopathology. To overcome this problem, physiotherapists who were working in mental health and psychiatry applied in 2011 for recognition as a subgroup within the World Confederation of Physical Therapy [6]. The main goal of this subgroup is to bring the different physiotherapy interventions in mental health and psychiatry together to clarify the role of physiotherapy in this field. For that reason, the International Organization of Physical Therapy in Mental Health (IOPTMH) [7, 8] adapted the recommendations of the WHO [1] concerning mental health care using physiotherapy language (see **Box 2**).

1. To improve [*physiotherapy*] mental health care
2. To organize specific [*physiotherapy*] care for different ages including children, adolescents and elderly and risk-related groups as persons with eating disorders, psychotic disorders, etc.
3. To ensure access to primary [*physiotherapy*] care for people with mental health problems
4. To provide treatment in 'community-based [*physiotherapy*] services for persons with severe mental health problems.

[adaptation]

Box 2: Recommendation for mental health care of the World Health Organisation [1] adapted by the IOPTMH.

4.1. Mental health in physiotherapy

Not all physiotherapists realize that mental health is all the business of physiotherapy. However, it is well illustrated in the following quotation: 'no health without mental health'.

As health care providers, physiotherapists are also involved in the prevention and promotion of health, including mental health. It is their responsibility to inform individuals adequately about mental health, eliminate misconceptions about mental illness and refer them when necessary to specialized professionals in mental health and psychiatry.

Consciously or unconsciously, colleagues will be confronted in their practice with individuals with frail mental health, chronic musculoskeletal disorders, chronic pain and psychosomatic disorders. In their stories, components of mental health are interwoven, and the patients deserve an appropriate physiotherapy intervention. In addition to these conditions, more severe physical diseases such as cardiovascular diseases, Parkinson's disease, rheumatoid arthritis, hypertension, Diabetes mellitus, metabolic syndrome, asthma, asthma/chronic obstructive pulmonary disorder (COPD), cerebrovascular diseases (stroke), obesity, epilepsy, cancer and other diseases are frequently accompanied with a 'rollercoaster' of emotions, feelings of anxiety and pain. After all, individuals with mental disorders have numerous physical health complaints (cardiovascular diseases, metabolic syndrome, obesity, osteoporosis, etc.) due to medication, sedentary behaviour or inactivity and consult primary health services.

In summary, it all adds up for the health care providers to optimize access to physiotherapy for people with mental illness, give them the most appropriate treatment [9] and give additional thought to the mental health dimension of their patients' physical conditions [10].

4.2. Physiotherapy in mental health care

In some countries, physiotherapists have a long tradition of using physiotherapy in mental health and developed specific approaches for common and severe disorders aimed at improving the quality of daily life. It is time to bring all the knowledge together to consolidate it and centralize the interventions with a view to offer appropriate care to a specific vulnerable but growing group in society. For these persons, specific interview, assessment and therapeutic skills are necessary. The interview is based on the principles of the bio-psychosocial and motivational interview [11]. The story, including the context, life events and chronic stressors in relation to the health of each patient, is mapped. The assessment focuses on lifestyle in relation to the health, mood and anxiety features, illness behaviour and psychological well-being.

5. Definition of physiotherapy in mental health

The IOPTMH developed a definition that generally describes the field of physiotherapy in mental health that is recognizable among most colleagues across the world. Physiotherapy in mental health is a specialty within physiotherapy. It is implemented in different health and mental health settings: psychiatry and psychosomatic medicine. It is Person-centered and provided for children, adolescents, adults and older people with common (mild, moderate) and severe, acute and chronic mental health problems, in primary and community care, inpatients and outpatients. Physiotherapists in mental health provide health promotion, preventive health care, treatment and rehabilitation for individuals, groups and in-group therapeutic settings. They create a therapeutic relationship to provide assessment and services specifically related to the complexity of mental health within a supportive environment applying a model including biological and psychosocial aspects. Physiotherapy in mental health aims to optimize well-being and empower the individual by promoting functional movement, movement awareness, physical activity and exercises, bringing together physical and mental aspects. It is based on the available scientific and best clinical evidence. Physiotherapists in mental health contribute to the multidisciplinary team and inter-professional care [12, 13].

6. The scope of physiotherapy in mental health

Depending upon the problem, the story of the patient, and the results of the observation/evaluation, the patient's treatment goals will be established, and the physiotherapist can choose a more health-related approach or psychotherapeutic physiotherapy (see **Figure 1**). *The physical health-related approach* aims to improve the global physical health of patients with psychiatric disorders. Physical activity can help to reduce cardiovascular disease and premature mortality in people with psychological problems. *The psychosocial-related approach* emphasizes the acquisition of mental and physical proficiencies related to the body in motion and support of personal development to enhance people's ability to function independently in society. *The psychotherapeutic-related approach uses the body in movement* as a gateway to ameliorate the social affective functioning of an individual. When using this approach, the physiotherapist creates a setting that favours the initiation and development of a process in the patient by employing specific working methods that aim to help patients to access their inner workings.

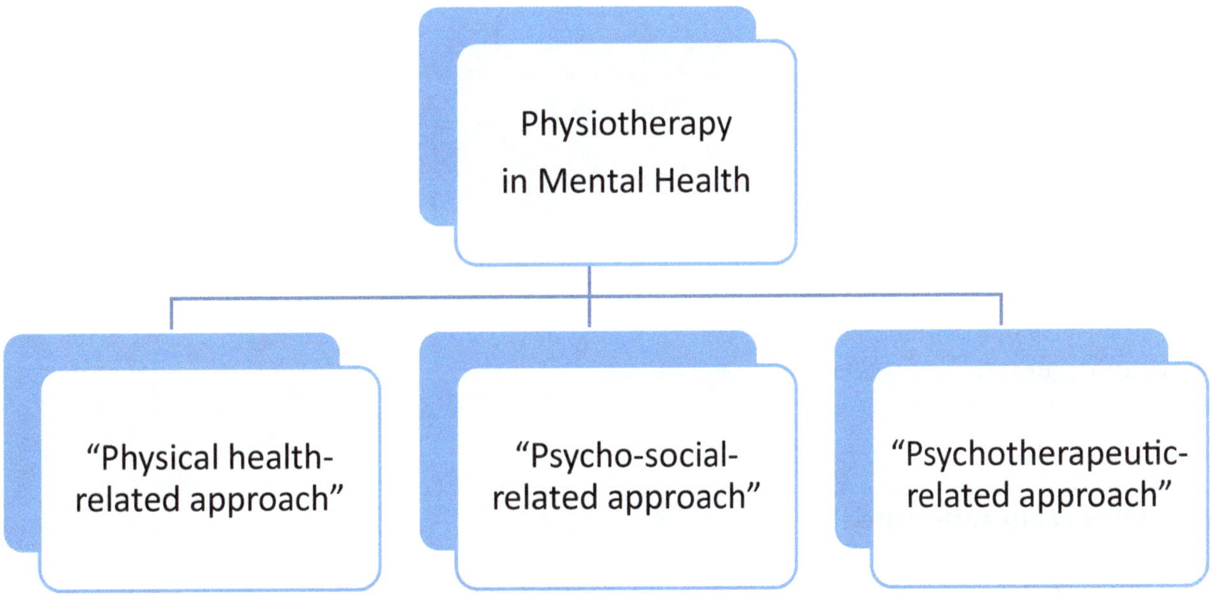

Figure 1. The scope of physiotherapy in mental health.

In physiotherapy in mental health, a rationale for applying psychological models (e.g. cognitive behavioural therapy, acceptance and commitment therapy, etc.) is offered as a tool to strengthen physiotherapy interventions in the treatment of a wide variety of disorders in children, adolescents, adults and the elderly. The cognitive behavioural physiotherapy treatment approach consists of the identification of current and specific problems related to the moving human being. The physiotherapy goals are based on the SMART principles (Specific, measurable, acceptable/attainable, realistic/relevant and time bound). The treatment is I think it is patient-centered and the ultimate physiotherapy goal is to change unhealthy habits and promoting an active lifestyle and healthy posture. The focus lays on self-management and relapse prevention. Different modalities (see **Figure 2**) such as cognitive techniques (cognitive restructuring, problem solving and cognitive functional training), behavioural (relaxation, pacing and graded exercise therapy and behavioural activation), supportive, educational and other techniques such as (bio-) feedback, movement and body awareness and relapse prevention for children and adults are integrated into this treatment [14]. The acceptance and commitment physiotherapy approach is supporting the patient to clarify his/her values and helping them to take the necessary steps towards living a meaningful life despite the discomfort [15].

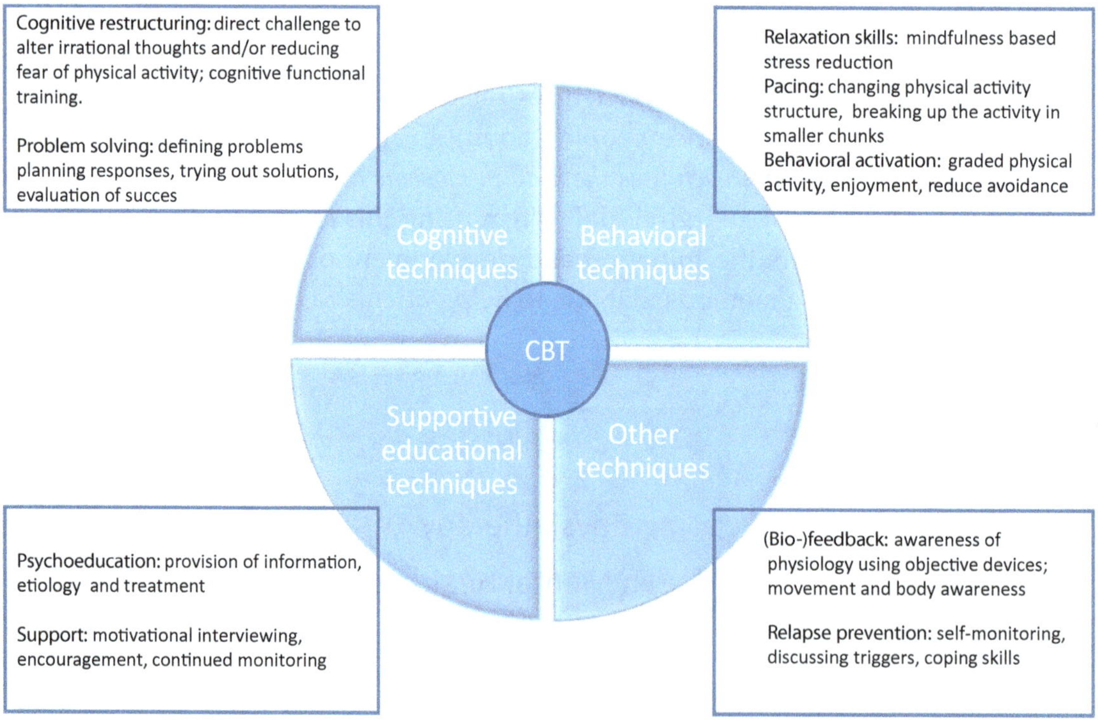

Figure 2. Cognitive behavioural techniques in physiotherapy.

6.1. 'Physical health-related' approach

The physical health-related approach aims to improve the global physical health of the person with mental health problems. Studies have shown that people with mental health problems are more susceptible to inactivity and are at risk of a sedentary lifestyle. In addition, the use of psychotropic drugs can result in the development of metabolic syndrome, obesity, osteoporosis and cardiovascular disease. The physical health-related approach is consistent with the recent recommendations of the World Health Organization (WHO) about the relationship between individuals' 'physical inactivity' and poor health and a serious threat to their quality of life [16].

Clinical practice has highlighted the importance of tailoring physical activity to each person's individual abilities to influence the quality of life. The challenge is to motivate people to stay active throughout their daily life. People who do not continue to exercise lose their independence and do not maximize their potential in life. The American College of Sport Sciences [17, 18] offers guidelines. It is the task of the physiotherapist to integrate and adapt these guidelines to fit the context of a person with mental health problems [19–22].

6.2. Psychosocial-related and psychophysiological approaches

The psychosocial-related approach emphasizes the acquisition of mental and physical skills related to the 'moving body' and support of people's ability to function independently in society and to improve their quality of life. The activities aim at learning, acquiring and training psychomotor, sensomotor, perceptual, cognitive, social and emotional proficiencies. Other elementary proficiencies are stressed, such as relaxation education, relaxation skills, stress management, breathing techniques, psychomotor and sensory skills and also cognitive, expression and social skills. Through exercises, patients acquire a broader perspective and can experience their own abilities. Moreover, the learning of the basic rules of communication is integrated [23]. The psychophysiological approach involves the use of physical activity to influence mental health problems such as in the treatment of depression and anxiety disorders [24–34]. In the literature, the benefits of physical activity for mental health are well accepted. Physical activity has a positive influence on mental well-being, self-esteem, mood and executive functioning. Through these effects, a downward spiral that leads to dejection can be stopped. Well-balanced and regularly executed endurance activities (walking, biking, jogging and swimming) power training (fitness training) and mindfulness-derived exercises) augment physical and mental resilience; improve the quality of sleep; enhance self-confidence, energy, endurance and relaxation; and, in general, decrease physical complaints.

6.3. Psychotherapeutic-oriented physiotherapy approach

The psychotherapeutic-oriented physiotherapy approach uses the motor domain as a gateway to ameliorate social affective functioning. This approach puts less emphasis on the acquisition of skills but more on the awareness of psychosocial functioning and facilitating a process of change. Using movement activities, the physiotherapist creates a setting that favours the initiation and development of a process aimed at helping patients to gain greater insight into their own functioning. During these activities, patients are invited to venture outside their comfort zone, think outside the box, experience new things, become more in touch with their inner self and cope with numerous emotions (depressive feelings, fear, guilt, anger, stress, feelings of unease, estrangement and dissatisfaction) and negative thoughts (intrusion, obsession, morbid preoccupations and worrying). Moreover, they are confronted with their behaviour (i.e. impulses and lack of abilities) or cognitive symptoms (i.e. derealisation and lack of concentration). Through psychomotor therapy, an alternative perspective on experiences can be proposed. Experiencing the possibility that an alternative may exist triggers new emotions and experiences, and a discrepancy between reality and the patient's perception of reality emerges. Consequently, it is important to note that it is not the physical activity itself but the patient's experiences and inner perception that play the central role. The careful guidance and encouragement of the physiotherapist and the opportunity to experience feelings in a safe environment allow the patient to develop behaviour, which would not have developed otherwise. Although the underlying problems are not necessarily resolved, the therapist tries to improve problem management of the patient. The patient shares his behaviour, feelings, and thoughts with the therapist initially and, eventually, with his peers. More emphasis is placed on experiences and how reactions to these experiences function as a dynamic source of power [23].

7. The content of physiotherapy in mental health

Physiotherapy is a specialized field in health care and is recognized as a conventional therapy. Physiotherapists who work in mental health are physiotherapists first and use interventions within the scope of general physiotherapy. In addition, due to the complex situation, physiotherapists who work in mental health require supplementary knowledge (e.g. psychopathology and psychological frames) and specific skills and competences (e.g. communication) to assess, treat, support and refer people with mental disorders effectively (see **Figure 3**).

7.1. Psychomotor therapy with children and adolescents

Psychomotor therapy is a type of body-oriented therapy. The cornerstones of this approach are body awareness, movement and physical activities. However, psychomotor therapy encompasses 'movement' or 'physical activity' in a strict sense. It is based on the holistic view and, therefore,

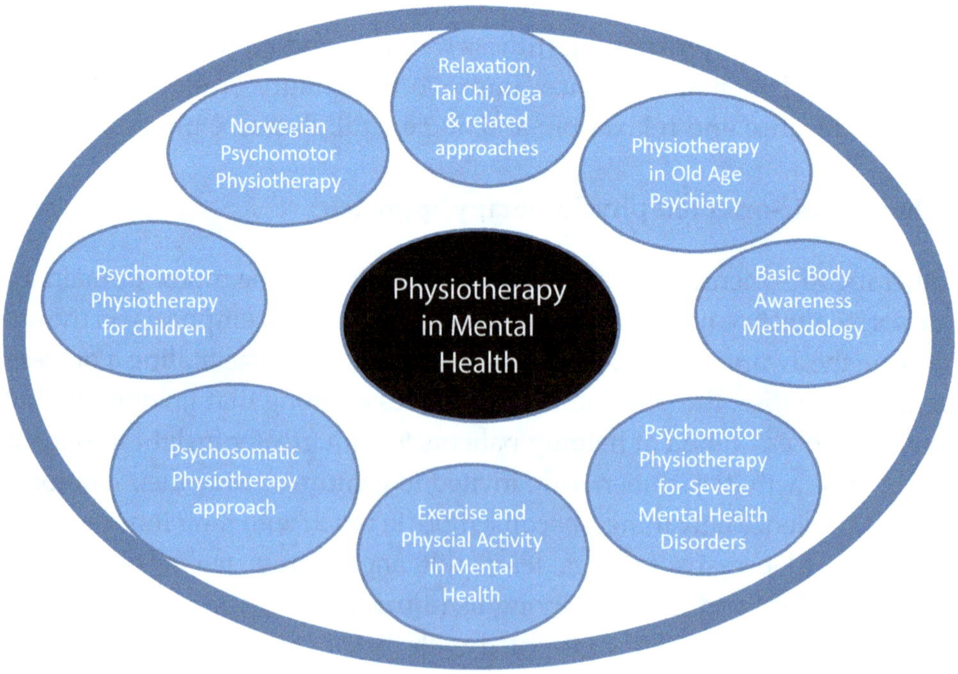

Figure 3. Overview of physiotherapy interventions in mental health.

integrates cognitive, emotional, social and motor aspects into an individual's development. The starting point is a strong acknowledgement of the continuous and complex interactions between the different developmental domains. Moreover, the functioning of a child is not only always integrated into but also dependent upon a certain context [35]. Psychomotor therapy is offered in different disciplines, including mental health care, child psychiatry, youth care, special education and rehabilitation, as well as private practice. The wide variety of psychomotor therapy interventions can be categorized into two main areas: psychomotor functional training and psychotherapeutic-oriented psychomotor therapy [35]. Although both approaches are aimed at supporting and aiding a child's personal development, the methods can be distinguished based upon the primary focus of the intervention. Psychomotor functional training is primarily aimed at improving the motor domain and includes activities that are aimed at learning, developing, practicing and training (psycho) motor, sensorimotor and perceptual abilities. In psychotherapeutic-oriented psychomotor therapy, the motor domain is employed as a gateway to ameliorate the social and affective development of individual functioning. More concretely, specific goals are formulated such as learning to recognize bodily signals, regulate aggression, play cooperatively, enhance self-confidence, reduce social anxiety, etc. The techniques that are employed include relaxation techniques [36], Sherborne Developmental Movement [37], movement and play situations, psychomotor family therapy [38, 39], physical activity, etc.

7.2. Norwegian psychomotor physiotherapy

The roots of Norwegian psychomotor physiotherapy began in the early 1950s and were the result of a collaboration between Trygve Braatøy, a psychoanalytically trained psychiatrist, and Aadel Bülow-Hansen, an orthopaedic physiotherapist [40–42]. In addition to its focus on how the past continues to influence the present, the psychoanalytic approach develops the client's awareness of what can be done to correct the harmful effects of the past [43]. Indications for this physiotherapy approach are conditions associated with strain and functional disturbances in the musculoskeletal system as well as psychosomatic disorders. Symptoms are viewed as an expression of a disturbance in posture, respiration, muscle tension or autonomic functions, which are often related to emotional conflicts or mental problems [44]. In Norwegian psychomotor physiotherapy, the case report and the examination are central to documenting and evaluating respiration, posture, function, muscles and other soft tissues as well as automatic functions and reactions. The patient's body and self-awareness are taken into consideration. These awareness concepts are based on the philosophy of phenomenology. The major finding of Braatøy and Bülow-Hansen was that the entire body needs to be examined and treated instead of using a local approach. The basis of the examination is the whole person, and the key is the body [44]. Relaxation treatment has yielded limited results, unless breathing is taken into consideration. Although breathing is an important cornerstone of the approach, breathing exercises are seldom used. The observation of how the patient breathes during massage and exercise is a guideline for the level of intensity of the therapy [45], allowing the therapist to adjust continually to the patient's reactions [44, 46]. Breathing and feelings are considered to be interdependent factors. The body is approached as an integrated physical-psychological phenomenon [44]. Changes in breathing could be a signal that the patient is reacting emotionally [44]. The patient's reaction to the examination also provides important information. In Norwegian psychomotor physiotherapy, the emphasis is on respiration because breathing can be viewed in relation to emotion and cognition. At the same time, breathing can contribute to the reduction of somatic disorders in stress-related and/or psychosomatic disorders [47]. In summary, Norwegian psychomotor physiotherapy aims to release respiration through an interaction among breathing, the musculoskeletal system and emotions [44] and to develop flexibility, versatility and the stability of the person [48]. The treatment is successful when a process of bodily changes is not separated from emotional changes [48–50]. A treatment session is mostly individual in nature and may be short, being composed of active exercises in standing, sitting or lying positions only, or it may be long, consisting of massage of the recumbent body only [49, 50].

7.3. Relaxation therapy and mind-body-related approaches

Relaxation as a therapeutic intervention is recommended in the treatment of stress and stress-related problems. The term relaxation therapy is used to describe a number of techniques that promote stress and anxiety reduction by decreasing tension throughout the body and creating a peaceful state of mind [51]. This valued therapeutic approach is frequently used in mental health care, and physiotherapists in mental health care apply relaxation training as one of their interventions. Relaxation is used as prevention (to protect the body), as a treatment (for instance, to relieve stress in individuals with hypertension, tension headache, insomnia and panic) or as a coping skill (to relax the mind and to promote clear and effective thinking). Relaxation therapy consists of three phases: (1) to learn the relaxation technique, (2) to evaluate if there is a relaxation response (physiological and psychological) after some training session, and (3) in the third phase and when the technique becomes automatic, to use relaxation in situations that induce stress. Although there are different techniques [52, 53], physiotherapists have primarily used the modified Jacobson's progressive relaxation method by Bernstein and Borkovec [54–56], applied relaxation of Öst [57], Mitchell method [58] and autogenic training [59].

Yoga, Tai Chi, mindfulness-related exercises and Pilates are also used to cope with stressful situations.

The **mindfulness-based stress reduction (MBSR) program**, which is centred on the principles and practice of mindfulness meditation and the use of stress-reduction skills, including sitting meditation, hatha yoga and a somatically focused technique called a 'body scan', which was developed to relieve suffering in patients with chronic pain [60, 61]. MBSR encourages the non-judgemental awareness of one's cognitive and somatic experiences on a moment-by-moment basis. This decentred stance is thought to disconnect cognitive and affective mental events in an adaptive manner and might reduce the negative impact of thoughts and sensations that are associated with chronic pain [60, 61].

Tai Chi has been practiced for centuries as a Chinese martial art that combines meditation, postures, slow and graceful movements, diaphragmatic breathing and relaxation. It can be regarded as an intervention that integrates physical, psychosocial, emotional, spiritual and behavioural elements and promotes mind-body interaction [62, 63].

Qi Gong (QG) is an ancient Chinese method that integrates body, energetic, respiratory and mental training with the aim of achieving optimal status of both the mind and the body. QG enhances physical, psychic and emotional rebalancing, thereby improving posture, respiration and concentration by low-impact movements [64].

Yoga is an mind-body therapy (MBT) that potentially fulfils the need for both exercise and coping skills in fibromyalgia syndrome (FMS) patients. Yoga varies greatly in terms of style and, beyond the physical poses that are identified with it, comprises meditation and breathing exercises [65–71].

The Pilates method, which was developed in the 1920s by J. H. Pilates (Germany, 1880–1967), is a low-impact, non-aerobic fitness programme (stretching and strengthening exercises) that also integrates physiotherapy [72]. The original exercises were influenced by the two gymnastic systems that dominated rehabilitation at that moment, namely the German (Friedrich Jahn) and the Swedish (Per Hendrik Ling) systems. Pilates became a form of movement that combines characteristics of Eastern (mind control during exercises, relaxation, increasing of elasticity, movement starting from body centre and balance) and Western (forming strength, endurance and exercises with both global and local effects) systems. Today, the applied form of Pilates has been influenced by other mind-body methods. Additionally, it involves not only the recovery of muscle strength and flexibility but also the correction of muscle imbalance and attention to body awareness, economical breathing, and neuromuscular coordination by executing fluent and precise movement. Pilates can lead to balancing of the body and the mind [72–75].

In some countries, the Mensendieck system [76] and the Feldenkrais method [77, 78] are integrated into the physiotherapy in mental health. They are seen as educational approaches, rather than interventions. The *Mensendieck system* focuses on teaching patients to understand the concepts of bodily functioning using pedagogically designed exercises and aims to enable them to change suboptimal patterns of movement. The *Feldenkrais method* is a somatic educational system that was designed to improve the movement repertoire, aiming to expand and refine the use of the self through awareness to reduce pain or limitations in movement and promote general well-being [77, 78].

7.4. Psychomotor physiotherapy for severe mental health problems

Psychomotor physiotherapy for severe mental health problems is a method of treatment that uses systematically a wide variety of (adapted) physical activities as well as movement, body and sensory awareness to stimulate and to integrate motor, cognitive and affective competences within the psychosocial context. This approach aims to realize clearly formulated consent goals, which are relevant to the patient's mental health problems (depression, anxiety, schizophrenia, autism, eating disorder, etc.). This approach is based on evidence-based research and 50 years of clinical practice. Today, it is an important standard adjunctive treatment for patients in residential treatment to optimize movement as well as the cognitive, affective and relational aspects of mind-body functioning (i.e. the relationships between physical movements and cognitive and social-affective aspects). The approach focuses on the somatic effects of physical activity and the physio-psychological effects as the core of the treatment. The goal is to stimulate a positive self-image and personal well-being in a balanced social relationship using movement activities. This approach is well described in inpatient settings as a different group approach and can be imbedded within diverse psychotherapy settings. On the one hand, the focus is on discovering the present healthy capabilities of the subject ('care') using the moving body as the core to influence psychological, social and somatic functioning. On the other hand, the physiotherapy addresses the dysfunctional part of the subject. Depending upon the goals and the competence level of the patient, the therapist can choose among a more health-related approach (to improve physical activity and to limit sedentary behaviour), a more psychosocial-related approach (to learn skills that are not only physical but also cognitive and communicative) or a more psychotherapeutic-related approach (to stimulate the patient to get in touch with his or her inner world). When persons with mental health problems are invited to (group) physical activities, they come out from their comfort zone and experience how they function. The combination of experience and insight drives changes and leads to new experiences. Specific approaches for eating disorders [78–83], schizophrenia [84–91], mood disorders [92–97] and depression and anxiety [23, 32–34] are developed.

7.5. Basic body awareness methodology

Body awareness is a term that is frequently used in mental health and psychiatry. It refers to the ability to pay attention to ourselves and feel our sensations and movements online, along with the motivational and emotional feelings that accompany them in the present moment, without the mediating influence of judgemental thoughts [98].

Body awareness is the subjective, phenomenological aspect of proprioception and interoception that enters conscious awareness and is modifiable by mental processes, including attention, interpretation appraisal, beliefs, memories, as well as conditioned attitudes and effect [99]. Different approaches, including those within physiotherapy and beyond, reportedly enhance body awareness (yoga, Tai Chi, mindfulness-based therapies, the Feldenkrais method, the Alexander method, different breathing therapies, etc.). Body awareness has become an umbrella term for different approaches. One such approach in physiotherapy is basic body awareness therapy [100].

Basic body awareness therapy was inspired by the French movement educator and psychotherapist J. Dropsy and further elaborated by Roxendal. The basic body awareness methodology (BBAM) is a Person-centered physiotherapeutic movement awareness training programme that is directed towards daily life movement [100–111]. It is used in multiple clinical settings, including primary health care, pain rehabilitation and psychiatric physical therapy, as well as in health promotion.

It is founded upon a three-dimensional approach to human movement: learning about and through movement and learning while being in movement [107]. Movement awareness in this methodology is defined as the sensitivity to movement nuances, awareness of one's own movements in relation to space, time and energy and identification of subtle movement reactions to internal and environmental conditions [100, 107]. Persons who are not aware or who have a lack of contact with the physical body and the emotional body (internal life) and who are not aware of the physical environment and their relationship to other people and persons who are cut off from reality, express this lack of awareness throughout their body. This can be observed as dysfunctional movements, for instance, movements that lack vitality, flow, rhythm and unity [100–102, 104–105]. From a broader perspective, the lack of awareness has negative consequences on movement quality, daily function, habits and health [100]. The phenomenological concepts of the body awareness methodology are relaxation, tension regulation, body contact, body consciousness, body image, body experience, body boundaries, body control, muscle consciousness, muscle control, body awareness and postural attunement [100, 111]. In general, body awareness combines a series of exercises that are related to posture, coordination, free breathing and awareness. Attending to both the patient's own performance and to the patient's experience during the exercises is a central element of body awareness that stimulates mental presence and awareness that aims to provide increased body consciousness. BBAT offers training situations that focus on healthy movement aspects, lying, sitting, walking, running, using the voice, relational movements and massage [105]. Embodied and mindful presence, awareness and movement quality represent keys to the therapeutic approach. Therapeutically, being in movement, exploring, experiencing, integrating, mastering and reflecting upon one's own movement coordination are critical to gaining more functional movement, strengthening the self and preparing for daily life [108]. It offers a strategy to equip the person to handle life more effectively. It is used in individual therapy but is foremost a group treatment. [100, 111]. Body awareness therapy refers to a group of movement awareness interventions that share a common perspective that focuses on the internal subjective experience of the body to promote physical, mental and emotional well-being [110, 111].

7.6. Psychosomatic physiotherapy approach

The psychosomatic approach differs from the somatic approach. The somatic approach involves the cells of the body and is based on the physical and biological aspects of the problem. The somatic approach is the traditional approach and usually addresses the symptoms of the problem. Psychosomatic means that a physical condition is caused or greatly influenced by psychological factors. The psychosomatic approach views illness as a form of communication between the conscious and the unconscious mind through the body. Illness is a person's way of adapting to the environment. It is a message that communicates a need for change. Based on the patient's perception, illness is consciously or unconsciously a legitimate way to avoid something unpleasant. Illness can be a subconscious defence mechanism. There are numerous situations that people would rather avoid than confront. The benefits of the illness are that they receive more attention, love and warmth from family members or friends when they are sick. Some patients are confronted with existential questions, including those relating to the purpose of life. Unable to answer these questions, some people turn their illness into their purpose in life. Everything begins to revolve around it. The scope of psychosomatic physiotherapy is broad, including the treatment of physical symptoms such as pain, fatigue, hyperventilation and distress in relation to psychosocial problems. Somatic symptoms and related disorders [4] are another category of illnesses that primarily are treated within psychosomatic physiotherapy. Medically unexplained symptoms are also categorized under this umbrella term. In all these cases, the therapist explores the relationships among social, psychological and behavioural factors with bodily processes and quality of life. It is obvious that the therapeutic relationship has an important role [112]. During this exploration, the patient is given the space to reflect on behavioural experiences and perceptions in a developmental process that focuses on the integration of thoughts, emotions and actions in relation to motor performance. With an awareness of the importance of addressing the physical complaint, the psychosomatic physiotherapist focuses specifically on the psychophysiological and behavioural characteristics of the client's motor performance-related problem. The aim is to recognize and gain insight into the complex relationship between motor and psychological performance within a psychosocial context and positively influence disrupted internal and external regulation mechanisms. The psychosomatic-oriented physiotherapist is inspired by cognitive behavioural interventions (see **Figure 2**) [113, 114], including graded activity and active pacing therapy. The therapist uses a number of specific awareness-raising methods such as relaxation techniques, breathing and communication methods, (bio-) feedback, problem solving strategies and stress management. The status of the patient is observed using the 'SCEGS model' (soma, cognitions, emotions, behaviour and social environment). Treatment objectives are formulated in terms of the SMART criteria. The relationships among the need for help as expressed by the patient, body language, body posture, movement and gestures are explored. In addition, verbal language is analysed. The balance between supporting load and supporting strength, tension and relaxation, and body and illness perception and reality is explored during the sessions.

7.7. Exercise and physical activity in mental health

Mental health problems are the leading predictor of years lived with disability worldwide. Furthermore, without more intensified prevention and management, the burden is estimated to increase to a greater extent [115]. The consequences of mental health problems are devastating for the person and society as a whole and are compounded by physical health comorbidities with which most people with mental health problems are confronted [115, 116]. Physical health comorbidities are a major cause of the reduced life expectancy of 15–20 years in this population [118–120]. The relationship between mental health and physical activity is supported by a growing number of articles [92]. There is rigorous evidence now that physiotherapy improves mental and physical health in this vulnerable population [121]. Unfortunately, these efforts are becoming integrated into clinical practice at a slow pace. Physical activity is not always considered to be a worthwhile strategy. The benefits of physical activity are twofold, as people with mental health problems are also at an increased risk of a range of physical health problems, including cardiovascular diseases, endocrine disorders and obesity [115–124]. Physical activity influences cognition [122] and cardiorespiratory fitness [123] and reduces dropout [121] due to a wide range of mental health problems. The relationship between physical activity and mental health has been widely investigated. The health benefits of regular exercise are improved cardiovascular fitness, improved sleep, better endurance, a positive influence on metabolic syndrome and diabetes, stress relief, improved mood, increased energy and reduced tiredness. Exercise reduces anxiety, depression, negative mood and social isolation and improves self-esteem, cognitive functions and quality of life [115–124].

7.8. Physiotherapy with the elderly in old age psychiatry

Old age psychiatry consists of two groups: dementia syndrome (Alzheimer, frontotemporal degeneration, vascular dementia) and functional psychiatric disorders (depression, addiction, mood disorders, personality disorders and schizophrenia). Elderly people experience declining physical activity levels and functional capabilities, loss of dependence, decreasing social contacts, increasing problems with mental health, loss of adaptive capabilities and quality of life. The most frequently observed characteristics in old age psychiatry are apathy (lack of motivation and interest), depression (fear, hopelessness, sad, low self-esteem, guilty,etc.), aggression (aggressive resistance, verbal and physical aggression), psychomotor agitation (aimless walking, pacing up and down, restlessness, repetitive actions and sleep disorders) and psychotic features (illusions, false identifications and hallucinations) [4].

Exercise helps to improve general daily activity, cognition and independency; increase cardiorespiratory fitness, strength and balance; reduce osteoporosis, sarcopenia, falls and risk factors for falls; increase quality of life and social activities; and reduce social isolation, loneliness, fear and institutionalization [125–127].

8. Conclusion

Today, there is a professional need in society for a physiotherapeutic approach to treat people who are suffering from chronic musculoskeletal and mental health problems. The general aims of physiotherapy in mental health are summarized in **Box 3**.

"Promoting, advising, teaching, warning, motivating maintaining, working, treating, assessing"

To promote human well-being and autonomy in people with physical health needs that are associated with a mental illness or learning disability and/or to use physical approaches safely to influence mental health.

To offer advice on the prevention of stress and physical problems as well as quality-improvement techniques.

To teach on topics relating to exercise, relaxation and communication.

To warn people about the side effects and to advise people on the use of quality-improvement techniques.

To motivate people to engage in healthy living habits.

To maintain (or to regain) physical mental and social skills to preserve the ability to function and the quality of life.

To work with the senses and motor skills of children with bodily and behavioural difficulties.

To treat physical and psychosomatic problems.

To assesstreatment effectiveness and patient satisfaction.

Box 3: General aims of physiotherapy in mental health.

In contrast to other fields in medicine, mental health consists of a labyrinth of conventional, complementary and alternative therapies and approaches [128]. A person with fluctuating mental health is more receptive to alternative approaches. Conventional health caregivers have to guide the patient in the search for optimal help. For that reason, physiotherapy interventions in mental health should at least satisfy four criteria. The nature of the interventions should be described clearly. The claimed benefits of the services must be stated explicitly. These benefits must be scientifically validated. Individual effects that might outweigh the benefits must be ruled out empirically. Collaboration and connections with other mental health care specialists within and outside physiotherapy are necessary to broaden the field of physiotherapy in mental health (see Box 3), avoid isolation, build a quality framework and cope with future challenges. In mental health care, boundaries between specialities have become increasingly more blurred. Intensive specialization of physiotherapy has been called into question. The demands to collaborate at the interdisciplinary (i.e. mutual contact between care providers) and transdisciplinary (various caregivers are at each other's domain) levels have increased. The inclusion of ideas from the social sciences and humanities in mental health care has become increasingly more important [129]. In the future, therapists will need to obtain informed consent for each treatment. Each therapist will need to explain that the proposed method has value for the patient and provide information about what, why, where, when and how he or she will proceed and what the potential outcomes are. Dialogue with the patient is important for the outcome and patient satisfaction. By definition, interventions in mental health are complex, given the nature of mental health and illness. Physiotherapists who work in mental health are well-trained therapists with knowledge of mental health (allegiance to theory) and motivation skills and have empathy (therapist-client alliance). The quality of the therapeutic relationship or alliance is important for the outcome of the physiotherapy treatment. Interventions require careful planning and sufficient resources to implement the programme as planned. Interventions are individually adapted according to the individual's psychophysical functioning, needs and wishes. The source of the most advanced knowledge of physiotherapy in mental health is a combination of scientifically derived knowledge and knowledge gained through years of experience (professional practice) (see **Box 3**). The different physiotherapy approaches are cost-effective and secure. Furthermore, they do not have side effects. They involve the patient and provide practical skills and insight for use in daily life. After a physiotherapy observational and/or evaluation assessment, the approaches focus on functional and (mental) health promotion. The patient's voice becomes increasingly more important. This chapter provides additional insight into why physiotherapy education needs to give more attention to the field of mental health in the curriculum. Currently, from the patient perspective, it is not acceptable for physiotherapists, as health care providers, to not have any or have limited courses on mental health during their education. Many excellent colleagues in primary care are not well prepared to work with persons with mental health, not because of their illness but because of their lack of information on how to address the illness.

Author details

Michel Probst

Address all correspondence to: michel.probst@kuleuven.be

KU Leuven, Department of Rehabilitation Sciences, Belgium

References

[1] World Health Organization (WHO). Promoting mental health: Concepts, emerging evidence, practice: report of the World Health Organization, Department of Mental Health

and substance abuse in collaboration with the Victorian Health Promotion Foundation and the University of Melbourne; 2005. Geneva: World Health Organization.

[2] Probst M, Skjaerven L. Editors. Physiotherapy in mental health and psychiatry: a scientific and clinical based approach. London: Elsevier; 2017, in press.

[3] Whittington J, Ruppert F. Changes in the prevalence of psychiatric disorder in a community are related to changes in the meal level of psychiatric symptoms. Psychological Medicine 1996; **26**:1253–1260.

[4] American Psychiatric Association. Diagnostic and statistical manual of mental disorders DSM-V (5th ed.). Washington, DC: APA Press; 2013.

[5] World Health Organization (WHO). International classification of diseases and related health problems ICD-10 10th revision; 2016. Fifth edition– Geneva: World Health Organization.

[6] WCPT. World Confederation of Physical Therapy [Internet]. 2016. Available from http://www.wcpt.org/

[7] ICPPMH. International conference of physiotherapy in psychiatry and mental health [Internet]. 2016. Available from http://www.icppmh.org/

[8] IOPTMH. International organization of physical therapy in mental health [Internet]. 2016. Available from http://www.wcpt.org/ioptmh

[9] Australian Physiotherapy Association. Position statement of mental health and physiotherapy [Internet]. 2016. Available from http://www.physiotherapy.asn.au

[10] Pope, C. Don't forget the mental aspects of your patients' health. Chartered society of physiotherapists [Internet]. 2013. Available from http://www.csp.org.uk/news/2013/10/09/don%E2%80%99t-forget-mental-aspects-your-patients%E2%80%99-health-says-president

[11] Miller WR, Rollnick S. Motivational interviewing, helping people change. 3rd revised edition. New York, NY: The Guildford Press; 2012.

[12] Probst M, Skjaerven LH, Parker A, Gyllensten AL, IJntema R, Catalán-Matamoros D. Do you support this definition of physiotherapy in mental health? Fisioterapia 2016; **38:**49.

[13] Probst M, Skjaerven LH, Parker A, Gyllensten AL, IJntema R, Catalán-Matamoros, D. International organization of physical therapy in mental health. Newsletter June [Internet]. 2015. Available from http://www.icppmh.org/

[14] Donaghy M, Nicol M, Davidson KM. Editors. Cognitive Behavioural Interventions in Physiotherapy and Occupational Therapy. London: Butterworth-Heineman; 2008. 194 p.

[15] Rovner G. Acceptance and commitment therapy in physiotherapy. In: Probst M, Skjaerven L. Editors. Physiotherapy in mental health and psychiatry: a scientific and clinical based approach. London: Elsevier; 2017, in press.

[16] World Health Organization (WHO). Global recommendations on physical activity for health; 2010. Geneva: World Health Organization.

[17] American College of Sports Medicine, editor. ACSM's health-related physical fitness assessment manual. New York: Lippincott Williams & Wilkins; 2013.

[18] Wilkins LW, Kaminsky LA, American College of Sports Medicine. 3rd ed. Philadelphia: Wolters Kluwer Health/Lippincott Williams & Wilkins Health; 2009.

[19] Vancampfort D, Stubbs B, Ward PB, Teasdale S, Rosenbaum S. "Why moving more should be promoted for severe mental illness. The Lancet Psychiatry 2015; **2:**295.

[20] Vancampfort D et al. "Health-related physical fitness in patients with bipolar disorder vs. Healthy controls: an exploratory study." Journal of Affective Disorders 2015; **177:**22–27.

[21] Vancampfort D. et al. "Cardiorespiratory fitness in severe mental illness: a systematic review and meta-analysis. Sports Medicine 2016; 2017, in press.

[22] Vancampfort D, Stubbs B, Ward PB, Teasdale S, Rosenbaum S. "Integrating physical activity as medicine in the care of people with severe mental illness." Australian & New Zealand Journal of Psychiatry 2015; **49:**681–682.

[23] Probst M, Knapen J, Poot G, Vancampfort D. Psychomotor therapy and psychiatry: what's in a name? The Open Complementary Medicine Journal 2010; **2:**105–113. oi.org/10.2174/1876391X010020010105

[24] Cooney GM et al. Exercise for depression. Advances in Psychiatric Treatment 2014**; 20:**2.

[25] Ekkekakis P. Honey, I shrunk the pooled SMD! Guide to critical appraisal of systematic reviews and meta-analyses using the cochrane review on exercise for depression as example. Mental Health and Physical Activity 2015; **8:**21–36.

[26] Cooney GM, Dwan K, Greig CA, Lawlor DA, Rimer J, Waugh FR, McMurdo M, Mead GE. Exercise for depression. Cochrane Database Systematic Review 2013; 9:CD004366. doi: 10.1002/14651858.CD004366.pub6.

[27] Josefsson T, Lindwall M, Archer T. Physical exercise intervention in depressive disorders: meta-analysis and systematic review. Scandinavian Journal of Medicine & Science in Sports 2013; **24:**259–272.

[28] Schuch FB, Vancampfort D, Richards J, Rosenbaum S., Ward PB, Stubbs B. Exercise as a treatment for depression: a meta-analysis adjusting for publication bias. Journal of Psychiatric Research 2016; **77:** 42–51.

[29] Richardson CR, Faulkner G, McDevitt J, Skrinar GS, Hutchinson DS, Piette JD. Integrating physical activity into mental health services for persons with serious mental illness. Psychiatric Services 2005; **56:**3.

[30] Craft LL, Landers DM. The effect of exercise on clinical depression and depression resulting from mental illness: a meta-analysis. Journal of Sport and Exercise Psychology 1998; **20**:339–357.

[31] Van de Vliet P, Auweele YV, Knapen J, Rzewnicki R, Onghena P, Van Coppenolle H. The effect of fitness training on clinically depressed patients: an intra-individual approach. Psychology of Sport and Exercise 2004; **5(2):**153–167.

[32] Knapen J et al. Comparison of changes in physical self-concept, global self-esteem, depression and anxiety following two different psychomotor therapy programs in non-psychotic psychiatric inpatients. Psychotherapy and Psychosomatics 2005; **74:**353–361.

[33] Knapen J, Vancampfort D, Moriën Y, Marchal Y. Exercise therapy improves both mental and physical health in patients with major depression. Disability and Rehabilitation 2015; **37:**1490–1495.

[34] Probst M. Vakttherapeutische interventies bij depressie. [Non-verbal interventions in depression]. In: Schene A, Sabbe B, Spinhoven P, Ruhe H. Editors. Handboek depressieve stoornissen. Utrecht: De Tijdstroom; 2016. pp. 465–482.

[35] Simons J. Introductie tot de psychomotorische therapie [Introduction of psychomotor therapy]. Leuven: Garant. p. 214

[36] Lehrer P M. Woolfolk RL, Sime W E. Principles and practice of stress management. 3th ed. New York/London: The Guilford Press; 2008.

[37] Sherborne V. Developmental movement for children. 2nd ed. London: Worth Publishing; 2001.

[38] Maurer J, Visser M, Albrechts B, Krot H. Psychomotorische gezinstherapie in de praktijk [psychomotor family therapy]. Kind & Adolescent Praktijk 200; **2**:60–66.

[39] Visser M, Albrechts B, Maurer J, Krot H. Een dialoog tussen systeemtherapeut, psychomotorisch therapeut en gezin. In: de Lange J. Psychomotorische Therapie. Amsterdam: Boom; 2010. pp. 115–131.

[40] Iansen B. Norwegian psychomotor physiotherapy. Movements of life. Trondheim: NPA; 2012.

[41] Ekerholt K, Bergland A. The first encounter with Norwegian p-sychomotor physiotherapy. Scandinavian Journal of Public Health 2004; **32**:403–410.

[42] Ekerholt K, Bergland A. Massage as interaction and a source of information. Advances in Physiotherapy 2006; **8**:137–144. DOI: 10.1080/14038190600836809

[43] Atkinson R, Smith E, Hilgard ER. Atkinson & Hilgard's introduction to psychology. Orlando, FL: Harcourt Brace & Company; 1999 ISBN: 9780155050693

[44] Thornquist E, Bunkan BH. What is psychomotor therapy? Oslo: Norwegian University Press; 1991.

[45] Bunkan, B.H. A comprehensive physiotherapy. In: Ekerholt K. ed. Aspects of psychiatric and psychosomatic physiotherapy. Oslo: Oslo University College; HiO-report 2010 no 3.

[46] Ekerholt K, Bergland A. Breathing: a sign of life and a unique area for reflection and action. Physical Therapy 2008; **88**:832–840. DOI: 10.2522/ptj.20070316

[47] Fried R. Breathing as clinical tool. In: Mostofsky DI, Barlow DH, editors. The management of stress and anxiety in medical disorders. 1st ed. Needham Heights, MA: Allyn & Bacon; 2000. ISBN: 978–0205287048

[48] Thornquist E. Psychomotor physiotherapy—principles, perspectives and potentials. In: Ekerholt K. Editor. Aspects of psychiatric and psychosomatic physiotherapy. Oslo: Oslo University College; HiO-report 2010 no 3.

[49] Ekerholt K. Awareness of breathing as a way to enhance the sense of coherence: patients' experiences in psychomotor physiotherapy. Body Movement and Dance in Psychotherapy Movement and Dance in Psychotherapy 2011; **6**:103–115. DOI:10.1080/17432979.2011.568762

[50] Ekerholt K, Schau G, Mathismoen KM, Bergland A. Body awareness—a vital aspect in mentalization: experiences from concurrent and reciprocal therapies. Physiotherapy Theory and Practice 2014; **30**:312–318. DOI: 10.3109/09593985.2013.876562st

[51] Van Damme T. Relaxation therapy. In: Probst M, Skjaerven L. Editors. Physiotherapy in mental health. London: Elsevier; 2017, in press.

[52] Payne R, Donaghy M. Payne's handbook of relaxation techniques. 4th Edition. A practical guide for the health care professional. London: Churchill Livingstone; 2010.

[53] Kerr K. Relaxation techniques: a critical review. Critical Reviews in Physical and Rehabilitation Medicine 2000; **12**:51–89.

[54] Bernstein DA, Borkovec T. Progressive relaxtion training. A manual for the helping professions. Champaign, IL: Research Press Company; 1973.

[55] Vancampfort D, Correll, CU, Scheewe TW, Probst M, De Herdt A, Knapen J, De Hert M. Progressive muscle relaxation in persons with schizophrenia: a systematic review of randomized controlled trials. Clinical Rehabilitation 2013; **27**:291–8.

[56] Georgiev A, Probst M, De Hert M, Genova V, Tonkova A, Vancampfort D. Acute effects of progressive muscle relaxation on state anxiety and subjective well-being in chronic bulgarian patients with schizophrenia. Psychiatria Danubina 2012; **24:**367–372.

[57] Öst LG. Applied relaxation. Manual for a behavioral coping technique. Stockholm: Stockholm University Press; 1992.

[58] Mitchell L. Simple relaxation: the Mitchell method for easing tension. 2nd edn. London: Murray; 1987.

[59] Kermani KS. Autogenic training. London: Souvenir Pressous; 1996.

[60] Baer RA. Mindfulness based treatment approaches. Clinician's guide to evidence base and applications. San Diego, CA: Academic Press; 2006.

[61] Kabat-Zinn J, Massion A, Kristeller J, Peterson l, Fletcher K, Pebert, l et al. Effectiveness of a meditation-base stress reduction program in the treatment of anxiety disorders. American Journal of Psychiatry 1992; **149**:936–943.

[62] Wang C, Schmid CH, Rones R, et al. A randomized trial of tai chi for fibromyalgia. New England Journal of Medicine 2010; **363**:743–54.

[63] Quinn MC, Ginnis P. Tai Chi. Complementary therapies for physical therapy. In: Deutsch J, Zambo Anderson E. Editors. A clinical Decision-making approach. Saint Louis: Saunders Elsevier; 2008. pp. 139–156.

[64] Gallager B, Lund R. Qigong. Complementary therapies for physical therapy. In: Deutsch J, Zambo Anderson E. Editors. A clinical Decision-making approach. Saint Louis: Saunders Elsevier; 2008. pp. 215–226.

[65] Khumar SS, Kaur P, Kaur S. Effectiveness of Shavasana on depression among university students. Indian Journal of Clinical Psychology 1993; **20**:82–87.

[66] Cramer H, Lauche R, Langhorst J, Dobos G. Yoga for depression: a systematic review and meta-analysis. Depression and Anxiety 2013; **30**:1068–1083.

[67] Janakiramaiah N, Gangadhar BN, Murthy PNV, Harish MG, Subbakrishna DK, Vedamurthachar A. Antidepressant efficacy of sudarshan kriya yoga in melancholia: a randomized comparison with electroconvulsive therapy and imipramine. Journal of Affective Disorders 2000; **57:**255–259.

[68] Duraiswamy G, Thirthalli J, Nagendra HR, Gangadhar BN. Yoga therapy as an add-on treatment in the management of patients with schizophrenia–a randomized controlled trial. Acta Psychiatrica Scandinavica 2007; **116**:226–32

[69] Bangalore NG, Varambally S. Yoga therapy for schizophrenia. International Journal of Yoga, 2012; **5**:85–91. doi: 10.4103/0973-6131.98212

[70] Vancampfort D, Vansteelandt K, Scheewe T, Probst M, Knapen J, De Herdt A, De Hert M. Yoga in schizophrenia: a systematic review of randomised controlled trials. Acta Psychiatrica Scandinavica 2012; **126:**12–20. DOI: 10.1111/j.1600-0447.2012.01865.x

[71] Galantino M, Musser J. Yoga. In: Deutsch J, Zambo Anderson E. Editors. Complementary therapies for physical therapy. A clinical Decision-making approach Saint Louis: Saunders Elsevier; 2008. p. 121–138.

[72] Patel NK, Newstead AH, Ferrer RL. The Effects of yoga on physical functioning and health related quality of life in older adults: a systematic review and meta-analysis. The Journal of Alternative and Complementary Medicine 2012; **18(10):**902–917. doi:10.1089/acm.2011.0473.

[73] Zambo Anderson E, Dickinson C. Pilates. Complementary therapies for physical therapy. In: Deutsch J, Zambo Anderson E. Editors. A clinical Decision-making approach Saint Louis: Saunders Elsevier; 2008. pp. 310–320.

[74] Latey P. The Pilates method: history and philosophy. The Journal **of** Bodywork and Movement Therapies 2001**;** **5**:275–282.

[75] Latey P. Upadating the principles of the pilates method – Part 2. The Journal **of** Bodywork and Movement Therapies 2002; **6**:094–101.

[76] Mętel S, Milert A, Szczygieł E. Pilates Based Exercise in Muscle Disbalances. In Zaslav KR. Editor. Prevention and treatment of sports injuries, an international perspective on topics

in sports medicine and sports injury. ISBN: 978-953-51-0005-8. InTech. Available from: http://www.intechopen.com/books/an-international-perspective-on-topics-in-sports-medicine-and-sportsinjury/ *2012*

[77] Soukup MG, Glomsröd B, Lönn JH, Bö K, Larsen S. The effect of a Mensendieck exercise program as secondary prophylaxis for recurrent low back pain. A randomized, controlled trial with 12-month follow-up. Spine 1999; **24**:1585–91; discussion 1592.

[78] Landi M. Il metodo Feldenkrais. [The Feldenkrais method] In Maddalie S, Bongi S. Riabilitazione reumatologica, approcciomultidisciplinare. Milano: Edra SPA; 2007. pp 339–364.

[79] Stephens J. Feldenkrais. Complementary therapies for physical therapy. In: Deutsch J, Zambo Anderson E. Editors. A clinical decision-making approach Saint Louis: Saunders Elsevier; 2008. pp. 273–286.

[80] Probst M, Coppenolle H, Vandereycken W. Body experience in anorexia nervosa patients: an overview of therapeutic approaches. Eating Disorders. 1995; **3**(2):145–157.

[81] Probst M, Majewski ML, Albertsen M, Catalan-Matamoros D, Danielsen M, De Herdt A, Duskova Zakova H, Fabricius S, Joern C, Kjolstad G, Patovirta M, Philip-Raverty S, Tyyska E, Vancampfort D. Physiotherapy for patients with anorexia nervosa. Advances in Eating Disorders;Theory, Research and Practice 2013; **1**:224–238. DOI: 10.1080/21662630.2013.798562

[82] Vancampfort D, Vanderlinden J, De Hert M, Adamkova M, Skjaerven LH, Catalan Matamoros D, Lundvik-Gyllensten A, Gomez Conesa A, IJntema R, Probst M. A systematic review on physical therapy interventions for patients with binge eating disorder. Disability and Rehabilitation 2013; **35**:2191–2196. DOI: 10.3109/09638288.2013.771707

[83] Soundy A, Stubbs B, Probst M, Gyllensten AL, Skjaerven LH, Catalan-Matamoros D, Vancampfort D. Considering the role of physical therapists within the treatment and rehabilitation of individuals with eating disorders: an international survey of expert clinicians. Physiotherapy Research International 2016; **21**:237–246. DOI: 10.1002/pri.1637

[84] Vancampfort D, Vanderlinden J, De Hert M, Soundy A, Adámkova M, Skjaerven LH, Catalán-Matamoros D, Lundvik Gyllensten A, Gómez-Conesa A, Probst M. A systematic review of physical therapy interventions for patients with anorexia and bulemia nervosa. Disability and Rehabilitation 2014; **36:**628–634. DOI: 10.3109/09638288.2013.808271

[85] Vancampfort D, Probst M, Skjaerven LH, Catalán-Matamoros D, Lundvik-Gyllensten A, Gómez-Conesa A, et al. Systematic review of the benefits of physical therapy within a multidisciplinary care approach for people with schizophrenia. Physical Therapy 2012; **92**:11–23. DOI: 10.2522/ptj.20110218

[86] Vera-Garcia E, Mayoral-Cleries F, Vancampfort D, Stubbs B, Cuesta-Vargas A. A systematic review of the benefits of physical therapy within a multidisciplinary care approach for people with schizophrenia: an update 2015. Psychiatry Research 2015; **229**:828–839. DOI: 10.1016/j.psychres.2015.07.083

[87] Stubbs B, Soundy A, Probst M, De Hert M, De Herdt A, Parker A, Vancampfort D. The assessment, benefits and delivery of physical activity in people with schizophrenia: a survey of members of the international organisation of physical therapists in mental health (IOPTMH). Physiotherapy Research International 2014; **19**:248–256. DOI: 10.1002/pri.1592

[88] Stubbs B, Soundy A, Probst M, Parker A, Skjaerven LH, Lundvik Gyllensten A, Vancampfort D. Addressing the disparity in physical health provision for people with schizophrenia: an important role for physiotherapists. Physiotherapy 2014; **100**:185–186. DOI: 10.1016/j.physio.2013.11.003

[89] Stubbs B, Soundy A, Probst M, De Hert M, De Herdt A, Vancampfort D. Understanding the role of physiotherapists in schizophrenia: An International perspective from members of the international organization of physical therapists in mental health (IOPTMH). Journal of Mental Health 2014, **23**:125–129. DOI: 10.3109/09638237.2013.869574

[90] Vancampfort D, De Herdt A, De Hert M, Probst M. There is a need for physiotherapists in the multidisciplinary treatment of schizophrenia. Fisioterapia: Revista de Salud, Discapacidad y Terapeutica Fisica 2013; **35**:239–242.

[91] Nyboe L, Vestergaard CH, Moeller MK, Lund H, Videbech P. Metabolic syndrome and aerobic fitness in patients with first-episode schizophrenia, including a 1-year follow-up. Schizophrenia Research 2015; **168(1–2)**:381–7. doi: 10.1016/j.schres.2015.07.053

[92] Nyboe L, Vestergaard CH, Lund H, Møller MK, Videbech P. Metabolic syndrome in first-time hospitalized patients with depression: a 1-year follow-up study. Acta Psychiatrica Scandinavica 2016; **133(3)**:241–8. doi: 10.1111/acps.12470

[93] Vancampfort D, De Hert M, Skjerven LH, Gyllensten AL, Parker A, Mulders N, Nyboe L, Spenser F, Probst M. International organization of physical therapy in mental health consensus on physical activity within multidisciplinary rehabilitation programmes for minimising cardio-metabolic risk in patients with schizophrenia. Disability and Rehabilitation 2012; **34**:1–12. DOI: 10.3109/09638288.2011.587090

[94] Vancampfort D, Rosenbaum S, Probst M, Connaughton J, du Plessis C, Yamamoto T, Stubbs B. Top 10 research questions to promote physical activity in bipolar disorders: a consensus statement from the international organization of physical therapists in mental health. Journal of Affective Disorders 2016; **195**:82–87.

[95] Vancampfort D, Sienaert P, Wyckaert S, De Hert M, Stubbs B, Kinyanda E, Probst M. The metabolic syndrome is associated with self-reported physical complaints in patients with bipolar disorder. Psychiatria Danubina 2016; **28**:139–145.

[96] Vancampfort D, Sienaert P, Wyckaert S, De Hert M, Stubbs B, Richards J, Mugisha J, Probst M. The functional exercise capacity is associated with global functioning in people with bipolar disorder. Journal of Nervous and Mental Disease 2016; **204**:673–677.

[97] Vancampfort D, Wyckaert S, Sienaert P, De Hert M, Soundy A, Rosenbaum S, Richards S, Probst M. Test-retest study of the six-minute walk test in people with bipolar disorder. Psychiatria Danubina 2016; **28**:39–44.

[98] Vancampfort D, Sienaert P, Wyckaert S, De Hert M, Stubbs B, Probst M. Sitting time, physical fitness impairments and metabolic abnormalities in people with bipolar disorder: an exploratory study. Psychiatry Research 2016; **242:**7–12.

[99] Fogel A. The psychophysiology of self-awareness: rediscovering the lost art of body sense. The norton series on interpersonal neurobiology. NY: W. W. Norton; 2009.

[100] Mehling W, Wrubel J, Daubenmier J, Price C, Kerr C, Silow T, Gopisetty V, Stewart, A. Body Awareness: a phenomenological inquiry into the common ground of mind-body therapies. Philos Ethics Humanit Med. 2011; **6**:6. doi: 10.1186/1747-5341-6-6

[101] Skjaerven, L. Basic Body awareness therapy. Promoting movement quality and health for daily life. Bergen: Bergen University College; 2013. p. 42.

[102] Dropsy J. Human expression: the coordination of mind and body. In: Skjaerven LH, Editor. Quality of movement: the art and health—lectures on philosophy, theory and practical implications to basic body awareness therapy. Bergen: Norway; 1998. pp. 21–34.

[103] Roxendal G. Body awareness therapy and the body awareness scale: treatment and evaluation in psychiatric physiotherapy [doctoral dissertation]. Göteborg: University of Göteborg; 1985.

[104] Mattsson M. Body awareness applications in physiotherapy [doctoral dissertation]. Umeå, Sweden: Umeå University; 1998.

[105] Lundvik Gyllensten A. Basic body awareness therapy [doctoral dissertation]. Lund, Sweden: Lund University; 2001.

[106] Lundvik Gyllensten A, Gard G, Salford E, Ekdahl C. Interaction between patient and physiotherapist: a qualitative study reflecting the physiotherapist's perspective. Physiotherapy Research International 1999; **4**:89–109.

[107] Lundvik Gyllensten A, Gard G, Hansson L, Ekdahl C. Interaction between patient and physiotherapist in psychiatric care: the physiotherapist's perspective. Advance Physiotherapy 2000; **2**:157–167.

[108] Skjaerven LH, Kristoffersen K, Gard G. How can movement quality be promoted in clinical practice? A phenomenological study of physical therapist experts. Physical Therapy 2010; **90**:1479–1492. DOI: 10.2522/ptj.20090059

[109] Skjaerven LH, Kristoffersen K, Gard G. An eye for movement quality: a phenomenological study of movement quality reflecting a group of physiotherapists' understanding of the phenomenon. Physiotherapy Theory and Practice 2008; **24**: 13–27. DOI: 10.1080/01460860701378042

[110] Gyllensten A, Skär L, Miller, M, Gard, G. Embodied identity—A deeper understanding of body awareness. Physiotherapy Theory and Practice 2010; **26**:439–446. DOI: 10.3109/09593980903422956

[111] Catalan-Matamoros D. 6th International Conference on Physiotherapy in Psychiatry and Mental Health, Madrid Fisioterapia 2016; **38:**219–223.

[112] Skjaerven L, Mattsson M, Parker A, Catalan-Matamoros D, Gard G, Gyllensten, A. Consensus on the theory of basic body awareness therapy – qualitative action research implemented into the movement awareness domain. Physiotherapy 2015; **101**:e1405–1406. DOI:10.1016/j.physio.2015.03.1357

[113] Hall AM, Ferreira PH, Maher CG, Latimer J, Ferreira, ML. The influence of the therapist-patient relationship on treatment outcome in physical rehabilitation: a systematic review. Physical Therapy 2010; **90**:1099–1110.

[114] Brunner E, Probst M, Meichtry A, Luomajoki H, Dankaerts W. Comparison of clinical vignettes and standardized patients as measures of physiotherapists' activity and work recommendations in patients with non-specific low back pain. Clinical Rehabilitation 2016;**30(1):**85–94. doi: 10.1177/0269215515570499.

[115] Brunner E, De Herdt A, Minguet P, Baldew SS, Probst M. Can cognitive behavioural therapy based strategies be integrated into physiotherapy for the prevention of chronic low back pain? A systematic review. Disability and Rehabilitation 2013 Jan; 35(1):1–10. doi: 10.3109/09638288.2012.683848.

[116] Whiteford HA, Degenhardt L, Rehm Jr, Baxter AJ, Ferrari AJ, Erskine HE, et al. Global burden of disease attributable to mental and substance use disorders: findings from the Global Burden of Disease Study 2010. The Lancet 2013; **382**:1575–1586.DOI: 10.1016/S0140-6736(13)61611-6

[117] Vancampfort D, Stubbs B, Mitchell AJ, De Hert M, Wampers M, Ward PB, et al. Risk of metabolic syndrome and its components in people with schizophrenia and related psychotic disorders, bipolar disorder and major depressive disorder: a systematic review and meta-analysis. World Psychiatry 2015; **14**:339–347. DOI: 10.1002/wps.20252

[118] Vancampfort D, Correll CU, Galling B, Probst M, De Hert M, Ward PB, et al. Diabetes mellitus in people with schizophrenia, bipolar disorder and major depressive disorder: a systematic review and large scale meta-analysis World Psychiatry 2016; **15**:166–174. DOI: 10.1002/wps.20309

[119] Lawrence D. Excess mortality, mental illness and global burden of disease. Epidemiology and Psychiatric Sciences 2015; **24**:141–143. DOI: 10.1017/S2045796014000742

[120] Pratt SI, Jerome GJ, Schneider KL, Craft LL, Buman MP, Stoutenberg M, et al. Increasing US health plan coverage for exercise programming in community mental health settings for people with serious mental illness: a position statement from the Society of Behavior Medicine and the American College of Sports Medicine. Translational Behavioral Medicine 2016; **6**:1–4. DOI: 10.1007/s13142-016-0407-7

[121] Stumbo SP, Yarborough BJH, Yarborough MT, Janoff SL, Stevens VJ, Lewinsohn M, et al. Costs of implementing a behavioral weight-loss and lifestyle-change program for individuals with serious mental illnesses in community settings. Translational Behavioral Medicine 2015; **5**: 269–276. DOI: 10.1007/s13142-015-0322-3

[122] Stubbs B, Probst M, Soundy A, Parker A, De Herdt A, De Hert M, Mitchell A, Vancampfort D. Physiotherapists can help implement physical activity programmes in clinical practice. British Journal of Psychiatry 2013; **204**:164–164. DOI: 10.1192/bjp.204.2.164.

[123] Firth J, Rosenbaum S, Stubbs B, Vancampfort D, Carney R, Yung A. Preferences and motivations for exercise in early psychosis. Acta Psychiatrica Scandinavica, 2016; **134**:83–84.

[124] Vancampfort D. Rosenbaum S, Schuch F, Ward PB, Probst M, Stubbs B. Prevalence and predictors of treatment dropout from physical activity interventions in schizophrenia: a meta-analysis. General Hospital Psychiatry 2016; **39:**S0163–8343(15)00243–1, 15–23.

[125] Kaur J, Masaum M, Bhatia MS. Psychophysiotherapy, the role of physiotherapy in mental health disorders. Delhi Psychiatry Journal 2013; **16**:404–408

[126] Zhu W, Wadley VG, Howard VJ, Hutto B, Blair SN, Hooker SP. Objectively measured physical activity and cognitive function in older adults. Medicine & Science in Sports & Exercise 2017; **49**:47–53. DOI: 10.1249/MSS.0000000000001079

[127] Gillespie LD, Robertson MC, Gillespie WJ, Sherrington C, Gates S, Clemson LM, Lamb SE. Interventions for preventing falls in older people living in the community. Cochrane Database Systematic Review 2012; **9**:CD007146. doi: 10.1002/14651858.CD007146.pub3.

[128] Vogel T, Brechat PH, Leprêtre PM, Kaltenbach G, Berthel M, Lonsdorfer J. Health benefits of physical activity in older patients: a review. International Journal of Clinical Practice 2009; **63**:303–20. doi: 10.1111/j.1742-1241.2008.01957.x.

[129] Liu- Ambrose T, Donaldson MG. Exercise and cognition in older adults: is there a role for resistance training programmes? British Journal of Sports Medicine 2009; **43(1):**25–7. doi: 10.1136/bjsm.2008.055616. Epub 2008 Nov 19.

8

Exercise Therapy for Physical Therapist

Naruemon Leelayuwat

Additional information is available at the end of the chapter

Abstract

This chapter describes exercise therapy in terms of definition, objectives, concept, techniques, mechanisms, and equipment. Mechanisms explaining the effect of exercise training on treatments for other diseases are included. In addition, new biomarkers capable of evaluating exercise performance capacity and progress in training and early detection of overtraining are provided. Very promising are mainly small non-coding microRNAs (miRNAs). Important background knowledge for exercise therapy is also provided. The knowledge covers the exercise for healthy and unhealthy people. The former includes sedentary and sport player. The latter includes patients with various diseases, for example, metabolic diseases, cardiovascular disease, orthopedics, etc. Importantly, all the knowledge was presented in latest information.

Keywords: physical activity, physical therapy, movement, oxidative stress, microRNA, sports, diseases

1. Introduction

Exercise therapy is defined as a regimen or plan of physical activities designed and prescribed to facilitate the patients to recover from diseases and any conditions, which disturb their movement and activity of daily life or maintain a state of well-being [1] through neuro re-education, gait training, and therapeutic activities. It is systemic execution of planned physical movements, postures, or activities intended to enable the patients to (1) reduce risk, (2) enhance function, (3) remediate or prevent impairment, (4) optimize overall health, and (5) improve fitness and well-being [2].

This therapy may relate specific muscles or parts of the body, to general and strenuous activities that can return a recovering patient to the peak of physical condition. It is highly repetitive and intensive and requires time and dedication on the part of the patients to encourage neuroplasticity. The therapy is performed by professionals with an educational background in exercise physiology, exercise science, or other similar degree. To succeed goal-oriented treatment, the personnel must [2].

1. Provide comprehensive and personalized patient/individual management.
2. Implement a variety of therapeutic interventions that are complementary (e.g., heat application before joint mobilization and passive stretch, followed by active exercise to use new mobility in a functional manner).
3. Rely on clinical decision-making skill.
4. Promote patients' independence whenever possible through the use of home management, self-management exercise programs, and patient-related instruction.

In-house physical therapy by family, friends, or caregivers to deliver the appropriate exercise therapy in the home can greatly decrease healthcare costs which may limit the intervention. Therefore, training and educating these persons are important in effective exercise therapy.

Exercise therapy can be called Activity-Based Therapy, Activity-Based Recovery Therapy, Neuro-based Therapy, and Restorative Therapy.

1.1. Important background knowledge to understand exercise therapy

Background knowledge needs to be understand [3].

Planes of movement

There are three planes of movement.

a) Movement in horizontal plane (transverse plane): This plane divides the body into upper and lower halves. Movements in transverse plane occur parallel to ground.
b) Movement in frontal plane (coronal plane): This plane divides side to side movements, for example, bringing the head to each of the shoulders.
c) Movement in vertical plane (sagittal plane): It is the plane that divides the body or body segment into the right and left parts. Movements in this plane include forward and backward motions such as nodding of the head.

Kinematics is the area of biomechanics that include description of motion without regard for the forces producing it. They include.

a) Types of motion. There are four types of motion:
    - Rotatory motion, which is the movement of an object around a fixed axis in a curved path.

- Translatory motion, which is the movement of an object in a straight line.
- Curvilinear motion, which is a combination of rotatory and translatory motions.
- General plane motion, which the object is segmented and free to move.

b) Location of motion: Motion at a joint may occur in transverse, frontal, or sagittal planes.

c) Direction of motion: Movement may occur either in clockwise or anticlockwise direction.

d) Magnitude of motion can be given either in degrees or radians.

Kinetics is biomechanics that concerned with the forces maintaining equilibrium or producing motion and are described as either external or internal forces.

Center of gravity (COG) is the point which the force of gravity acts effectively independently on position of body. The COG of human body lies approximately at S2, anterior to sacrum.

Line of gravity (LOG) is the line that lies vertically through center of gravity.

Base of support is the area which is supported.

Equilibrium results when the forces acting upon a body are balanced and the body remains at rest.

Fixation and stabilization: Fixation is the state of immobility, and stabilization is the state of relative immobility.

Force is that which alters the state of rest of a body or its uniform motion in a straight line

Lever is a rigid bar that rotates around on axis.

Mechanical advantage is efficacy of force in relation to lever depends on two factors.

Pulley is a grooved wheel which rotates about a fixed axis by a rope that passes round it. The axis is supported by a frame work or block. There are two types of pulleys: (1) fixed pulleys and (2) movable pulleys.

Starting position is the first posture before the following movement during the exercise therapy. There are five fundamental starting positions: standing, kneeling, sitting, lying, and hanging. Equilibrium and stability are maintained in these positions by balance of forces acting upon the body.

2. Objectives of exercise therapy

The objectives of exercise therapy are as following;

a) Promote activity and minimize the effects of inactivity, increased independence

b) Increase the normal range of motion.

c) Improve strength the weak muscles.

d) Improve the performance in daily activities.

e) Enable ambulation.

f) Release contracted muscles, tendons, and fascia.

g) Improve circulation.

h) Improve respiratory capacity.

i) Improve coordination.

j) Reduce rigidity.

k) Improve balance.

l) Promote relaxation.

m) Increased motor or sensory function.

n) Reduction of medication, reduction of hospital visits, and increased overall health.

The most important goal of exercise therapy is an optimal level of physical fitness by the end of the intervention. The physical fitness a state characterized by good muscle strength combined with good endurance.

3. Concept

Exercise therapy based on the independent movement which depends on individual goals. It aims to improve the ability to achieve optimal daily functioning. To achieve the goal of exercise therapy, the practitioner needs to understand the disablement process which include [4]

The disablement process

a) Impairment: A loss or abnormality of anatomic, physiologic, or psychologic structure or function.

b) Functional limitation: A limitation of the whole person performance, task in an efficient, typically expected, or competent manner, or a physical action activity.

c) Disability: The inability or a limitation to perform the performance of actions, or tasks.

There are three models of the disablement process:

a) World Health Organization's (WHO) International Classification of Impairments, Disabilities, and Handicaps (IDICH) [5].

b) NAGI scheme [6].

c) Modified disablement model [2]. This model exhibits the complexity of the relationships among pathology, impairments, functional limitations, disability, risk factors, interventions, quality of life, and prevention, wellness, and fitness.

4. Patient management

Physical therapist's approach to patient management involves examination, evaluation, diagnosis, prognosis, and intervention [2].

4.1. Therapeutic exercise intervention model

A three-dimensional model has been created to assist the clinician in the clinical decision-making process regarding exercise prescription. The model includes

Elements of the movement system: These elements relate to the purpose of each activity or technique

a) Support

b) Base

c) Modulator

d) Biomechanics

e) Cognitive/affective

The specific activity or technique chosen

a) Posture

b) Mode

c) Movement

The specific dosage

a) Type of contraction

b) Intensity

c) Speed

d) Duration

e) Frequency

f) Sequence

g) Environment

h) Feedback

The therapist must continually monitor the exercise to determine the need for modification to increase or decrease difficulty to ensure continual progress is being made with minimal setbacks. In addition, exercise therapy can be complemented with adjunctive interventions if the additional intervention can lead to a higher level of functional outcome in a short time.

5. Techniques

The techniques of exercise therapy used in treatment may be classified as follows [7].

5.1. Passive movement

Passive movements

Passive movements (Motion Therapy, Continuous Passive) provide continuous passive motion to the applied joint. The apparatus can be used immediately after the operation to improve the range of motion, reduce pain, discomfort, and healing. This machine is adjustable, easily controlled, versatile, and usually electrically operated.

a) Relaxed passive movements

The physiotherapist performed these movements for the patients. The physiotherapist needs knowledge of the anatomy of joints. The same direction and range of the movements are the same as those performed in the active movements. The physiotherapist moves the joint d through the existing free range and within the limits of pain.

b) Accessory movements

These movements are parts of any normal joint movement but may be absent or limited in abnormal joint conditions. They consist of rotational or gliding movements which cannot be separately performed as a voluntary movement but can be performed by the physiotherapist.

Passive manual mobilization techniques

a) Mobilizations of joints

The physiotherapist performed these movements which are usually small repetitive oscillatory, rhythmical, localized functional, or accessory in various amplitudes within the available range. These can be done quite strongly or very gently and are graded according to the part of the available range in which they are performed.

b) Manipulations of joints

- Physiotherapists

The movements are performed by the physiotherapist. They are accurately localized, single, quick decisive movements, which have small amplitude and high velocity completed before the patient can stop it.

- Surgeon/physician

The movements are performed by a surgeon under anesthesia or physician to receive further range. The maintaining of the increase in movement must be performed by the physiotherapist.

c) Controlled sustained stretching of tightened structure:

The increase in range of movement can be done by passive stretching of muscles and other soft tissues. The stretching adhesions in these structures and lengthening of muscle increase the movement by inhibition of the tendon protective reflex.

5.2. Active exercise

Movement performed or controlled by the voluntary action of muscles, working in opposition to an external force

Voluntary

a) Assisted active exercise

In this type of exercise, the patient tries to perform the movement by himself/herself. However, his/her muscular action is insufficient for the production or control of full range of movement. To complete it, an external force needs to be added. If the muscle power increases, the assistance given must decrease.

b) Free exercise

Free exercises are those which are performed by the patient's own muscular efforts without the assistance or resistance of any external force, other that of gravity.

c) Assisted-resisted exercise

This type of exercise constitutes a combination of assistance and resistance during a single movement.

d) Resisted exercise

The external force may be applied to the body levers to oppose the force of muscular contraction and there will be increase in muscle power and hypertrophy.

Resisted exercise technique is classified into six major categories:

- Endurance training
- Resistance training
- Muscle stretching exercises (flexibility training)
- Balance training
- Coordination training
- Agility training
- Body mechanics and awareness training
- Enhance function
- Gait and locomotion training
- Plyometric exercise (power training)

Exercise preparation

Before exercise training, a patient should be evaluated by a physician. It is important to exclude patients with ventricular hypertrophy, valvular heart disease, dangerous arrhythmias, and malignant hypertension. Other cardiac cases, and patients at risk, such as those with exercise-induced asthma, obesity, or diabetes, should perform an exercise stress test under careful medical supervision. Blood pressure and heart rate and the electrocardiogram (ECG) must be monitored throughout the exercise to confirm their cardiovascular function.

Aerobic or endurance training

In endurance training program, there are three important variables, including frequency, intensity, and duration. The recommendations by the American College of Sports Medicine (ACSM) are as follows:

- Frequency—Appropriate frequency of the aerobic exercise should be 3–5 days per week.
- Intensity of training—64/70—94% of maximum heart rate (HR max), or 40/50—85% of maximum oxygen uptake reserve (VO_2R) or heart rate reserve (HRR).
- Duration of training—The appropriate duration of training should be intermittent or continuous aerobic exercise for 20–60 min (minimum of 10-min bouts accumulated throughout the day).

The duration of training is dependent on the intensity of the exercise. Thus, lower-intensity exercise should be performed over longer duration (≥30 min), and conversely, higher levels of intensity should be performed at least 20 min or longer. Moderate-intensity exercise of longer duration is recommended for untrained adults, because total fitness is more readily attained with exercise sessions of longer duration and because potential hazards and adherence problems are associated with high-intensity activity.

Exercise for healthy individuals

Continuously aerobic exercises that use large muscle groups are recommended including western and eastern style:

Western style

- Cycling
- Swimming
- Walking
- Running
- Jogging
- Aerobic dance/exercise classes
- Dancing
- Stair climbing
- Rowing
- Skating
- Jumping rope
- Cross-country skiing

Eastern style

- Tai chi
- Yoga
- Arm swing exercise (**Figure 1**)
- Wand exercise (**Figure 2**)

The maximal HR can be calculated by the following formula: HR max = 220 – age.

The exercise session should consist of three periods. Starting with a warm-up period of approximately 10 min which combines calisthenic-type stretching exercises (without equipment). This follows by progressive aerobic activity that should increase the heart rate close to the prescribed heart rate for the session. Then, endurance training at the targeted heart rate for 20–60 min is performed and following by a cool-down period of 5–10 min.

Exercise for patients

A less strenuous exercise training regimen must be used, with the training heart rate not exceeding 50–60% of maximum O_2uptake (VO_{2max}) or a heart rate of 130 beats per minute (/min). In elderly patients and patients at risk, the intensity, frequency, and duration of therapeutic exercise should be established for each patient individually with medical evaluation before.

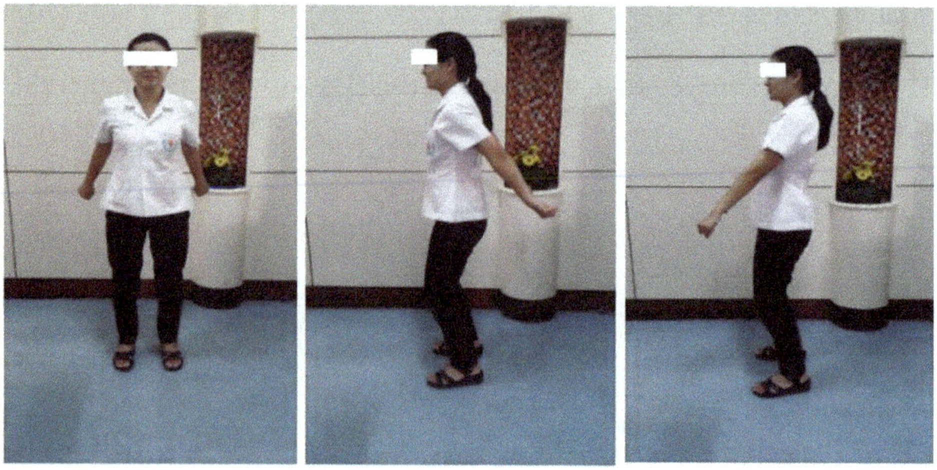

Figure 1. Arm swing exercise.

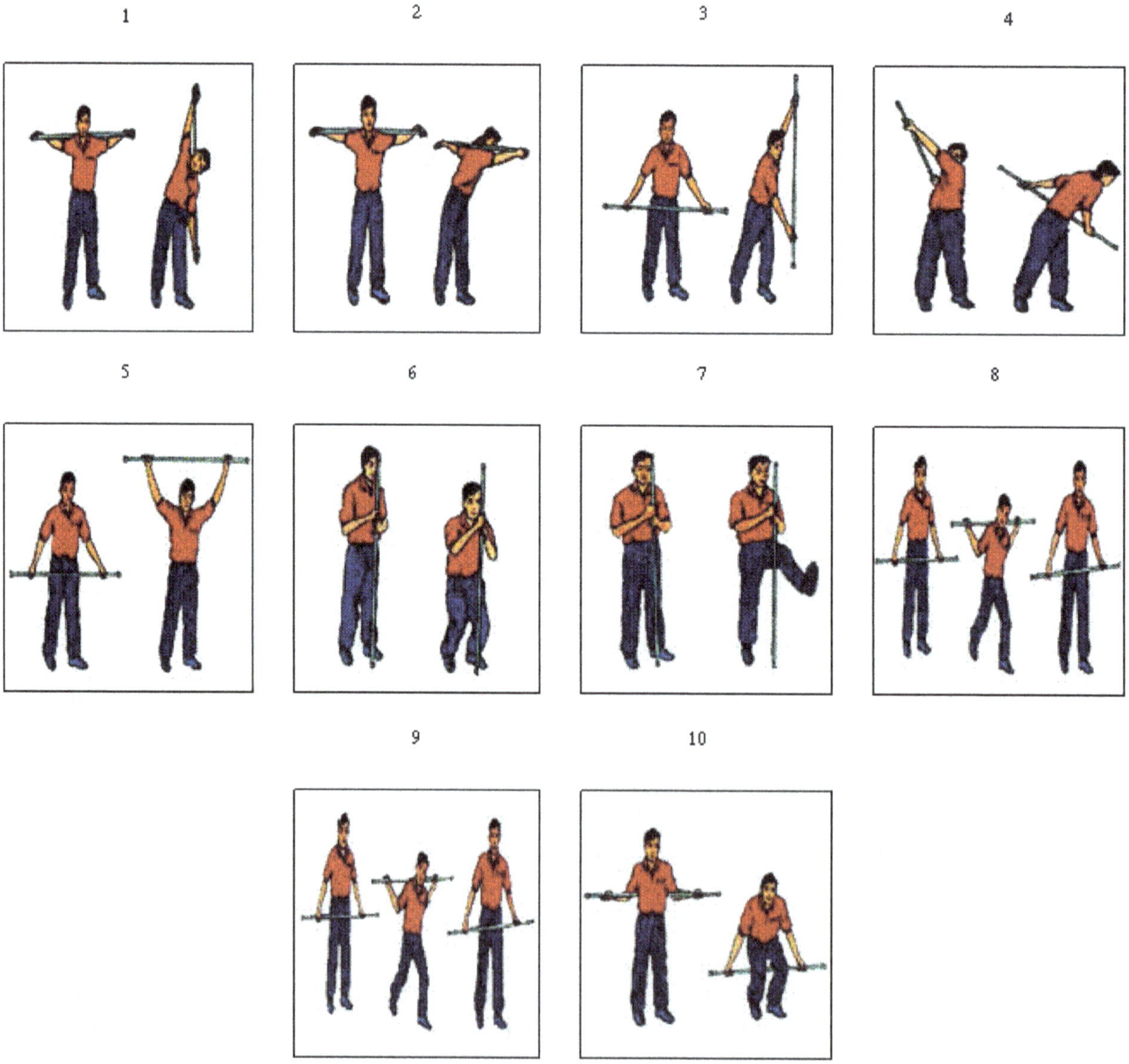

Figure 2. Wand exercise.

Karvonen method should be employed to determine the target heart rate for the ill or elderly patient: Target HR = (220 — age — resting heart rate × % intensity selected) + resting HR.

Progression

In endurance training, progression can happen by increasing the intensity or the duration. Several factors affecting the suitable rate of progression including age, current activity levels, exercise goals, and physiologic limitations should be considered. Most importantly, progression rate should be used that results in long-term participation. Being too aggressive can increase dropout rates because of injuries and/or perceived excessive discomfort. In addition, a progression of balance ability can be enhanced more by the exercise on the unstable support surface than exercise on the stable support surface.

a) Special techniques There are many special techniques used in exercise therapy [6]

- Frenkel's exercises are used to treat the incoordination which results from many other diseases, for example, disseminated sclerosis. Dr. H.S. Frenkel was Medical Superintendent of the Sanatorium "Freihof" in Switzerland toward the end of the last century.
- Proprioceptive neuromuscular facilitation (PNF) is an approach in which treatment is directed at a total human being, not just at a specific problem or body segment. This method was developed by Dr. Herman Kabat and Ms. Margaret Knott in 1946 and 1951 [7].
- Hydrotherapy refers to the use of multi-depth immersion pools or tanks that facilitate the application of various established therapeutic interventions including stretching, joint mobilization, strengthening, etc.
- Breathing exercises are designed to retrain the muscles of respiration, improve ventilation, lessen the work of breathing, and improve gaseous exchange and patient's overall function in daily living activities.

6. Mechanisms

Uptodate, there are many mechanisms explaining the beneficial effects of exercise therapy. These include enhancing antioxidant defenses. Very promising are mainly small non-coding microRNAs (miRNAs).

6.1. Mechanisms that enhance antioxidant defenses

An important mechanism that contributes to many disease is oxidative stress [8], although exhaustive and/or unaccustomed exercise in both aerobic and anaerobic exercise can generate excessive reactive oxygen species (ROS) according to mitochondrial enzymes, NADPH oxidases, and xanthine oxidases. This results in oxidative stress-related tissue damages and impaired muscle contractility. Moderate exposure to ROS is needed to induce adaptive responses of the body such as the activation of antioxidant defense mechanisms [9]. Regular exercise is well known to benefit health by enhancing antioxidant defenses in the body [10], thereby leading to a reduced generation of free radicals both at rest and in response to exercise stress. Therefore, exercise training-induced antioxidant activity decreases risk of many diseases.

In the elderly, sarcopenia is characterized by structural, biochemical, molecular and functional muscle changes. An imbalance between anabolic and catabolic intracellular signaling pathways and an increase in oxidative stress both play important roles in muscle abnormalities.

Regular exercise is promoted as a therapeutic strategy for age-associated endothelial dysfunction. However, sex was shown to affect the antioxidant response in the elderly. Improvements in endothelial function are found with endurance exercise in older men, but are reduced or absent in older women. This may be due to sex hormones modulating vascular adaptations to exercise training by influencing antioxidant defense systems, mitochondrial function, oxidative stress, and intracellular signaling [11].

6.2. Mechanisms that decrease the risk of developing cancer

In addition, exercise is known to be one of several lifestyle factors that lower the risk of cancer and is associated with lower relapse rates and better survival. The indirect effects included changes in vitamin D, weight reduction, sunlight exposure and improved mood. The direct effects included insulin-like growth factor, epigenetic effects on gene expression and DNA repair, vasoactive intestinal peptide, and antioxidant pathways, heat shock proteins, testosterone, irisin, immunity, chronic inflammation and prostaglandins, energy metabolism and insulin resistance [12].

6.3. Mechanisms that are responsible to cardioprotection

Importantly, exercise protects cardiovascular system through the modulation of

a) cardiac performance directly,

b) endothelial and vascular functions,

c) systemic risk factors. Both moderate- and high-intensity exercise training were shown to improve aerobic capacity of metabolic syndrome patients [13].

Moreover, Wand Exercise which is Thai mode of exercise significantly reduced body mass, total fat mass, waist and hip circumferences and increased flexibility, functional capacity (determined by 6MWD), physical health dimension and vitality of mental health dimension of the QOL [14]. The results showed that Thai Wand Exercise training decreased obesity, improved physical health status, and vitality. Therefore, this easy and low impact exercise program is a good approach to reduce cardiovascular risks. Data on cardioprotective effects of low-intensity exercise are controversial. This could be due to the fact that low-intensity exercise may not meet the recommended minimum threshold of exercise intensity form improving cardiorespiratory endurance [15]. However, our research group found that low-intensity exercise improved aerobic capacity of overweight and normal weight sedentary young adults [16]. Exercise also mediated improvement in hyperglycemia-induced cardiovascular dysfunction in patients with type 2 diabetes [10]. Exercise training also improved insulin resistance-induced lipotoxicity, mediated protection against pro-inflammatory cytokines and improved pro-survival signaling cascade. An appropriate duration and intensity of exercise can decrease myocardial dysfunction through the improvement of maximum oxygen consumption (VO2max), left ventricular ejection fraction (LVEF), LV diastolic and systolic volumes, ventilatory threshold, cardiac output and diastolic function (E/A ratio) [13, 17–25].

6.4. Mechanisms that improve respiratory function

Exercise training has been shown to improve pulmonary function in patients with type 2 diabetes [26]. Exercise training improves exercise tolerance and health-related quality of life in patients with very severe COPD [27]. RME training led to a significant increase in respiratory muscle endurance in children with CF [28]. In addition, pulmonary rehabilitation reduced expiratory flow limitation (EFL) in COPD patients [29].

6.5. Mechanisms that treat orthopedic patients

A systematic review revealed that short-term Traditional Chinese exercise (TCE) was potentially beneficial in terms of reducing pain, improving physical function and alleviating stiffness for patient [30]. In individuals operated with total knee arthroplasty, the 12-month progressive home exercise program starting 2 months after the operation comparing to usual care improved maximal gait velocity, cadence and stance time [31]. This may be due to exercise loading in the cartilage-subchondral bone (SB) unit in attenuation of post-traumatic osteoarthritis development [32].

6.6. Mechanisms that mediate differential expression of microRNAs

MicroRNA is a non-coding RNA which is increasingly interesting from scientists in many fields including Physical therapist [33]. It has been shown to regulate many process in our body, for example, muscle-specific miRs (miR-1, miR-133 and miR-499), the vascular wall of the vascular smooth muscle cells miR-222, EC miR-126, and the pathophysiology of Diabetic heart disease.

Exercise training, both acute endurance and resistance in healthy male volunteers, was shown to enhance miR-133 expression in the vastus lateralis muscles [34, 35]. Moreover, endurance exercise elevated circulating levels of miR-133 in healthy individuals after either an acute bout of aerobic exercise, or endurance training [36, 37]. Marathon training also increased miR-133 level which is appeared to be associated with improved VO_{2max} [38]. Similarly, T2DM mice which did a 10-week swimming exercise had increased miR-133 expression in cardiac tissue. Their contractile function improved and matrix metallopeptidase-9 (MMP-9), an extracellular matrix regulator protein decreased [39]. Since miR-133 is reported to be expressed and enriched in both cardiac and skeletal muscles [40], it is possible that miR-133 is secreted from skeletal muscle into the circulation after a bout of exercise, which then travels to the cardiomyocytes to suppress fibrotic markers and reduce cardiac hypertrophy.

6.7. Mechanisms that treat neurological patients

In Parkinson's disease patients, aerobic exercise training [28] may be altering central nervous system pathways that regulate the physiologic or cognitive processes controlling olfaction [41]. In spinal cord injury patients, the exercise training has been considered to improve spinal cord function not only through enhancement, compensation, and replacement of the remaining function of nerve and muscle but also improve the function in different levels from end-effector organ such as skeletal muscle to cerebral cortex through reshaping skeletal muscle structure and muscle fiber type, regulating physiological and metabolic function of motor neurons in the spinal cord and remodeling function of the cerebral cortex [42].

7. New biomarkers capable of evaluating exercise performance capacity and progress in training

1. Blood biomarkers—include glutamine, glutamate, cortisol, IL-6, testosterone, cholesterol, glucose, leptin, cortisol, ACTH, hematocrit, hemoglobin, norepinephrine, epinephrine, immunological parameters, and creatinine kinase.
2. Physiological measurements—include resting heart rate, resting systolic blood pressure, and resting diastolic blood pressure but not heart rate variability.
3. Psychological measurements—include mood states for tension, fatigue, confusion, reaction time, vigor, anger, and depression. Such parameters may reflect a highly individual nature of the psychological response to overtraining. However, a trend for impaired sleep patterns, increased wakefulness, decrements and stability in sleep quality and increased levels of stress may be observed.

miRNAs meet most of the requirements for good biomarkers, such as easily accessible sample collection, minimally invasive and remarkable stability in body fluids. In addition, miRNAs affect many processes and play a crucial role not only in cell differentiation, proliferation and apoptosis, but also affect extracellular matrix composition and maintaining processes of homeostasis. They play significant role in the regulation of physiological adaptation to exercise, such as skeletal muscle and cardiomyocyte hypertrophy, mitochondrial biogenesis, vascular angiogenesis and metabolic processes [33].

8. Early detection of overtraining

Some patients may perform the prescribed exercise program too hard leading to overtraining [43, 44]. Such overload can result in fatigue and acute decreases in performance either directly after a single intense training session, or following the training. However, in the normal course of training and recovery, this overload then leads to a positive response, adaptation, and consequent improvement in performance. If the balance between overload and recovery is not managed properly, a positive training response does not occur and performance is not enhanced. To reach a true diagnosis of overtraining syndrome, it is necessary to exclude the presence of non-communicable diseases (e.g., disorders involving the thyroid or adrenal gland, anemia, diabetes, and iron deficiency), infectious diseases (e.g., hepatitis, myocarditis and glandular fever), and other major disorders or feeding behaviors (e.g., bulimia and anorexia nervosa). In addition, Psychomotor speed: possibly a new marker for overtraining syndrome.

Additional information

However, up-to-date there has been slight improvement in the tools available for the diagnosis of overtraining syndrome [45, 46]

9. Equipment

There are many kinds of equipment for exercise therapy including [7]:

a) Hydrotherapy equipment (tank, bath, chair).

b) Electrotherapy (shortwave medical diathermy, muscle stimulator, interferential therapy unit, ultrasound therapy unit, transcutaneous nerve stimulation.

c) Heat and cold therapy equipment (paraffin wax bath, moist heat therapy unit, moist heat therapy unit, stream/hot pack, infrared lamp).

d) Treatment equipment (massage cum treatment table, hi-low mat platform, tilt table, activity mattress, continuous passive motion unit, medicine ball, parallel bar, equilibrium board).

e) Multi exercise therapy unit (complex exercising unit).

f) Shoulder, arm, hand, leg, knee, foot exercise unit.

g) Suspension unit.

h) Mobility aids (Walkers, crutch, cane).

i) Massage: Massage signifies a group of procedures, which are usually done with hand on the external tissue of the body in a variety of ways either with a curative, palliative or hygienic point of view.

- To improve mobility of the soft tissues.
- To reduce muscle spasm and pain under abnormal conditions.

- To reduce edema.
- To increase circulation.
- To mobilize secretions in the lung.
- To induce local and general relaxations.

Acknowledgements

I appreciate Khon Kaen University for providing me a grant, opportunity, and facility to write this chapter. I thank Exercise and Sport Sciences Development and Research Group for the financial support for this chapter. Moreover, I also thank all participants for their excellent participation in my researches.

Author details

Naruemon Leelayuwat

Address all correspondence to: naruemon.leelayuwat@gmail.com

Department of Physiology, Faculty of Medicine, Khon Kaen University, Khon Kaen, Thailand; Exercise and Sport Sciences Development and Research Group, Khon Kaen University, Khon Kaen, Thailand

References

[1] Kottke FJ, Stillwell GK, Lehmann JF, editors. Krusen's Handbook of Physical Medicine and Rehabilitation. 3rd ed. Philadelphia, Pa: WB Saunders Co; 1982

[2] Hall CM, Brody LT. Therapeutic Exercise: Moving Toward Function. 2nd ed. Philadelphia: Lippincott Williams & Wilkins; 2005

[3] http://bie.telangana.gov.in/Pdf/Biomechonics.pdf [Accessed: December 12, 2016]

[4] American Physical Therapy Association. A guide to Physical Therapist practice, I: A description of patient management. Physical Therapy. 1995;**75**:709–764

[5] World Health Organization. International classification of impairments, disabilities, and handicaps: a manual of classification relating to the consequences of disease, published in accordance with resolution WHA29.35 of the Twenty-ninth World Health Assembly, May 1976. Geneva 1980

[6] Nagi SZ. Disability, and Rehabilitation. Columbia, OH: Ohio State University Press; 1969

[7] Nagavani C. Textbook of Biomechanics and Exercise Therapy. Available from: https://static1.squarespace.com/static/554d3c40e4b04605cb444b18/t/5550e0f2e4b0e93349b5e684/1431363828551/ [Accessed: December 12, 2016]

[8] Alfadda AA, Sallam RM. Reactive oxygen species in health and disease. Journal of Biomedicine and Biotechnology. 2012;2012:936486. DOI: 10.1155/2012/9364862012

[9] He F, Li J, Liu Z, et al. Redox mechanism of reactive oxygen species in exercise. Frontiers in Physiology. 2016;7:486. DOI: 10.3389/fphys.2016.00486

[10] Leelayuwat N, Tunkumnerdthai O, Donsom M, et al. An alternative exercise and its beneficial effects on glycaemic control and oxidative stress in subjects with type 2 diabetes. Diabetes Research and Clinical Practice. 2008;**82**:e5–8. Epub 2008 Sep 23

[11] Moreau KL, Ozemek C. Vascular adaptations to habitual exercise in older adults: Time for the sex talk. Exercise and Sport Sciences Reviews. 2017;45:116-123 Jan 13. DOI: 10.1249/ JES.0000000000000104. [Epub ahead of print]

[12] Thomas RJ, Kenfield SA, Jimenez A. Exercise-induced biochemical changes and their potential influence on cancer: A scientific review. British Journal of Sports Medicine. 2016;0:1-8. pii: bjsports-2016-096343. DOI: 10.1136/bjsports-2016-096343. [Epub ahead of print]

[13] Tjonna AE, Lee SJ, Rognmo O, et al. Aerobic interval training versus continuous moderate exercise as a treatment for the metabolic syndrome: A pilot study. Circulation. 2008;**118**:346–54

[14] Puengsuwan P, Promdee K, Sruttabul W, et al. Effectiveness of Thai Wand Exercise training on health-related quality of life in sedentary older adults. Chulalongkorn Medical Journal. 2008;**52**:120–122

[15] Albright A, Franz M, Hornsby G, et al. American College of Sports Medicine position stand: Exercise and type 2 diabetes. Medicine & Science in Sports & Exercise. 2000;**32**:1345–1360. DOI: 10.1097/00005768-200007000-00024. [PubMed] [Cross Ref]

[16] Prasertsri P, Boonla O, Phoemsapthawee J, et al. Arm swing exercise improves exercise capacity and oxygen consumption in overweight and normal weight sedentary young adults. JEPonline 2017;20(1):111–124

[17] Brassard P, Legault S, Garneau C, et al. Normalization of diastolic dysfunction in type 2 diabetics after exercise training. Medicine & Science in Sports & Exercise. 2007;**39**:1896–1901

[18] Hafstad AD, Boardman NT, Lund J, et al. High intensity interval training alters substrate utilization and reduces oxygen consumption in the heart. Journal of Applied Physiology. 2011;**111**:1235–1241

[19] Lee S, Park Y, Zhang C. Exercise training prevents coronary endothelial dysfunction in type 2 diabetic mice. American Journal of Biomedical Sciences. 2011;**3**:241–252

[20] Dunstan DW, Daly RM, Owen N, et al. High-intensity resistance training improves glycemic control in older patients with type 2 diabetes. Diabetes Care. 2002;**25**:1729–1736

[21] Byrkjeland R, Njerve IU, Anderssen S, et al. Effects of exercise training on HbA1c and VO_2 peak in patients with type 2 diabetes and coronary artery disease: A randomised clinical trial. Diabetes and Vascular Disease Research. 2015;**12**:325–333

[22] DeBlieux PM, Barbee RW, McDonough KH, et al. Exercise training improves cardiac performance in diabetic rats. Proceedings of the Society for Experimental Biology and Medicine. 1993;**203**:209–213

[23] Broderick TL, Poirier P, Gillis M. Exercise training restores abnormal myocardial glucose utilization and cardiac function in diabetes. Diabetes/Metabolism Research and Reviews. 2005;**21**:44–50

[24] De Angelis KL, Oliveira AR, Dall'Ago P, et al. Effects of exercise training on autonomic and myocardial dysfunction in streptozotocin-diabetic rats. Brazilian Journal of Medical and Biological Research. 2000;**33**:635–641

[25] Rodrigues B, Jorge L, Mostarda CT, et al. Aerobic exercise training delays cardiac dysfunction and improves autonomic control of circulation in diabetic rats undergoing myocardial infarction. Journal of Cardiac Failure. 2012;**18**:734–744

[26] Tunkamnerdthai O, Auvichayapat P, Donsom M, et al. Arm swing exercise improved the pulmonary function of the patients with type 2 diabetes. Journal of Physical Therapy Science. 2015;**27**:649–654

[27] Paneroni M, Simonelli C, Vitacca M, et al. Aerobic exercise training in very severe chronic obstructive pulmonary disease: A systematic review and meta-analysis. American Journal of Physical Medicine & Rehabilitation. 2017 Jan 17. DOI: 10.1097/PHM.0000000000000667. [Epub ahead of print]

[28] Bieli C, Summermatter S, Boutellier U, et al. Respiratory muscle training improves respiratory muscle endurance but not exercise tolerance in children with cystic fibrosis. Pediatric Pulmonology. 2017; 52: 331-336. DOI: 10.1002/ppul.23647. [Epub ahead of print]

[29] Theodorakopoulou EP, Gennimata SA, Harikiopoulou M, et al. Effect of pulmonary rehabilitation on tidal expiratory flow limitation at rest and during exercise in COPD patients. Respiratory Physiology & Neurobiology. 2017; 238: 47-54. pii: S1569-9048(16)30260-9. DOI: 10.1016/j.resp.2017.01.008. [Epub ahead of print]

[30] Zhang Y, Huang L, Su Y, et al. The effects of traditional Chinese exercise in treating knee osteoarthritis: A systematic review and meta-analysis. PLoS One. 2017;**12**(1):e0170237. DOI: 10.1371/journal.pone.0170237. eCollection 2017

[31] Anneli H, Nina SK, Arja H, et al. Effect of total knee replacement surgery and postoperative 12 month home exercise program on gait parameters. Gait and Posture. 2017;**53**:92–97. DOI: 10.1016/j.gaitpost.2017.01.004. [Epub ahead of print]

[32] Iijima H, Ito A, Nagai M, et al. Physiological exercise loading suppresses post-traumatic osteoarthritis progression via an increase in bone morphogenetic proteins expression in an experimental rat knee model. Osteoarthritis Cartilage. 2016 Dec 10. pii: S1063-4584(16)30468-X. DOI: 10.1016/j.joca.2016.12.008. [Epub ahead of print]

[33] Polakovičová M, Musil P, Laczo E, et al. Circulating microRNAs as potential biomarkers of exercise response. International Journal of Molecular Sciences. 2016 Oct 5;**17**(10). pii: E1553

[34] Russell AP, Lamon S, Boon H, et al. Regulation of miRNAs in human skeletal muscle following acute endurance exercise and short-term endurance training. The Journal of Physiology. 2013;**591**:4637–53

[35] Nielsen S, Scheele C, Yfanti C, et al. Muscle specific microRNAs are regulated by endurance exercise in human skeletal muscle. The Journal of Physiology. 2010;**588**:4029–37

[36] Nielsen S, Akerstrom T, Rinnov A, et al. The miRNA plasma signature in response to acute aerobic exercise and endurance training. PLoS One. 2014;**9**:e87308

[37] Uhlemann M, Mobius-Winkler S, Fikenzer S, et al. Circulating microRNA-126 increases after different forms of endurance exercise in healthy adults. European Journal of Preventive Cardiology. 2014;**21**:484–491

[38] Mooren FC, Viereck J, Kruger K, et al. Circulating microRNAs as potential biomarkers of aerobic exercise capacity. American Journal of Physiology. Heart and Circulatory Physiology. 2014;**306**:H557–H563

[39] Mishra PK, Awe O, Metreveli N, et al. Exercise ameliorates diabetic cardiomyopathy by inducing beta2adrenergic receptors and miR-133a, and attenuating MMP-9. The FASEB Journal. 2011;**25**:1032–1034

[40] Rawal S, Manning P, Katare R. Cardiovascular microRNAs: As modulators and diagnostic biomarkers of diabetic heart disease. Cardiovascular Diabetology. 2014;**13**:44

[41] Rosenfeldt AB, Dey T, Alberts JL. Aerobic exercise preserves olfaction function in individuals with parkinson's disease. Parkinson's Disease. 2016;**2016**:9725089. DOI: 10.1155/2016/9725089. Epub 2016 Nov 23

[42] Fu J, Wang H, Deng L, et al. Exercise training promotes functional recovery after spinal cord injury. Neural Plasticity. 2016;**2016**:4039580. DOI: 10.1155/2016/4039580. Epub 2016 Dec 6

[43] Kreher JB, Schwartz JB. Overtraining syndrome: A practical guide. Sports Health. 2012 Mar;**4**:128–138

[44] Nederhof E, Lemmink KA, Visscher C, et al. Psychomotor speed: Possibly a new marker for overtraining syndrome. Sports Medicine. 2006;**36**:817–828

[45] Urhausen A, Kindermann W. Diagnosis of overtraining: What tools do we have? Sports Medicine. 2002;**32**(2):95–102

[46] Meeusen R, Duclos M, Foster C, et al. European College of Sport Science; American College of Sports Medicine. Prevention, diagnosis, and treatment of the overtraining syndrome: Joint consensus statement of the European College of Sport Science and the American College of Sports Medicine. Medicine & Science in Sports & Exercise. 2013 Jan;**45**:186–205. DOI: 10.1249/MSS.0b013e318279a10a

9

Physical Therapy in Patients with Cancer

Shinichiro Morishita and Atsuhiro Tsubaki

Additional information is available at the end of the chapter

Abstract

Physical therapists often treat cancer patients. Cancer treatment includes chemotherapy, radiotherapy, and surgery, which are being continuously developed and thus increase survival of patients with each cancer diagnosis. More specifically, 5-year survival rates increase with each cancer diagnosis. Cancer patients have many problems including muscle weakness, pulmonary dysfunction, fatigue, and pain. In the end, patients with cancer tend to have a decline in activities of daily living (ADL) and quality of life (QOL). Additionally, cancer patients often have progressive disease, depression, and anxiety. Physical therapy often helps patients regain strength and physical function and improve their QOL and independence of daily living that they may have lost due to cancer or its treatment. Physical therapy has an important role in increasing physical function of cancer patients, cancer survivors, and children with cancer. In the future, physical therapy may be progressively needed for management of cancer patients.

Keywords: physical therapy, cancer, cancer survivor, ADL, QOL

1. Introduction

Cancer and its treatments are associated with a wide range of distressing physical and psychological symptoms that can affect patients for many years following treatment [1]. Many cancer patients also have physical dysfunction and experience deficits in muscle strength, flexibility, and endurance as a result of chemotherapy, radiation therapy, and surgery [2]. Physical therapy is a comprehensive, multidisciplinary approach to the evaluation and treatment of patients diagnosed with various forms of cancer. Physical therapy can improve functional problems such as weakness, soft tissue tightness, joint stiffness, fatigue, and swelling or edema [3, 4]. Physical therapy allows experts to find the best ways for cancer patients to stay active. Physical therapy-led exercise is clinically effective and can help cancer patients improve their quality of life (QOL) [5]. Physical therapy includes stretching, strengthening, and aerobic exercises for the inpatients, outpatients, and cancer survivors. It often helps patients regain strength, physical functioning, quality of life, and independence in activities of daily living (ADL) that they may have lost due to cancer or its treatment. Physical therapists are available in multiple treatment settings, including preoperative, postoperative, acute care, nursing home, and inpatient and outpatient rehabilitation. Physical therapists also work in conjunction with the rehabilitation team to design components of a survivorship care plan in order to optimize overall functional outcomes (**Figure 1**) [6]. Cancer has four stages, and cancer patients have differences in disease and disabilities during each stage (**Table 1**). Physical therapists often use four cancer rehabilitation stages and identify the stage before physical therapy for cancer patients (**Table 2**) [7]. There are different approaches for therapy of cancer patients during each stage.

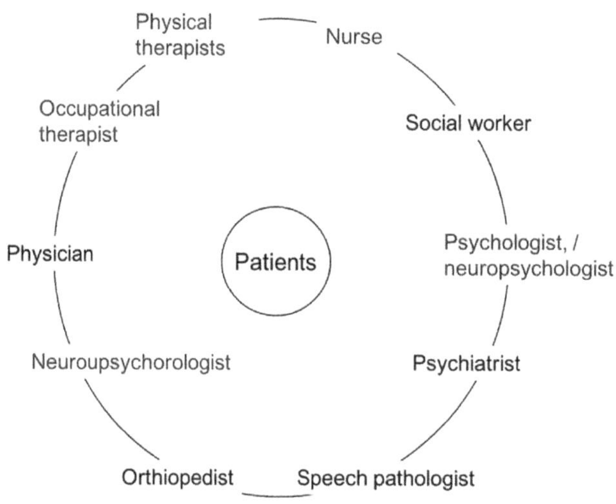

Figure 1. Rehabilitation team for cancer patients.

Stage	Characteristics
Stage 1	Cancer is relatively small and contained within the organ it originated from. This stage describes cancer in situ, which means "in place." Stage 1 cancers have not spread to nearby tissues. This stage of cancer is often highly curable, usually by removing the entire tumor with surgery
Stage 2	Cancer has not started to spread into surrounding tissue but the tumor is larger than in Stage 1. Sometimes, Stage 2 means that cancer cells have spread into lymph nodes close to the tumor. At this stage, cancer or tumor is relatively small and has not grown deeply into the nearby tissues. It also has not spread to the lymph nodes or other parts of the body. It is often called an early-stage cancer
Stage 3	Cancer is larger. It may have started to spread into surrounding tissues, and cancer cells may be present in the lymph nodes of the area. This stage indicates larger cancers or tumors
Stage 4	Cancer has spread from where it started to another organs or parts of the body. This is also called a secondary, advanced, or metastatic cancer

Table 1. Cancer stage.

Stage
(1) Preventive
Intervention focused on improving the patient's level of function prior to the onset of the effects of the cancer and its treatment, patient education, and psychological support
(2) Restorative rehabilitation
Intervention focused on returning the patient to a previous level of function and addressing impairments from cancer and its treatment
(3) Supportive rehabilitation
Intervention is meant to assist the cancer patient to function at the highest level within the context of his or her impairments, activity limitations, and participation restrictions
(4) Palliative rehabilitation
Intervention focused on minimizing complications such as pressure ulcers, contractures, and muscle deconditioning ensuring adequate pain control and emotional support for the family

Table 2. Four cancer rehabilitation stages.

This chapter introduces overview, treatment, common dysfunctions, physical therapy assessment, physical therapy, key points in diagnosis, and palliative care of following cancer types: breast cancer, gynecologic cancers, brain tumor, head and neck cancer, lung cancer, esophagus cancer, bone cancer, and blood cancer. This chapter also shows the important role of physical therapy in cancer patients.

2. General concept of physical therapy

Physical therapists must undergo assessment based on the International Classification of Functioning, Disability and Health (ICF) model before, during, and after physical therapy for each cancer patient (**Figure 2**). ICF enables physical therapist to provide cancer patients with therapy. Cancer patients have many problems caused by cancer treatment or cancer itself. Physical therapy assessment should include manual muscle testing (MMT), range of motion (ROM), balance test, endurance test, and ADL test. Performance status (PS; **Table 3**) [8], Palliative Performance Scale (PPS; **Table 4**) [9], Barthel index (BI) [10], functional independence measure (FIM) [11, 12], and QOL are also used as assessment tools for cancer patients. Physical therapists should be aware that cancer patients are exposed to various risks such as infectious diseases due to immunosuppressive effects of the treatment. Thus, physical therapists must manage risks that are related to cancer and its treatment (**Table 5**) [13]. Additionally, physical therapists must recognize that cancer is a progressive disease. In general, cancer patients have a gradual decline in their physical function. Once a goal is set, physical therapists must be aware of cancer progression and patients' prognosis [14]. Physical therapists also must know a variety of other problems that occur in cancer patients. Cancer patients might not only have physical function problems but may also develop depression and anxiety in the future [15]. Cancer patients might feel the fear of cancer recurrence or death. Physical therapy may be effective in reducing fatigue, increasing muscle strength and exercise capacity, and improving QOL in various cancer patients.

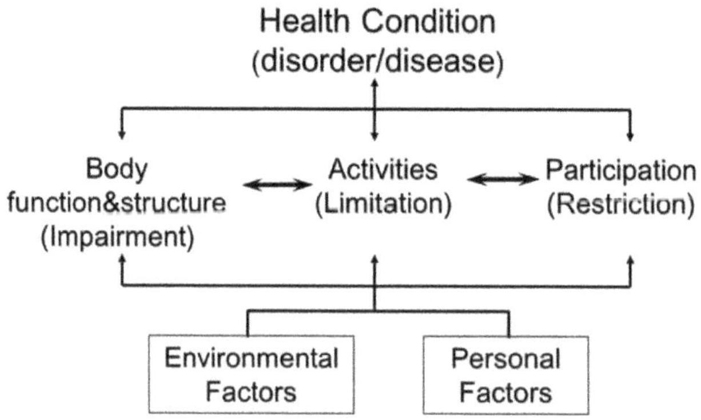

Figure 2. International Classification of Functioning, Disability, and Health.

Grade	ECOG performance status
0	Fully active, able to carry on all pre-disease performance without restriction
1	Restricted in physically strenuous activity but ambulatory and able to carry out work of a light or sedentary nature, e.g., light house work, office work
2	Ambulatory and capable of all self-care but unable to carry out any work activities. Up and about more than 50% of waking hours
3	Capable of only limited self-care, confined to bed or chair more than 50% of waking hours
4	Completely disabled. Cannot carry on any self-care. Totally confined to bed or chair
5	Dead

Table 3. Performance status (PS).

PPS level	Ambulation	Activity and evidence of disease	Self-care	Intake	Conscious level
100	Full	Normal activity and work no evidence of disease	Full	Normal	Full
90	Full	Normal activity and work Some evidence of disease	Full	Normal	Full
80	Full	Normal activity with effort Some evidence of disease	Full	Normal or reduced	Full
70	Reduced	Unable normal job/ work Significant disease	Full	Normal or reduced	Full
60	Reduced	Unable hobby/house work Significant disease	Occasional assistance necessary	Normal or reduced	Full or confusion

PPS level	Ambulation	Activity and evidence of disease	Self-care	Intake	Conscious level
50	Mainly sit/lie	Unable to do any work Extensive disease	Considerable assistance required	Normal or reduced	Full or confusion
40	Mainly in bed	Unable to do most activity Extensive disease	Mainly assistance	Normal or reduced	Full or drowsy ± confusion
30	Totally bed bound	Unable to do any activity Extensive disease	Total care	Normal or reduced	Full or drowsy ± confusion
20	Totally bed bound	Unable to do any activity Extensive disease	Total care	Minimal to sips	Full or drowsy ± confusion
10	Totally bed bound	Unable to do any activity Extensive disease	Total care	Mouth care only	Drowsy or coma ± confusion
0	Death				

[1]PPS scores are determined by reading horizontally at each level to find a "best fit" for the patient who is then assigned as the PPS% score.

[2]Begin at the left column, read downward until the appropriate ambulation level is reached, and then read across to the next column and downward again until the activity/evidence of disease is located. These steps are repeated until all five columns are covered before assigning the actual PPS for that patient. In this way, "leftward" columns (columns to the left of any specific column) are "stronger" determinants and generally take precedence over others.

[3]PPS scores are in 10% increments only. Sometimes, there are several columns easily placed at one level but one or two which seem better at a higher or lower level. One then needs to make a "best fit" decision. Choosing a "halfwit" value of PPS 45%, for example, is not correct. The combination of clinical judgment and "leftward precedence" is used to determine whether 40% or 50% is the more accurate score for that patient.

Table 4. Palliative Performance Scale (PPSv2).

1. Hematologic profile: hemoglobin <7.5 g, platelets <20,000, white blood cell count <3000
2. Metastatic bone disease
3. Compression of a hollow viscous (bowel, bladder, or ureter) vessel or spinal cord
4. Fluid accumulation in the pleura, pericardium, abdomen, or retroperitoneum associated with persistent pain, dyspnea, or problems with mobility
5. CNS depression or coma or increased intracranial pressure
6. Hypokalemia/hyperkalemia, hyponatremia, or hypocalcemia/hypercalcemia
7. Orthostatic hypotension
8. Heart rate in excess 110 beat/min or ventricular arrhythmia
9. Fever greater than 101°F

Table 5. Precaution rehabilitation for cancer patients.

3. Physical therapy in cancer patients

3.1. Breast cancer

3.1.1. Overview

Breast cancer is the most common invasive cancer in women worldwide [16]. Breast cancer alone accounts for 25% of all cancer cases and 15% of all cancer deaths among women [17]. Breast cancer starts when cells in the breast begin to grow out of control. These cells usually form a tumor that can be often seen on an X-ray or felt as a lump. Breast cancer can develop following changes in genetic material leading to cellular changes that causes cells to start multiplying in an uncontrolled fashion, forming lumps or nodules.

3.1.2. Treatment

In general, breast cancer patients have few treatment options such as surgery (breast-conserving surgery and mastectomy), radiation therapy, chemotherapy, and hormone therapy [18, 19]. In some cases, lymph nodes located close to the affected breast need to be surgically removed.

3.1.3. Common dysfunctions in breast cancer

Muscle weakness around the shoulder joint, decline of ADL using upper extremities, dizziness, loss of appetite, shortness of breath, depression are present in a substantial majority of patients during or after their initial treatment (surgery, radiation, and/or chemotherapy) [20, 21]. Physical therapists must pay attention to the occurrence of musculoskeletal disorders and lymph vascular disorders following breast surgery. Musculoskeletal disorders include postsurgical pain, rotator cuff disease, and adhesive capsulitis [22]. Lymph vascular disorders are common after removal of lymph nodes [23]. As a result, breast cancer patients have limited range of motion, muscle weakness, pain, and ADL decline such as difficulties while brushing hair or taking off the jacket. In some cases of breast cancer, cellulitis occurs that can become a potentially serious bacterial skin infection [21, 24].

3.1.4. Physical therapy assessment

Physical therapy assessment of cancer patients includes the ICF, examination of shoulder ROM, MMT, pain levels, fatigue, upper limb volume, an upper limb disability questionnaire, and QOL evaluation. Additionally, in the cases of breast cancer patients, physical therapists assess exercise tolerance.

3.1.5. Physical therapy

Many previous studies showed that physical therapy has effectiveness in breast cancer patients [25, 26]. In general, combined physical therapy is effective to treat postoperative lymphedema, pain, and impaired ROM after treatment for breast cancer [26]. Physical therapy for breast cancer patients includes lymphatic drainage massage, vantage, manual stretching, myofascial therapy, relaxation massage, stretching, strengthening, resisted exercise, proprioceptive neuromuscular facilitation (PNF) exercises, isometric exercises, aerobic exercises, transcutaneous electrical nerve stimulation (TENS), heat and cold, patient education, and behavioral training. Breast cancer patients also receive ADL training such as bathing, showering (washing the body), and dressing.

3.1.6. Key points

Physical therapists should improve mobility of upper extremities with a reduction of their volume. This should be followed by an attempt to recover upper limb function in ADL.

3.2. Gynecologic cancers

3.2.1. Overview

Gynecologic cancers accounted for 19% of the 5.1 million estimated new cancer cases and 13 million 5-year prevalent cancer cases among women in the world in 2002 [27]. Gynecologic cancer is described as the uncontrolled growth and spread of abnormal cells originating in the female reproductive organs. They are found in different places within a woman's pelvis, which is the area below the stomach and in between the hip bones. Five main types of gynecologic cancers are present: cervical, ovarian, uterine, vaginal, and vulvar.

3.2.2. Treatment

In general, gynecologic cancers can be cured with aggressive treatment involving surgery, chemotherapy, and/or radiation. Treatment goal in recurrent and metastatic cancer is to decrease progression of the disease [28, 29].

3.2.3. Common dysfunctions in gynecologic cancer

Weakness of pelvic floor muscles, decline in ADL, dizziness, loss of appetite, shortness of breath, depression are the symptoms present in a substantial majority of patients during or after their initial treatment (surgery, radiation, and/or chemotherapy) [30]. Lower extremity weakness often occurs in gynecologic cancer patients; thus, locomotion disability is common [31]. Physical therapists must pay attention to occurrence of musculoskeletal and lymph vascular disorders at the lower extremities following gynecologic surgery [32]. Lymphovascular disorders cause problems after removal of lymph nodes [33]. As a result, patients experience limited ROM, muscle weakness, pain, and decline in ADL.

3.2.4. Physical therapy assessment

First, physical therapists should assess pelvic floor muscle strength as gynecologic cancers have urinary incontinence after the treatment [34, 35]. Second, physical therapists should assess ICF category: lower extremities such as hip, knee, and ankle ROM; MMT; assessment of pain levels; fatigue; upper limb volume; locomotion ability such as gait speed; balance function; QOL; ADL; and sexual function [36]. Additionally, physical therapists should assess exercise tolerance.

3.2.5. Physical therapy

A few previous reports showed that physical therapy has a positive effect on gynecologic cancer patients [37]. Physical therapists should perform pelvic floor physical therapy as a tool to aid in addressing pelvic floor symptoms [37]. In general, physical therapy for gynecologic cancer patients includes locomotion ability exercises such as standing and walking, lymphatic drainage massage, vantage, manual stretching, myofascial therapy, relaxation massage, stretching, strengthening, resisted exercise, PNF, aerobic exercise, TENS, patient education, and behavioral training.

3.2.6. Key points

Physical therapists should improve muscle strength of lower extremities and reduce their volume as soon as possible. This should be followed by acquiring locomotion.

3.3. Brain tumor

3.3.1. Overview

The worldwide cancer incidence of a malignant brain tumor is 3.4 per 100,000 for men and 3.0 per 100,000 for women [38]. Brain tumor is the most common neurological complication related to cancer [39]. Brain tumors can originate from the patient's brain (primary brain tumors) or from other parts of the patient's body (secondary or metastatic brain tumors) [40, 41]. Brain tumors can destroy brain cells, increase inflammation, and elevate brain pressure. Brain tumors may cause a wide range of neurological dysfunctions, including disorders of the nervous system.

3.3.2. Treatment

In general, treatment options include surgery, radiation therapy, chemotherapy, targeted biological agents, or a combination of these [42]. Surgical resection is commonly the first recommended treatment in order to rapidly reduce brain pressure.

3.3.3. Common dysfunctions in brain tumor

Brain tumor patients commonly experience weakness, sensory loss, and abnormal muscle tone. These include spasticity, visuospatial deficits, hemi-neglect or bilateral visual deficits, ataxia, cognitive deficits (thought processes, memory changes, apraxia, etc.), speech difficulties, dysphagia, bowel and bladder dysfunction, psychological problems, and fatigue. As a result, ADL decline and lower QOL are common in brain tumor patients [43, 44].

3.3.4. Physical therapy assessment

Physical therapists often assess ICF category, Glasgow Coma Scale, Mini-Mental State Examination, Fugl-Meyer, Motor Assessment Scale, Motricity Index, Berg Balance Assessment, Beck Depression Inventory (BDI), and Hospital Anxiety and Depression Scale (HADS). They examine pain levels and locomotion ability such as gait speed, QOL, and sexual function. Additionally, physical therapists should assess exercise tolerance in brain tumor patients [45, 46].

3.3.5. Physical therapy

To date, no previous study has reported positive effects of physical therapy in adult brain tumor patients. However, a few reports showed that physical therapy may be effective in pediatric brain tumor patients [47]. In general, physical therapy performed in brain tumor patients is also performed in stroke patients [48]. It includes neurofacilitation techniques such as Bobath, PNF, Brunnstrom, motor relearning, functional electrical stimulation (FES), biofeedback, balance retraining, gait reeducation, and use of supportive equipment. Physical therapists must be aware of the progress of paralysis in brain tumor patients as a result of increasing tumor size. Physical therapists should know how to improve convalescence of the brain. Additionally, cognitive dysfunction, apraxia, and aphasia should be assessed [49].

3.3.6. Key points

Physical therapists should aim to treat paralysis and improve ADL as soon as possible. Attention should be paid to progressive paralysis in brain tumor patients.

3.4. Head and neck cancer

3.4.1. Overview

Overall, the annual incidence of head and neck cancer worldwide is more than 550,000 cases with around 300,000 deaths [50]. Men are affected significantly more than women [51]. Head and neck cancer includes cancers of the mouth, nose, sinuses, salivary glands, throat, and lymph nodes in the neck. Most originate from the moist tissues that line the mouth, nose, and throat. Head and neck cancers can also originate within the salivary glands. Salivary glands contain many different types of cells that can become cancerous leading to many different types of salivary gland cancers.

3.4.2. Treatment

Treatment options include surgery, radiation therapy, chemotherapy, and targeted therapy [52]. Surgery or radiation therapy alone or a combination of these treatments may be part of a patient's treatment plan [53]. Tracheostomy is performed when there are concerns about breathing due to airway obstruction associated with a throat cancer or treatment side effects [54]. Nutritional status of patients declines following tracheostomy. As patients are not able to eat, they usually receive intravenous feeding.

3.4.3. Common dysfunctions in head and neck tumor

Aspiration pneumonia after concurrent chemoradiation therapy and surgery is seen in head and neck cancer patients [55]. Most patients have dysphagia and are at increased risk of having aspiration and subsequent pneumonia [56]. Additionally, physical therapists must be aware of the decline in nutritional status after surgery or chemoradiation in these patients [57]. Paralysis of accessory nerve that causes trapezius muscle dysfunction is often seen following neck dissection [58]. This dysfunction leads to shoulder syndrome with adhesive capsulitis. Muscle weakness, decline of ADL, dizziness, loss of appetite, shortness of breath, depression are observed in a substantial majority of patients during or after their initial treatment (surgery, radiation, and/or chemotherapy) [59]. Upper and lower extremities tend to be weaker following long-term bedridden and sedentary treatment.

3.4.4. Physical therapy assessment

General pulmonary function tests are performed: spirometry; breathing pattern and cough; breath sounds including wheezing, coarse crackles, fine crackles, and rhonchi; and posture deformities in the chest or the spine; dysphagia evaluation; and ADL. Additionally, physical therapists should perform exercise tolerance test in gynecologic cancer patients. Furthermore, physical therapists should assess shoulder function including strength, mobility, and pain after surgery or chemoradiotherapy. Physical therapists often assess ICF category and lower and upper joint ROM; perform MMT; and evaluate pain levels, fatigue, and locomotion ability such as gait speed, balance function, and QOL.

3.4.5. Physical therapy

Physical therapy of the arms is performed to improve locomotion and pulmonary dysfunction. Some previous reports showed that physical therapy has effectiveness in head and neck cancer patients [60, 61]. When patients have paralysis of the accessory nerve, physical therapists perform exercises for the trapezius muscle to reduce its dysfunction [62]. Additionally, physical therapy of head and neck cancer patients includes locomotion ability exercises such as standing and walking, massage, manual stretching, myofascial therapy, relaxation massage, stretching, strengthening, resisted exercise, PNF, aerobic exercise, TENS, patient education, and behavioral training [63, 64]. However, if patients are fasting and have aspiration, they may have lower nutritional status requiring physical function recovery to be delayed.

3.4.6. Key points

Physical therapists must recognize that head and neck cancer patients tend to experience decline of the pulmonary function and paralysis of accessory nerve following the neck surgery. Physical therapists should recover pulmonary and shoulder function and improve ADL in such patients.

3.5. Lung cancer

3.5.1. Overview

Lung cancer is the most frequently diagnosed cancer worldwide with about 1.35 million new cases diagnosed each year [65]. Lung cancer starts with uncontrollable growth of abnormal cells in the lung. These cells can invade nearby tissues and form tumors. Lung cancer can start anywhere in the lungs and affect any part of the respiratory system. Cancer cells can spread, or metastasize, to the lymph nodes and other parts of the body. There are two main types of lung cancer: small-cell lung cancer (SCLC) and non-small-cell lung cancer (NSCLC). Small-cell lung cancers usually grow quicker and are more likely to spread to other body parts. Non-small-cell lung cancer accounts for about 85% of all lung cancer cases, whereas small-cell lung cancer accounts for about 15% of all lung cancer cases [50, 66].

3.5.2. Treatments

Lung cancer treatment depends on its type. Small-cell lung cancer is mostly treated with chemotherapy [67]. Non-small-cell lung cancer can be treated with surgery, chemotherapy, radiotherapy, or a combination of these depending on the stage at which the cancer is diagnosed [68, 69].

3.5.3. Common dysfunctions in lung cancer

When lung cancer treatment involves chemotherapy only, patients experience a decrease in physical function including decreased muscle strength and flexibility, which is also observed before the treatment. However, if lung cancer patients receive surgery, they encounter more problems than without the surgery. These problems include pulmonary dysfunction and decline of locomotion and ADL. Additionally, lung cancer patients experience pain of a surgical wound following thoracotomy and costectomy. Muscle weakness, decline of ADL, dizziness, loss of appetite, shortness of breath, and depression occur in a substantial majority of patients during or after their initial treatment (surgery, radiation, and/or chemotherapy). Upper and lower extremity and trunk muscle strength decreases following long-term bedridden and sedentary treatment.

3.5.4. Physical therapy assessment

General pulmonary function tests include spirometry; breathing pattern and cough; breath sounds like wheezing, coarse crackles, fine crackles, and rhonchi; postural deformities in the chest or the spine; and dysphagia evaluation on ADL [70, 71]. Additionally, physical therapists should assess exercise tolerance and shoulder function including its strength, mobility, and pain following surgery or chemoradiotherapy in patients with lung cancer. Physical therapists often assess ICF category and lower and upper joint ROM; perform MMT; and assess pain levels, fatigue, and locomotion ability such as gait speed, balance function, and QOL.

3.5.5. Physical therapy

Physical therapy of the arms is done in order to improve locomotion and pulmonary dysfunction after the treatment [72]. Some previous studies reported that preoperative physical therapy has effectiveness in lung cancer patients [73, 74]. Intensive physical therapy appears to increase oxygen saturation, reduce hospital stay, and change ventilation/perfusion distribution in lung cancer patients [73]. Following surgery with resection, physical therapists promote mobilization starting at the intensive care unit (ICU) because lung cancer patients tend to be sedentary leading to progressive decline in their physical function. Physical therapy for lung cancer patients includes massage, manual stretching, myofascial therapy, relaxation massage, stretching, strengthening, resisted exercise, PNF, aerobic exercise, TENS, patient education, and behavioral training.

3.5.6. Key points

Physical therapists should prevent development of further weakness after the treatment. Following surgery, physical therapists must make lung cancer patients perform pulmonary and mobilization exercises as soon as possible.

3.6. Esophageal cancer

3.6.1. Overview

Esophageal carcinoma affects more than 450,000 people worldwide, and the incidence is rapidly increasing [75]. Esophageal cancer is a disease in which malignant (cancer) cells form in the tissues of the esophagus. The most common types of esophageal cancer are squamous cell carcinoma and adenocarcinoma. Smoking and heavy alcohol use increase the risk of esophageal squamous cell carcinoma [76]. Esophageal cancer is often diagnosed at an advanced stage because there are no early signs or symptoms. A cancerous tumor is malignant, meaning it can grow and spread to other parts of the body. Esophageal cancer can also spread into the lungs, liver, stomach, and other parts of the body.

3.6.2. Treatment

Chemotherapy, radiotherapy, and surgery are often used as treatments for esophageal cancers [77]. Chemotherapy by itself rarely is effective. It is often combined with radiation therapy. Chemoradiation is often used before the surgery aiming to remove the cancer and some of the normal surrounding tissues. In some cases it might be combined with other treatments, such as chemotherapy and/or radiation therapy [78].

3.6.3. Common dysfunctions in esophageal cancer

If esophageal cancer patients receive chemotherapy or radiotherapy alone, they tend to have decreased physical function including loss of muscle strength and flexibility which is also observed before treatment. However, if surgery is performed, patients have more problems than without surgery, including pulmonary dysfunction and decline of locomotion and ADL. Following surgery, patients have to stay in ICU for few days. During this period, patients may develop a decline in pulmonary function and as a result, they may be intubated for a long time. Additionally, fasting is common for a few weeks until patients can eat food without aspiration. Muscle weakness, decline of ADL, dizziness, loss of appetite, shortness of breath, depression are observed in a substantial majority of patients during or after their initial treatment (surgery, radiation, and/or chemotherapy). Upper and lower extremity and trunk muscle strength decreases following long-term bedridden and sedentary treatment.

3.6.4. *Physical therapy assessment*

General pulmonary function tests should be performed in cancer patients. This includes spirometry; breathing pattern and cough; breath sounds like wheezing, coarse crackles, fine crackles, and rhonchi; and postural deformities in the chest or the spine. Evaluation of dysphagia on ADL should be also often assessed. Additionally, physical therapists should assess exercise tolerance in esophageal cancer patients and shoulder function including strength, mobility, and pain after surgery or chemoradiotherapy in patients with esophageal cancers. Physical therapists often assess ICF category and lower and upper joint ROM; perform MMT; and assess pain levels, fatigue, and locomotion ability such as gait speed, balance function, and QOL [79].

3.6.5. *Physical therapy*

To date, there are no previous studies reporting that physical therapy is effective in esophageal cancer patients. In general, physical therapy has few aims in these patients. First, performance of pulmonary exercises including positioning and breathing exercises promotes weaning of the ventilator and extubating. Second, improvement of locomotion promotes mobilization in patient's bedside [80]. Third, physical therapy aims to improve muscle strength and exercise tolerance during hospitalization. Physical therapy often includes massage, manual stretching, myofascial therapy, relaxation massage, stretching, strengthening, resisted exercise, PNF, aerobic exercise, TENS, patient education, and behavioral training.

3.6.6. *Key points*

Physical therapists should aim to prevent further weakness after the treatment. Following surgery, physical therapists must make patients perform pulmonary exercise and mobilization as soon as possible.

3.7. Bone cancer

3.7.1. *Overview*

The age-adjusted incidence rate of primary malignant bone tumors in the United States is 0.9 per 100,000 persons per year, accounting for approximately 0.2% of all malignancies [81]. Bone cancer is a rare form of cancer that can affect any bone in the body. Bone cancer is a cancer that arises from the cells that make up the bones. When cancer is detected in the bone, it most often has started somewhere else (e.g., in another organ) and then spread to the bones. This is known as cancer that has metastasized to the bone and is named after the site where the original cancer began. Bone cancer can vary widely from person to person depending on its location and size. The most common type of malignant bone tumor is osteosarcoma, which most often develops in the bones of the arms, legs, and pelvis. Other types of bone cancer include the following: chondrosarcoma, Ewing's tumor, chordoma, fibrosarcoma, giant cell tumor, and malignant fibrous histiocytoma [82].

3.7.2. Treatment

Treatment includes surgery, chemotherapy, and radiation therapy [83, 84]. Amputation may be necessary if limb-sparing surgery is not possible or had no positive outcomes [85].

3.7.3. Common dysfunctions in bone cancer

Chemotherapy or radiotherapy alone results in and improvement of physical function including muscle strength and flexibility. However, if bone cancer patients received surgery, they could develop some problems. Patients may have pain and weakness of the affected limb and may have restricted weight bearing and movement of limbs or the spine. In addition, when amputation of the arm, leg, hand, or foot is performed, patients become more physically disabled. Bone cancer patients with spine tumor, paraplegia, or quadriplegia have declined motor and sensory function in addition to bladder and bowel dysfunction [86].

3.7.4. Physical therapy assessment

Physical therapists should often assesses ICF category; pain levels; affected bone tumor; ROM; MMT; fatigue; ADL; and locomotion ability such as gait speed, balance function, and QOL. Physical therapists should be aware of motion and weight-bearing restrictions that occur after the surgery. In case of amputation, physical therapists should assess phantom limb pain, muscle strength, and mobility of the affected limb. Patients with spine tumor have paralysis; hence, physical therapists should use the American Spinal Injury Association (ASIA) scores for evaluation of sensory function, strength, mobility, and pain after the surgery or chemoradiotherapy.

3.7.5. Physical therapy

To date, there are no previous studies reporting that physical therapy is effective in bone cancer patients. In general, physical therapists must pay attention to fragile bones. Bone tumors make bones easy to fracture with vigorous movements. Physical therapy differs depending on the treatment of bone cancer. When bone cancer patients receive chemotherapy and radiotherapy only, muscle strengthening and endurance exercises are performed. However, when patients receive surgery, physical therapists must pay attention to contraindicative exercises. When patients receive amputation, limb prosthetics should be considered by the physiotherapist together with a prosthetist and an orthotist. In bone cancer patients with paraplegia such as bone tumor in the spinal cord, physical therapy is carried out in accordance with physical therapy of spinal cord injury. Otherwise, physical therapy often includes stretching, strengthening, resisted exercise, PNF, aerobic exercise, patient education, and behavioral training.

3.7.6. Key points

Physical therapists must know the location and progression of bone tumor as it is an important factor allowing improvement of physical function after treatment.

3.8. Blood cancer including hematopoietic stem cell transplantation (HSCT)

3.8.1. Overview

The number of new cases of leukemia is 4.5–9.1 per 100,000 men and 3.6–6.0 per 100,000 women per year [50]. Blood cancer affects the blood and lymph systems. Bone marrow has a function of producing blood cells such as red blood cells, white blood cells, and platelets. Bone marrow is a flexible soft tissue found in the hollow interior of the bones. Blood cancer may begin in blood-forming tissue (e.g., bone marrow) or in the cells of the immune system. There are different types of hematological cancers including leukemia, non-Hodgkin lymphoma, Hodgkin lymphoma, and multiple myeloma. Leukemia is a cancer that originates in the white blood cells and affects people of all ages [87].

3.8.2. Treatment

In general, blood cancer treatment includes chemotherapy, corticosteroids, radiation, and HSCT.

3.8.3. Common dysfunctions in blood cancer

First, blood cancer patients that have received chemotherapy experience a decrease in physical function including muscle strength and endurance capacity. Second, if complete remission is not achieved after chemotherapy, HSCT has to be chosen. In this case, patients experience even more decreased muscle strength and endurance capacity as they have to stay in a hospital for a few weeks [88, 89]. Hospitalized patients often have graft-versus-host disease (GVHD). GVHD normally affects the skin, liver, and gastrointestinal system resulting in further dysfunctions. Furthermore, following HSCT treatment, patients must stay in the isolation room to prevent infection; hence, a decrease in physical activity during these days will occur [90].

3.8.4. Physical therapy assessment

Physical therapists should assess muscle strength, body composition, mobility, and endurance capacity in blood cancer patients. Physical therapists often assess ICF category, lower and upper joint ROM, balance function, MMT, fatigue, and locomotion ability such as gait speed, balance function, and QOL [91–94].

3.8.5. Physical therapy

Physical therapy focused on the arms is performed in order to improve locomotion and muscle strength after treatment. Some previous reports showed that physical therapy is effective in pediatric leukemia patients [95, 96]. Additionally, some previous reports showed that physical therapy is effective in patients with HSCT [90, 97]. Following HSCT, physical therapists must wear a mask, plastic grove, and apron during physical therapy. The most common physical therapy of blood cancer includes massage, manual stretching, myofascial therapy, relaxation massage, stretching, strengthening, resisted exercise, PNF, aerobic exercise, balance training, TENS, patient education, and behavioral training.

3.8.6. Key points

Physical therapists should aim to increase muscle strength and exercise capacity in blood cancer patients. Additionally, physical therapists must be aware that patients may have myelosuppression as a result of chemotherapy. Physical therapy should be performed in such a way that it prevents infection in these patients.

3.9. Palliative care in cancer

Palliative care helps people cope with the symptoms of cancer and cancer treatment [98]. Palliative care aims to improve the quality of life of patients who have serious or life-threatening diseases [99]. The goal of palliative care is to prevent or treat the symptoms and side effects of the disease and its treatment in addition to related psychological, social, and spiritual problems [100]. However, the main goal is not to cure patients [101]. When many different treatments have been tried and showed no control over cancer, it could be the time to weigh the benefits and risks of continuing trying new treatments. Palliative care provides patients of any age or disease stage with relief from symptoms, pain, and stress and should be provided along curative treatment. Palliative care focuses on helping people get relief from symptoms caused by serious illness (e.g., nausea, pain, fatigue, or shortness of breath) [102].

3.9.1. Treatment

Palliative treatment is designed to relieve symptoms and often includes medication, nutritional support, relaxation techniques, spiritual support, emotional support, and other therapies [103, 104]. Palliative treatment improves patient's quality of life. It can be used at any stage of an illness and also if there are troubling symptoms such as pain or sickness. Palliative treatment can also mean using medicines to reduce or control side effects of cancer treatments.

3.9.2. Common dysfunctions in palliative care in cancer patients

Cancer patients have many problems making palliative care a good additional treatment option. Patients have many symptoms including pain, fatigue, loss of appetite, nausea, vomiting, shortness of breath, insomnia, thirst, dry mouth, bad taste, and difficulty swallowing. Gradually, patients may become bedridden and sedentary. Patients usually have a bigger decrease in muscle strength, pulmonary function, ADL, and locomotion after they received palliative care. In some cases, cancer patients have lymphedema. Unfortunately, patients may die in a few weeks or months.

3.9.3. Physical therapy assessment

Physical therapists should often assess ICF category, pain levels, ROM, MMT, fatigue, ADL, and QOL. Additionally, physical therapists should perform pulmonary function tests including spirometry; breathing pattern; cough; breath sounds such as wheezing, coarse crackles, fine crackles, and rhonchi; and postural deformities in the chest or the spine and evaluate dysphagia on ADL. If cancer patients become bedridden for a long time, physical therapists should assess pressure ulcers at the sacrum and coccyx.

3.9.4. Physical therapy

A few previous reports showed that physical therapy may be effective in cancer patients who receive palliative care [105, 106]. In general, physical therapy helps to maintain mobility and improves body movements [7, 107]. Physical therapists improve locomotion ability by exercises that include standing and walking, massage, manual stretching, strengthening, resisted exercises, aerobic exercises, patient education, and behavioral training. If patients have severe pain related to cancer, physical therapy includes myofascial therapy, relaxation massage, TENS, heat and cold, and positioning. If patients are bedridden or sedentary for a long time, physical therapists should relieve pressure to prevent pressure ulcers on bones such as the sacrum and coccyx.

3.9.5. Key points

Physical therapists must be aware that cancer patients experience more fatigue and pain while improving their locomotion. When cancer patients cannot receive progressive physical therapy, physical therapists should use myofascial therapy, relaxation massage, TENS, heat and cold, and positioning to relieve pain.

4. Summary and conclusion

Cancer patients have some physical impairment. Physical therapy is helpful and contributes to patients' recovery. Cancer patients are exposed to some risk factors during physical therapy. Therefore, physical therapists must pay attention and manage those risk factors. Cancer survivors increase 5 years of survival in various cancer diseases. Physical therapy may have an important role to improve physical function, ADL, and QOL of cancer patients and cancer survivors.

Author details

Shinichiro Morishita* and Atsuhiro Tsubaki

*Address all correspondence to: ptmorishin@yahoo.co.jp

Institute for Human Movement, Medical Sciences, Niigata University of Health and Welfare, Niigata, Japan

References

[1] de Haes JC, van Knippenberg FC, Neijt JP: Measuring psychological and physical distress in cancer patients: structure and application of the Rotterdam Symptom Checklist. Br J Cancer 1990, 62(6):1034–1038.

[2] Fialka-Moser V, Crevenna R, Korpan M, Quittan M: Cancer rehabilitation: particularly with aspects on physical impairments. J Rehabil Med 2003, 35(4):153–162.

[3] Fernández-Lao C, Cantarero-Villanueva I, Fernández-de-Las-Peñas C, del Moral-Ávila R, Castro-Sánchez AM, Arroyo-Morales M: Effectiveness of a multidimensional physical therapy program on pain, pressure hypersensitivity, and trigger points in breast cancer survivors: a randomized controlled clinical trial. Clin J Pain 2012, 28(2):113–121.

[4] Carmeli E, Bartoletti R: Retrospective trial of complete decongestive physical therapy for lower extremity secondary lymphedema in melanoma patients. Support Care Cancer 2011, 19(1):141–147.

[5] Swenson KK, Nissen MJ, Knippenberg K, Sistermans A, Spilde P, Bell EM, Nissen J, Chen C, Tsai ML: Cancer rehabilitation: outcome evaluation of a strengthening and conditioning program. Cancer Nurs 2014, 37(3):162–169.

[6] Kirschner KL, Eickmeyer S, Gamble G, Spill GR, Silver JK: When teams fumble: cancer rehabilitation and the problem of the "handoff". PM R 2013, 5(7):622–628.

[7] Silver JK, Raj VS, Fu JB, Wisotzky EM, Smith SR, Kirch RA: Cancer rehabilitation and palliative care: critical components in the delivery of high-quality oncology services. Support Care Cancer 2015, 23(12):3633–3643.

[8] Oken MM, Creech RH, Tormey DC, Horton J, Davis TE, McFadden ET, Carbone PP: Toxicity and response criteria of the Eastern Cooperative Oncology Group. Am J Clin Oncol 1982, 5(6):649–655.

[9] Lau F, Maida V, Downing M, Lesperance M, Karlson N, Kuziemsky C: Use of the palliative performance scale (PPS) for end-of-life prognostication in a palliative medicine consultation service. J Pain Symptom Manage 2009, 37(6):965–972.

[10] Collin C, Wade DT, Davies S, Horne V: The Barthel ADL index: a reliability study. Int Disabil Stud 1988, 10(2):61–63.

[11] Hamilton BB, Laughlin JA, Fiedler RC, Granger CV: Interrater reliability of the 7-level functional independence measure (FIM). Scand J Rehabil Med 1994, 26(3):115–119.

[12] Linacre JM, Heinemann AW, Wright BD, Granger CV, Hamilton BB: The structure and stability of the functional Independence measure. Arch Phys Med Rehabil 1994, 75(2):127–132.

[13] Vargo MM, Gerber LH: Rehabilitation for patients with cancer diagnosis. In: Physical medicine and rehabilitation: principles and practice. edn. Edited by Delisa JA, Gans BM, Walsh NE. Philadelphia: Lippincott Williams & Wilkins; 2005: 1771–1794.

[14] Gerber LH, Stout NL, Schmitz KH, Stricker CT: Integrating a prospective surveillance model for rehabilitation into breast cancer survivorship care. Cancer 2012, 118(8 Suppl):2201–2206.

[15] Buffart LM, van Uffelen JG, Riphagen II, Brug J, van Mechelen W, Brown WJ, Chinapaw MJ: Physical and psychosocial benefits of yoga in cancer patients and survivors, a systematic review and meta-analysis of randomized controlled trials. BMC Cancer 2012, 12:559.

[16] Parkin DM, Bray F, Ferlay J, Pisani P: Global cancer statistics, 2002. CA Cancer J Clin 2005, 55(2):74–108.

[17] Torre LA, Bray F, Siegel RL, Ferlay J, Lortet-Tieulent J, Jemal A: Global cancer statistics, 2012. CA Cancer J Clin 2015, 65(2):87–108.

[18] Yadav BS, Sharma SC, Singh R, Singh G: Patterns of relapse in locally advanced breast cancer treated with neoadjuvant chemotherapy followed by surgery and radiotherapy. J Cancer Res Ther 2007, 3(2):75–80.

[19] Mannino M, Yarnold JR: Local relapse rates are falling after breast conserving surgery and systemic therapy for early breast cancer: can radiotherapy ever be safely withheld? Radiother Oncol 2009, 90(1):14–22.

[20] Rietman JS, Dijkstra PU, Hoekstra HJ, Eisma WH, Szabo BG, Groothoff JW, Geertzen JH: Late morbidity after treatment of breast cancer in relation to daily activities and quality of life: a systematic review. Eur J Surg Oncol 2003, 29(3):229–238.

[21] Chan DN, Lui LY, So WK: Effectiveness of exercise programmes on shoulder mobility and lymphoedema after axillary lymph node dissection for breast cancer: systematic review. J Adv Nurs 2010, 66(9):1902–1914.

[22] Stubblefield MD, Custodio CM: Upper-extremity pain disorders in breast cancer. Arch Phys Med Rehabil 2006, 87(3 Suppl 1):S96–S99; quiz S100–101.

[23] Armer J, Fu MR, Wainstock JM, Zagar E, Jacobs LK: Lymphedema following breast cancer treatment, including sentinel lymph node biopsy. Lymphology 2004, 37(2):73–91.

[24] Stuiver MM, ten Tusscher MR, Agasi-Idenburg CS, Lucas C, Aaronson NK, Bossuyt PM: Conservative interventions for preventing clinically detectable upper-limb lymphoedema

in patients who are at risk of developing lymphoedema after breast cancer therapy. Cochrane Database Syst Rev 2015(2):CD009765.

[25] Cho Y, Do J, Jung S, Kwon O, Jeon JY: Effects of a physical therapy program combined with manual lymphatic drainage on shoulder function, quality of life, lymphedema incidence, and pain in breast cancer patients with axillary web syndrome following axillary dissection. Support Care Cancer 2016, 24(5):2047–2057.

[26] De Groef A, Van Kampen M, Dieltjens E, Christiaens MR, Neven P, Geraerts I, Devoogdt N: Effectiveness of postoperative physical therapy for upper-limb impairments after breast cancer treatment: a systematic review. Arch Phys Med Rehabil 2015, 96(6):1140–1153.

[27] Sankaranarayanan R, Ferlay J: Worldwide burden of gynaecological cancer: the size of the problem. Best Pract Res Clin Obstet Gynaecol 2006, 20(2):207–225.

[28] Bhoola S, Hoskins WJ: Diagnosis and management of epithelial ovarian cancer. Obstet Gynecol 2006, 107(6):1399–1410.

[29] Fader AN, Rose PG: Role of surgery in ovarian carcinoma. J Clin Oncol 2007, 25(20): 2873–2883.

[30] Gonzalez BD, Manne SL, Stapleton J, Myers-Virtue S, Ozga M, Kissane D, Heckman C, Morgan M: Quality of life trajectories after diagnosis of gynecologic cancer: a theoretically based approach. Support Care Cancer 2017, 25(2):589–598.

[31] Abu-Rustum NR, Rajbhandari D, Glusman S, Massad LS: Acute lower extremity paralysis following radiation therapy for cervical cancer. Gynecol Oncol 1999, 75(1):152–154.

[32] Deura I, Shimada M, Hirashita K, Sugimura M, Sato S, Oishi T, Itamochi H, Harada T, Kigawa J: Incidence and risk factors for lower limb lymphedema after gynecologic cancer surgery with initiation of periodic complex decongestive physiotherapy. Int J Clin Oncol 2015, 20(3):556–560.

[33] Lagoo AS, Robboy SJ: Lymphoma of the female genital tract: current status. Int J Gynecol Pathol 2006, 25(1):1–21.

[34] Yang EJ, Lim JY, Rah UW, Kim YB: Effect of a pelvic floor muscle training program on gynecologic cancer survivors with pelvic floor dysfunction: a randomized controlled trial. Gynecol Oncol 2012, 125(3):705–711.

[35] Rutledge TL, Rogers R, Lee SJ, Muller CY: A pilot randomized control trial to evaluate pelvic floor muscle training for urinary incontinence among gynecologic cancer survivors. Gynecol Oncol 2014, 132(1):154–158.

[36] Thorsen L, Nystad W, Stigum H, Hjermstad M, Oldervoll L, Martinsen EW, Hornslien K, Strømme SB, Dahl AA, Fosså SD: Cardiorespiratory fitness in relation to self-reported physical function in cancer patients after chemotherapy. J Sports Med Phys Fitness 2006, 46(1):122–127.

[37] Huffman LB, Hartenbach EM, Carter J, Rash JK, Kushner DM: Maintaining sexual health throughout gynecologic cancer survivorship: A comprehensive review and clinical guide. Gynecol Oncol 2016, 140(2):359–368.

[38] Ferlay J, Soerjomataram I, Dikshit R, Eser S, Mathers C, Rebelo M, Parkin DM, Forman D, Bray F: Cancer incidence and mortality worldwide: sources, methods and major patterns in GLOBOCAN 2012. Int J Cancer 2015, 136(5):E359–E386.

[39] Williams BJ, Suki D, Fox BD, Pelloski CE, Maldaun MV, Sawaya RE, Lang FF, Rao G: Stereotactic radiosurgery for metastatic brain tumors: a comprehensive review of complications. J Neurosurg 2009, 111(3):439–448.

[40] Sontheimer H: Ion channels and amino acid transporters support the growth and invasion of primary brain tumors. Mol Neurobiol 2004, 29(1):61–71.

[41] Yamamoto M, Ueno Y, Hayashi S, Fukushima T: The role of proteolysis in tumor invasiveness in glioblastoma and metastatic brain tumors. Anticancer Res 2002, 22(6C):4265–4268.

[42] Bouffet E, Tabori U, Huang A, Bartels U: Possibilities of new therapeutic strategies in brain tumors. Cancer Treat Rev 2010, 36(4):335–341.

[43] Schiff D, Lee EQ, Nayak L, Norden AD, Reardon DA, Wen PY: Medical management of brain tumors and the sequelae of treatment. Neuro Oncol 2015, 17(4):488–504.

[44] Correa DD: Cognitive functions in brain tumor patients. Hematol Oncol Clin North Am 2006, 20(6):1363–1376.

[45] Giordana MT, Clara E: Functional rehabilitation and brain tumour patients. A review of outcome. Neurol Sci 2006, 27(4):240–244.

[46] Vargo M: Brain tumor rehabilitation. Am J Phys Med Rehabil 2011, 90(5 Suppl 1):S50–S62.

[47] Panossian A: Facial paralysis reconstruction in children and adolescents with central nervous system tumors. J Pediatr Rehabil Med 2014, 7(4):295–305.

[48] Van Peppen RP, Kwakkel G, Wood-Dauphinee S, Hendriks HJ, Van der Wees PJ, Dekker J: The impact of physical therapy on functional outcomes after stroke: what's the evidence? Clin Rehabil 2004, 18(8):833–862.

[49] Day J, Gillespie DC, Rooney AG, Bulbeck HJ, Zienius K, Boele F, Grant R: Neurocognitive deficits and neurocognitive rehabilitation in adult brain tumors. Curr Treat Options Neurol 2016, 18(5):22.

[50] Jemal A, Bray F, Center MM, Ferlay J, Ward E, Forman D: Global cancer statistics. CA Cancer J Clin 2011, 61(2):69–90.

[51] Gupta B, Johnson NW, Kumar N: Global epidemiology of head and neck cancers: a continuing challenge. Oncology 2016, 91(1):13–23.

[52] Merlano M, Mattiot VP: Future chemotherapy and radiotherapy options in head and neck cancer. Expert Rev Anticancer Ther 2006, 6(3):395–403.

[53] Nelke KH, Pawlak W, Gerber H, Leszczyszyn J: Head and neck cancer patients' quality of life. Adv Clin Exp Med 2014, 23(6):1019–1027.

[54] Siddiqui AS, Dogar SA, Lal S, Akhtar S, Khan FA: Airway management and postoperative length of hospital stay in patients undergoing head and neck cancer surgery. J Anaesthesiol Clin Pharmacol 2016, 32(1):49–53.

[55] Nguyen NP, Smith HJ, Dutta S, Alfieri A, North D, Nguyen PD, Lee H, Martinez T, Lemanski C, Ludin A et al.: Aspiration occurrence during chemoradiation for head and neck cancer. Anticancer Res 2007, 27(3B):1669–1672.

[56] Eisbruch A, Schwartz M, Rasch C, Vineberg K, Damen E, Van As CJ, Marsh R, Pameijer FA, Balm AJ: Dysphagia and aspiration after chemoradiotherapy for head-and-neck cancer: which anatomic structures are affected and can they be spared by IMRT? Int J Radiat Oncol Biol Phys 2004, 60(5):1425–1439.

[57] Prevost V, Joubert C, Heutte N, Babin E: Assessment of nutritional status and quality of life in patients treated for head and neck cancer. Eur Ann Otorhinolaryngol Head Neck Dis 2014, 131(2):113–120.

[58] McGarvey AC, Chiarelli PE, Osmotherly PG, Hoffman GR: Physiotherapy for accessory nerve shoulder dysfunction following neck dissection surgery: a literature review. Head Neck 2011, 33(2):274–280.

[59] van Wilgen CP, Dijkstra PU, van der Laan BF, Plukker JT, Roodenburg JL: Shoulder and neck morbidity in quality of life after surgery for head and neck cancer. Head Neck 2004, 26(10):839–844.

[60] Murphy BA, Deng J: Advances in supportive care for late effects of head and neck cancer. J Clin Oncol 2015, 33(29):3314–3321.

[61] Tacani PM, Franceschini JP, Tacani RE, Machado AF, Montezello D, Góes JC, Marx A: Retrospective study of the physical therapy modalities applied in head and neck l ymphedema treatment. Head Neck 2016, 38(2):301–308.

[62] McGarvey AC, Osmotherly PG, Hoffman GR, Chiarelli PE: Scapular muscle exercises following neck dissection surgery for head and neck cancer: a comparative electromyographic study. Phys Ther 2013, 93(6):786–797.

[63] Guru K, Manoor UK, Supe SS: A comprehensive review of head and neck cancer rehabilitation: physical therapy perspectives. Indian J Palliat Care 2012, 18(2):87–97.

[64] Espitalier F, Testelin S, Blanchard D, Binczak M, Bollet M, Calmels P, Couturaud C, Dreyer C, Navez M, Perrichon C et al.: Management of somatic pain induced by treatment of head and neck cancer: postoperative pain. Guidelines of the French oto-rhino-laryngology—head and neck surgery Society (SFORL). Eur Ann Otorhinolaryngol Head Neck Dis 2014, 131(4):249–252.

[65] Dela Cruz CS, Tanoue LT, Matthay RA: Lung cancer: epidemiology, etiology, and prevention. Clin Chest Med 2011, 32(4):605–644.

[66] Herbst RS, Heymach JV, Lippman SM: Lung cancer. N Engl J Med 2008, 359(13):1367–1380.

[67] Noonan KL, Ho C, Laskin J, Murray N: The influence of the evolution of first-line chemotherapy on steadily improving survival in advanced non-small-cell lung cancer clinical trials. J Thorac Oncol 2015, 10(11):1523–1531.

[68] Xu YP, Li B, Xu XL, Mao WM: Is there a survival benefit in patients with stage IIIA (N2) non-small cell lung cancer receiving neoadjuvant chemotherapy and/or radiotherapy prior to surgical resection: a systematic review and meta-analysis. Medicine (Baltimore) 2015, 94(23):e879.

[69] Vandenbroucke E, De Ryck F, Surmont V, van Meerbeeck JP: What is the role for surgery in patients with stage III non-small cell lung cancer? Curr Opin Pulm Med 2009, 15(4):295–302.

[70] Rivas-Perez H, Nana-Sinkam P: Integrating pulmonary rehabilitation into the multidisciplinary management of lung cancer: a review. Respir Med 2015, 109(4):437–442.

[71] Nazarian J: Cardiopulmonary rehabilitation after treatment for lung cancer. Curr Treat Options Oncol 2004, 5(1):75–82.

[72] Nici L: The role of pulmonary rehabilitation in the lung cancer patient. Semin Respir Crit Care Med 2009, 30(6):670–674.

[73] Pehlivan E, Turna A, Gurses A, Gurses HN: The effects of preoperative short-term intense physical therapy in lung cancer patients: a randomized controlled trial. Ann Thorac Cardiovasc Surg 2011, 17(5):461–468.

[74] Morano MT, Araújo AS, Nascimento FB, da Silva GF, Mesquita R, Pinto JS, de Moraes Filho MO, Pereira ED: Preoperative pulmonary rehabilitation versus chest physical therapy in patients undergoing lung cancer resection: a pilot randomized controlled trial. Arch Phys Med Rehabil 2013, 94(1):53–58.

[75] Pennathur A, Gibson MK, Jobe BA, Luketich JD: Oesophageal carcinoma. Lancet 2013, 381(9864):400–412.

[76] Peng Q, Chen H, Huo JR: Alcohol consumption and corresponding factors: A novel perspective on the risk factors of esophageal cancer. Oncol Lett 2016, 11(5):3231–3239.

[77] Carcaterrra M, Osti MF, De Sanctis V, Caruso C, Berardi F, Enrici RM: Adjuvant radiotherapy and radiochemotherapy in the management of esophageal cancer: a review of the literature. Rays 2005, 30(4):319–322.

[78] Siersema PD, van Hillegersberg R: Treatment of locally advanced esophageal cancer with surgery and chemoradiation. Curr Opin Gastroenterol 2008, 24(4):535–540.

[79] Gimigliano R, Bertella M, Gimigliano F, Iolascon G: Rehabilitation in esophageal cancer. Rays 2005, 30(4):295–298.

[80] Aceto P, Congedo E, Cardone A, Zappia L, De Cosmo G: Postoperative management of elective esophagectomy for cancer. Rays 2005, 30(4):289–294.

[81] Franchi A: Epidemiology and classification of bone tumors. Clin Cases Miner Bone Metab 2012, 9(2):92–95.

[82] Bertoni F, Bacchini P: Classification of bone tumors. Eur J Radiol 1998, 27 Suppl 1:S74–S76.

[83] O'Toole GC, Boland P: Metastatic bone cancer pain: etiology and treatment options. Curr Pain Headache Rep 2006, 10(4):288–292.

[84] Anderson P, Salazar-Abshire M: Improving outcomes in difficult bone cancers using multimodality therapy, including radiation: physician and nursing perspectives. Curr Oncol Rep 2006, 8(6):415–422.

[85] Bekkering WP, Vliet Vlieland TP, Fiocco M, Koopman HM, Schoones JW, Nelissen RG, Taminiau AH: Quality of life, functional ability and physical activity after different surgical interventions for bone cancer of the leg: a systematic review. Surg Oncol 2012, 21(2):e39–e47.

[86] Baines MJ: Spinal cord compression—a personal and palliative care perspective. Clin Oncol (R Coll Radiol) 2002, 14(2):135–138.

[87] Dores GM, Devesa SS, Curtis RE, Linet MS, Morton LM: Acute leukemia incidence and patient survival among children and adults in the United States, 2001–2007. Blood 2012, 119(1):34–43.

[88] Morishita S, Kaida K, Yamauchi S, Wakasugi T, Ikegame K, Kodama N, Ogawa H, Domen K: Early-phase differences in health-related quality of life, psychological status, and physical function between human leucocyte antigen-haploidentical and other allogeneic haematopoietic stem cell transplantation recipients. Eur J Oncol Nurs 2015, 19(5):443–450.

[89] Morishita S, Kaida K, Yamauchi S, Sota K, Ishii S, Ikegame K, Kodama N, Ogawa H, Domen K: Relationship between corticosteroid dose and declines in physical function among allogeneic hematopoietic stem cell transplantation patients. Support Care Cancer 2013, 21(8):2161–2169.

[90] Morishita S, Kaida K, Setogawa K, Kajihara K, Ishii S, Ikegame K, Kodama N, Ogawa H, Domen K: Safety and feasibility of physical therapy in cytopenic patients during allogeneic haematopoietic stem cell transplantation. Eur J Cancer Care (Engl) 2013, 22(3):289–299.

[91] Morishita S, Kaida K, Aoki O, Yamauchi S, Wakasugi T, Ikegame K, Ogawa H, Domen K: Balance function in patients who had undergone allogeneic hematopoietic stem cell transplantation. Gait Posture 2015, 42(3):406–408.

[92] Morishita S, Kaida K, Yamauchi S, Wakasugi T, Yoshihara S, Taniguchi K, Ishii S, Ikegame K, Kodama N, Ogawa H et al.: Gender differences in health-related quality of life, physical function and psychological status among patients in the early phase following allogeneic haematopoietic stem cell transplantation. Psychooncology 2013, 22(5):1159–1166.

[93] Morishita S, Kaida K, Ikegame K, Yoshihara S, Taniguchi K, Okada M, Kodama N, Ogawa H, Domen K: Impaired physiological function and health-related QOL in patients before hematopoietic stem-cell transplantation. Support Care Cancer 2012, 20(4):821–829.

[94] Morishita S, Kaida K, Tanaka T, Itani Y, Ikegame K, Okada M, Ishii S, Kodama N, Ogawa H, Domen K: Prevalence of sarcopenia and relevance of body composition, physiological function, fatigue, and health-related quality of life in patients before allogeneic hematopoietic stem cell transplantation. Support Care Cancer 2012, 20(12):3161–3168.

[95] Vercher P, Hung YJ, Ko M: The effectiveness of incorporating a play-based intervention to improve functional mobility for a child with relapsed acute lymphoblastic leukaemia: a case report. Physiother Res Int 2016, 21(4):264–270.

[96] Esbenshade AJ, Friedman DL, Smith WA, Jeha S, Pui CH, Robison LL, Ness KK: Feasibility and initial effectiveness of home exercise during maintenance therapy for childhood acute lymphoblastic leukemia. Pediatr Phys Ther 2014, 26(3):301–307.

[97] van Haren IE, Timmerman H, Potting CM, Blijlevens NM, Staal JB, Nijhuis-van der Sanden MW: Physical exercise for patients undergoing hematopoietic stem cell transplantation: systematic review and meta-analyses of randomized controlled trials. Phys Ther 2013, 93(4):514–528.

[98] Armes J, Crowe M, Colbourne L, Morgan H, Murrells T, Oakley C, Palmer N, Ream E, Young A, Richardson A: Patients' supportive care needs beyond the end of cancer treatment: a prospective, longitudinal survey. J Clin Oncol 2009, 27(36):6172–6179.

[99] Peters L, Sellick K: Quality of life of cancer patients receiving inpatient and home-based palliative care. J Adv Nurs 2006, 53(5):524–533.

[100] Jocham HR, Dassen T, Widdershoven G, Halfens R: Quality of life in palliative care cancer patients: a literature review. J Clin Nurs 2006, 15(9):1188–1195.

[101] Gattellari M, Voigt KJ, Butow PN, Tattersall MH: When the treatment goal is not cure: are cancer patients equipped to make informed decisions? J Clin Oncol 2002, 20(2):503–513.

[102] Dy SM, Harman SM, Braun UK, Howie LJ, Harris PF, Jayes RL: To stent or not to stent: an evidence-based approach to palliative procedures at the end of life. J Pain Symptom Manage 2012, 43(4):795–801.

[103] Mansky PJ, Wallerstedt DB: Complementary medicine in palliative care and cancer symptom management. Cancer J 2006, 12(5):425–431.

[104] True G, Phipps EJ, Braitman LE, Harralson T, Harris D, Tester W: Treatment preferences and advance care planning at end of life: the role of ethnicity and spiritual coping in cancer patients. Ann Behav Med 2005, 30(2):174–179.

[105] Kumar P, Casarett D, Corcoran A, Desai K, Li Q, Chen J, Langer C, Mao JJ: Utilization of supportive and palliative care services among oncology outpatients at one academic cancer center: determinants of use and barriers to access. J Palliat Med 2012, 15(8):923–930.

[106] López-Sendín N, Alburquerque-Sendín F, Cleland JA, Fernández-de-las-Peñas C: Effects of physical therapy on pain and mood in patients with terminal cancer: a pilot randomized clinical trial. J Altern Complement Med 2012, 18(5):480–486.

[107] Olson E, Cristian A: The role of rehabilitation medicine and palliative care in the treatment of patients with end-stage disease. Phys Med Rehabil Clin N Am 2005, 16(1):285–305, xi.

10

The Function of Scapular Muscle

Tomohito Ijiri

Additional information is available at the end of the chapter

Abstract

In shoulder rehabilitation, it is important to evaluate scapular stability. However, it is not revealed how the mechanism runs for scapular stability. Additionally, the contribution of scapular muscles for scapular stability remains a matter of debate. Wherefore, I suggest some studies in this section to understand the function of scapulothoracic joint and the mechanism of scapular stability in detail. In the results of these studies, it was revealed that each scapular muscle activation is different for shoulder isometric contraction, and the exercise for a scapular muscle increases only the shoulder muscle strength of specific movement direction. If we can consider each scapular muscle individually by utilizing these results, we can provide more effective rehabilitation program.

Keywords: scapular muscle, muscle activity, scapular stability, shoulder disease, muscle strength

1. Introduction

The shoulder complex is constituted with some joint. It is understood that glenohumeral joint (GHJ) and scapulothoracic joint (STJ) are important for shoulder complex and they make up a large fraction of shoulder movement. Especially, scapulothoracic joint has been focused recently. It was reported that patients with shoulder disease show abnormal scapular movement and scapular muscle activation during shoulder motion, so to normalize the scapular movement, it is important to improve the symptom [1–3]. Clinically, the therapist usually prescribes the scapular exercise to the patients. So, we will be able to provide the more effective rehabilitation program if we understand more about the scapulothoracic joint. Some functions of the scapula were reported in previous studies. These include contributing to the range of shoulder motion synchronizing the motion of humerus, supporting the humerus, keeping the muscle tension, maintaining the appropriate muscle length on glenohumeral joint, and getting off the impingement raising the glenoid fossa [4]. However, not only these, scapulothoracic joint is also related to the "exertion of muscle power" on shoulder joint, so we have to consider keeping rehabilitation in mind. However, there remain some ambiguities regarding the function of scapular muscle. In previous studies, scapular muscles with high activation during specific exercises for scapular muscles [5, 6] have been reported. And it was reported that the combination of standard rehabilitation interventions and scapulothoracic joint control training exercises were effective treatments for the shoulder joint dysfunction [7, 8]. But the change of shoulder muscle strength by only one scapular muscle exercise is not examined in exact detail, not by a number of exercises. In other words, the evidence is not enough to choose the best exercise from a number of exercises for each patient. Additionally, it is not revealed how the mechanism runs for scapular stability. Wherefore, which exercise is the best for the improvement of scapular movement for each patient remains a matter of research. And so, I suggest some studies in this section to understand the function of scapulothoracic joint. From this, I expect upgrading your ability about the clinical rehabilitation.

2. The study

2.1. The changes of muscle strength on shoulder joint after strengthening of serratus anterior

The muscle weakness is usually involved in the rehabilitation of patients with shoulder disease. So, we have to have the skill to improve this. The reason for muscle weakness on shoulder joint is not only due to glenohumeral joint like the weakness on deltoid and rotator cuff muscle but due to scapular instability with scapular muscle weakness. The patient with scapular instability usually have "winging scapula." The winging scapula was also caused by long thoracic nerve paralysis and the patients with this have weakness of shoulder muscle strengths. Serratus anterior innervated by long thoracic nerve is scapular protractor muscle and it plays a prominent role in scapular stability in consort with trapezius. Clinically, the exercise for serratus anterior has an effect on improved strength on shoulder joint. But the study which investigated how the change in the muscle strength on shoulder joint by the strengthening for serratus anterior is modest in size. Wherefore, I examined the changes of muscle strength on shoulder joint after the exercise for serratus anterior.

2.1.1. Materials and methods

Thirty-six healthy young men who had no orthopedic and neurological abnormality participated in this study. The subjects were separated into two groups randomly, one was the training group where members were exercised for serratus anterior, and the other was the control group where members did not exercise. The mean anthropometric characteristics ± standard deviation (SD) of the training group were age, 22.1 ± 1.5 years; height, 172.2 ± 6.5 cm; and weight, 62.7 ± 8.7 kg. Those of the control group were age, 21.6 ± 1.5 years; height, 171.4 ± 5.6 cm; and weight, 62.4 ± 6.3 kg.

First, the subjects in the training group and control group were measured for muscle strength. Then, in the training group, they performed exercise every day for a week. The exercise was established at the modified elbow pushup plus, which was known as the typical exercise for serratus anterior. In control group, they spent without exercise. After 1 week, they were measured for the muscle strength in common for the first time.

The measurement of muscle strength was composed by the muscle strengths of scapular protraction, shoulder flexion, abduction, external rotation, and internal rotation. The measurement was done using handheld-dynamometer (MicroFET2, Hoggan Health Industries, Inc., USA). Regarding the muscle strength of shoulder flexion, abduction, external rotation, and internal rotation, the measurement values (*N*) were multiplied by the lever arm length (m), and the muscle strength was represented by torque values (Nm). The measurement position of shoulder flexion and abduction was the same as manual muscle testing, and that of shoulder external and internal rotation was at 0° abduction. The measurement position of scapular protraction was defined at supine and 90° shoulder flexion and 90° elbow flexion (**Figure 1**). From this position, the subjects thrusted their upper limb vertically upwards. The measurer measured the power by handheld - dynamometer on olecranon. The measurement of each muscle strength was done three times and the average was adopted as the muscle strength value.

The exercise was established at the modified elbow pushup plus (**Figure 2**). The pushup plus indicated high serratus anterior activity by Decker et al. and Moseley et al. [9, 10]. The basic position of this exercise was on elbow, and the femoral area was grounded. Then, the subjects moved their scapula to maximum scapular retraction position like moving their body close to the floor. And they moved their scapular to the maximum scapular protraction position like getting their body away from the floor. Additionally, they returned to the maximum scapular retraction position and this process was defined one time. The subjects in the training group performed this exercise in three sets: one set was 20 times, each day for 1 week.

Each muscle strength for the first time was normalized as 100% and the muscle strengths after 1 week were computed as percentage. The muscle strengths between the first time and after 1 week were compared for each group using paired *t*-test.

2.1.2. Results

The result is shown in **Table 1**. Representative value is as follows. The muscle strength of scapular protraction in the right side was 113 ± 14%, shoulder flexion 106 ± 9%, abduction 110 ± 10%, external rotation 104 ± 8%, and internal rotation 112 ± 12% in the training group. In the control group, scapular protraction 99 ± 4%, shoulder flexion 101 ± 6%, abduction 100 ± 5%, external rotation 101 ± 5%, and internal rotation 101 ± 6%. The same tendency was indicated in the left side on both groups.

In the training group, the muscle strengths of scapular protraction, shoulder flexion, shoulder abduction, and internal rotation after 1 week were significantly higher than the first time on both sides. The muscle strength of shoulder external rotation was not increased. On the other hand, the muscle strength in the control group was not changed after 1 week.

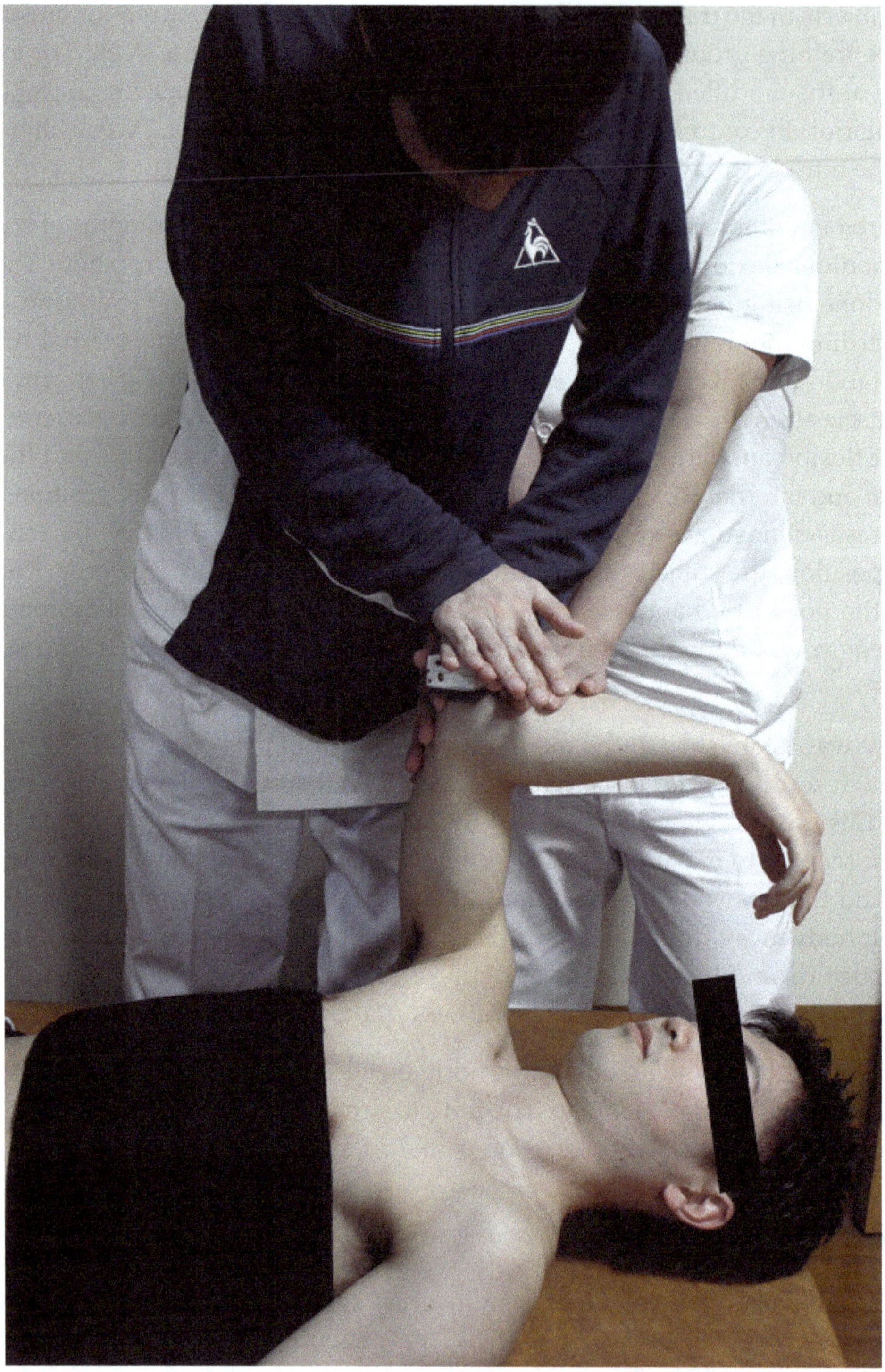

Figure 1. The measurement position of scapular protraction. The measurement position of scapular protraction was defined at supine and 90° shoulder flexion and 90° elbow flexion. From this position, the subjects thrusted their upper limb for vertical upward.

2.1.3. Discussion

In this study, the muscle strength of scapular protraction was higher after 1 week in the training group. So, the exercise was effective for serratus anterior. And it was indicated that the exercise for serratus anterior can increase the shoulder muscle strength, but the direction is

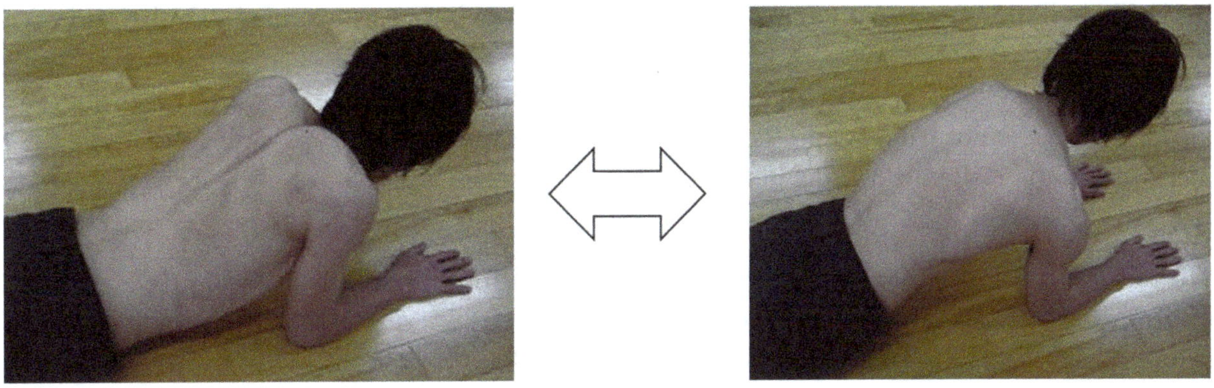

Figure 2. The modified elbow pushup plus. The basic position of this exercise was on elbow, and femoral area was grounded. They moved their scapular to maximum scapular protraction position like getting their body away from the floor.

not all limited. We have to gain consciousness of this fact. In the rehabilitation of shoulder disease patients, we usually assess the scapular position and scapular movement. If the therapist infers that abnormal scapular position and movement encumber the normal motion, then we will treat for the scapular abnormality. Additionally, the reason for the scapular abnormality is assessed in the impairment of functional level. We assess the scapular muscle strength, like manual muscle testing for scapula. In this assessment, even if the weakness of serratus anterior is found, it is not always effective for the chief complaint motion. From this study, serratus anterior must influence the motion which consists of shoulder flex, abduction, and internal rotation, but does not influence the motion which does not consist of their movements. So, we have to consider the task characteristically and calculate the weakness of serratus anterior

	Right	Left
Training group		
Scapular protraction	113 ± 14*	112 ± 12*
Shoulder flexion	106 ± 9*	107 ± 9*
Shoulder abduction	110 ± 10*	109 ± 11*
Shoulder external rotation	104 ± 8	103 ± 8
Shoulder internal rotation	112 ± 12*	109 ± 11*
Control group		
Scapular protraction	99 ± 4	99 ± 5
Shoulder flexion	101 ± 6	101 ± 5
Shoulder abduction	100 ± 5	99 ± 4
Shoulder external rotation	101 ± 5	102 ± 4
Shoulder internal rotation	101 ± 6	100 ± 4

*$p < 0.01$.

Table 1. The muscle strength after 1 week.

for improved motion. As a matter of fact, the relationship between scapular stability and each scapular muscle strength remains unclear, and the therapist often confuses oneself. Therapists usually believe that one scapular muscle can contribute to scapular stability of all motion. However, this is not true. As previously noticed, therapists need to consider the movement direction of the task and make a decision about the muscle's influence to the task. This decision is important.

The reason that the exercise for serratus anterior led to an increase in the muscle strength of shoulder flexion, abduction, and internal rotation will relate to interlocking between humerus and scapula. Shoulder joint is constituted with glenohumeral joint and scapulothoracic joint and so on. Every shoulder motion involves scapular movement. Shoulder flexion includes scapular upward rotation and posterior tilt, shoulder abduction includes scapular upward rotation, and internal rotation includes scapular protraction (**Figure 3**). The function of serratus anterior is scapular upward rotation, protraction, and posterior tilt, so the scapular movements of shoulder flexion, abduction, and internal rotation, where muscle strengths were increased in this study, agree with the functions of serratus anterior. Wherefore, I conclude that the increasing of serratus anterior muscle strength conduced the increasing of these shoulder muscle strengths. On the other hand, shoulder external rotation includes scapular retraction, which does not agree with the function of serratus anterior. Therefore, I suspect that the muscle strength of shoulder external rotation did not increase in this study.

In this study, it is revealed that the muscle strength at scapulothoracic joint influences the muscle strength at shoulder complex, but not all movement directions. The muscle strength of the only shoulder movement direction having the scapular movement agrees with the function of strengthened muscle which will be increased. From this reflection, if the scapular retractor, like middle trapezius, was strengthened, the muscle strength of shoulder external

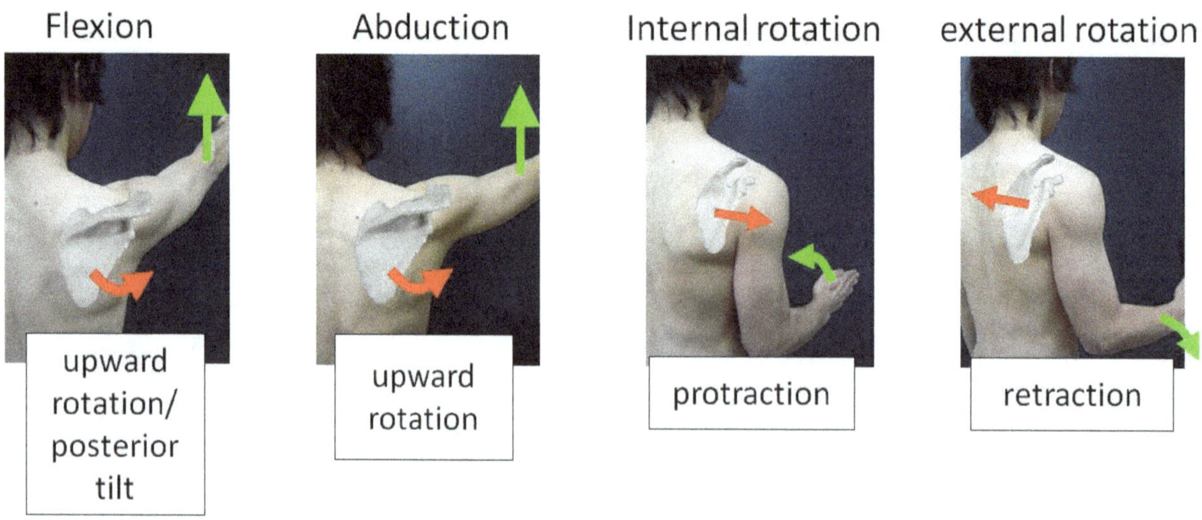

Figure 3. Scapular movement of each shoulder motion. Shoulder flexion includes scapular upward rotation and posterior tilt, shoulder abduction includes scapular upward rotation, and internal rotation includes scapular protraction. These scapular movements agree in the functions of serratus anterior.

rotation will be increased because external rotation at 0° abduction is associated with scapular retraction.

2.2. The changes of muscle strength on shoulder joint after strengthening of scapular retractor muscles

In a previous study, the muscle strengths of shoulder flexion, abduction, and internal rotation were increased after exercise for serratus anterior. And it was thought that the reason for this change must be related to the scapular movement during each motion. Contrary to previous study, if the exercise for scapular retractor was done, the muscle strength of external rotation will be increased. So, I examined the change of muscle strength on shoulder joint after exercise for scapular retractor, mainly on the middle trapezius.

2.2.1. Materials and methods

Thirty healthy men participated in this study. These subjects were divided into two groups, training group and control group, randomly. The mean anthropometric characteristics of 15 subjects in the training group were age, 23.3 ± 2.8 years; height, 172.1 ± 5.8 cm; and weight, 65.7 ± 8.5 kg. Those of the control group were age, 22.5 ± 1.6 years; height, 170.7 ± 5.3 cm; and weight, 63.7 ± 11.5 kg. There were no significant differences between two groups regarding anthropometric characteristics.

The subjects in the training group and control group were measured for muscle strength on the first day. Then, in the training group, they performed exercise every day for a week. The exercise was scapular retraction exercise at 0° shoulder abduction. In the control group, they spent without the exercise. After 1 week, they were measured for the muscle strength in common for the first time.

The muscle strengths on scapulothoracic retraction, shoulder flexion, abduction, external rotation, and internal rotation were measured. The measurement of muscle strength on shoulder flexion, abduction, external rotation, and internal rotation was the same as above-referenced previous study. The measurement of muscle strength on scapular retraction was on prone. The subject performed scapular retraction at 90° shoulder abduction and 90° elbow flexion (**Figure 4**). At that time, the muscle strength was measured by resisting their movement at the point of 3 cm inside from the axilla using handheld-dynamometer (MicroFET2, Hoggan Health Industries, Inc., USA).

The exercise was scapular retraction at 0° shoulder abduction consulted from the report by Andrews and Wilk [11] (**Figure 5**). The subjects performed scapular retraction with shoulder internal rotation for preventing to strengthen external rotator muscles by external rotation accompanied by scapular retraction. And they returned to neutral position. This process was defined one time. The subjects in the training group performed this exercise in three sets: one set was 20 times, each day for 1 week.

Each muscle strength for the first time was normalized as 100% and the muscle strengths after 1 week were computed as percentage. The muscle strengths between the first time and after 1 week were compared for each group using paired *t*-test.

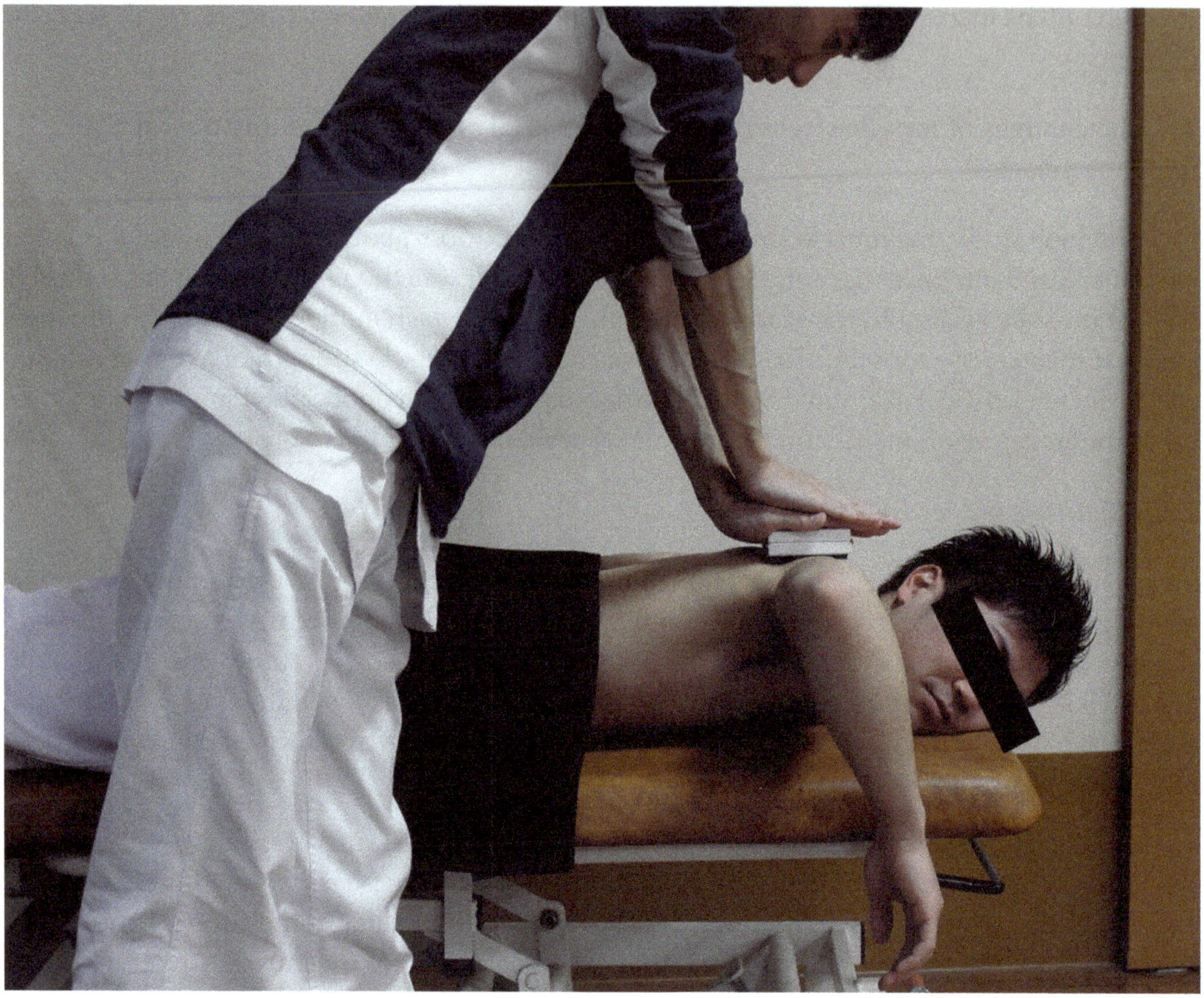

Figure 4. The measurement position of scapular retraction. The subject performed scapular retraction at 90° shoulder abduction and 90° elbow flexion. At that time, the muscle strength was measured by resisting their movement at the point of 3 cm inside from the axilla using handheld-dynamometer.

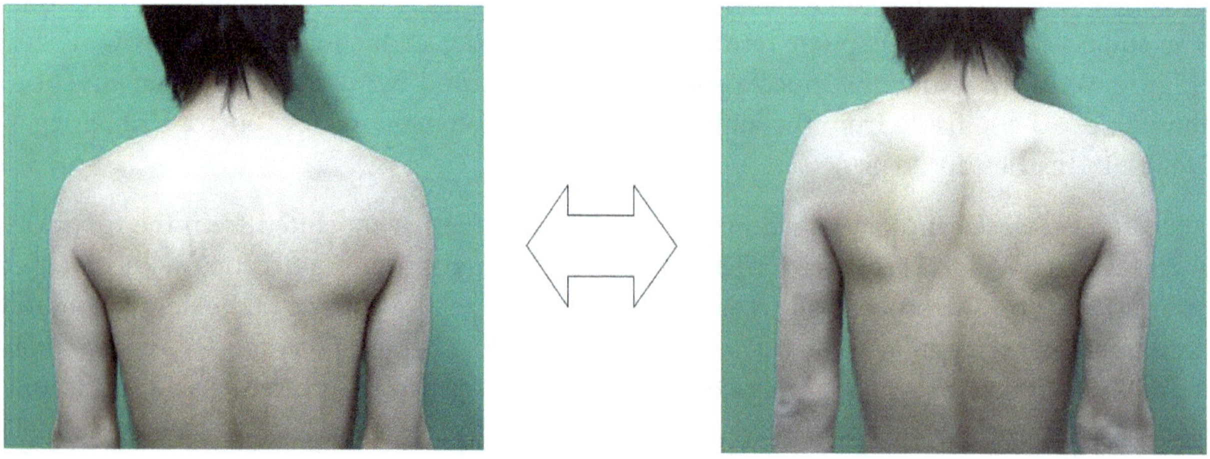

Figure 5. Scapular retraction exercise. The subjects performed scapular retraction with shoulder internal rotation for preventing to strengthen external rotator muscles by external rotation accompanied by scapular retraction. And they returned to neutral position.

2.2.2. Results

The results are shown in **Table 2**. The muscle strength of scapular retraction in the right side was 106 ± 8%, shoulder flexion 101 ± 4%, abduction 103 ± 6%, external rotation 105 ± 6%, and internal rotation 103 ± 7% in the training group. In the control group, scapular retraction 101 ± 9%, shoulder flexion 100 ± 6%, abduction 101 ± 5%, external rotation 101 ± 5%, and internal rotation 100 ± 6%. The same tendency was indicated in the left side on both groups.

In the training group, the muscle strengths of scapular retraction and shoulder external rotation after 1 week were significantly higher than the first time on both sides. The muscle strengths of shoulder flexion, abduction, and internal rotation were not increased. On the other hand, the muscle strength in control group was not changed after 1 week.

2.2.3. Discussion

In this study, the exercise for middle trapezius led to an increase in the muscle strength of scapular retraction and shoulder external rotation. From this result, the hypothesis was proved to be correct. The reason regarding increasing the muscle strength of shoulder external rotation will be the same as the previous study of exercise for serratus anterior. Shoulder external rotation includes scapular retraction. The function of middle trapezius is scapular retraction. This homology must be the reason about increasing the muscle strength of shoulder external rotation.

Considering these two studies, the muscle strength of serratus anterior must have a part of muscle strength of shoulder flexion, abduction, and internal rotation, and that of middle trapezius

	Right	Left
Training group		
Scapular retraction	106 ± 8*	109 ± 12*
Shoulder flexion	101 ± 4	101 ± 6
Shoulder abduction	103 ± 6	98 ± 6
Shoulder external rotation	105 ± 6*	106 ± 5*
Shoulder internal rotation	103 ± 7	100 ± 8
Control group		
Scapular protraction	101 ± 9	102 ± 9
Shoulder flexion	100 ± 6	99 ± 5
Shoulder abduction	101 ± 5	100 ± 9
Shoulder external rotation	101 ± 5	101 ± 4
Shoulder internal rotation	100 ± 6	99 ± 4

*$p < 0.01$.

Table 2. The results about the changing muscle strength.

must have a part of shoulder external rotation. In fact, the muscle strength of shoulder complex will combine the muscle strength of glenohumeral joint and scapulothoracic joint. Therefore, muscle weakness occurred either on glenohumeral joint or on scapulothoracic joint, and the muscle strength of shoulder complex will decrease (**Figure 6**). Winging scapula by long thoracic nerve palsy decreases the shoulder muscle strength, and this case is an easy-to-follow typical example. It is necessary to consider the function of not only glenohumeral joint but also scapulothoracic joint during the measurement of muscle strength. And we have to make a hypothesis about specific scapular muscle weakness when shoulder muscle strength is decreased.

2.3. The activities of scapular muscles during isometric contraction

I indicated the characteristic about scapular muscle strengthening in the previous paragraphs. From this, it was shown that scapular muscle strength relates with the muscle strength of shoulder complex. During daily living and sports situation, there are many opportunities requiring powerful force, for example, transfer the burden and have a frying pan. In contact sports, they require continuing their performance resisting external force. In these cases, which scapular muscle is important? I thought that it is necessary to investigate the scapular muscle activity during shoulder isometric contraction to clear the question. From previous studies, to have all scapular muscle activities during shoulder isometric contraction is hard to imagine and I predicted the characteristic muscle-active pattern. Therefore, I investigated each scapular muscle activity during isometric shoulder abduction, internal rotation, and external rotation.

2.3.1. Materials and methods

Seventeen healthy men participated in this study. The mean anthropometric characteristics were age, 26.0 ± 3.6 years; height, 172.9 ± 4.3 cm; and weight, 65.8 ± 9.1 kg.

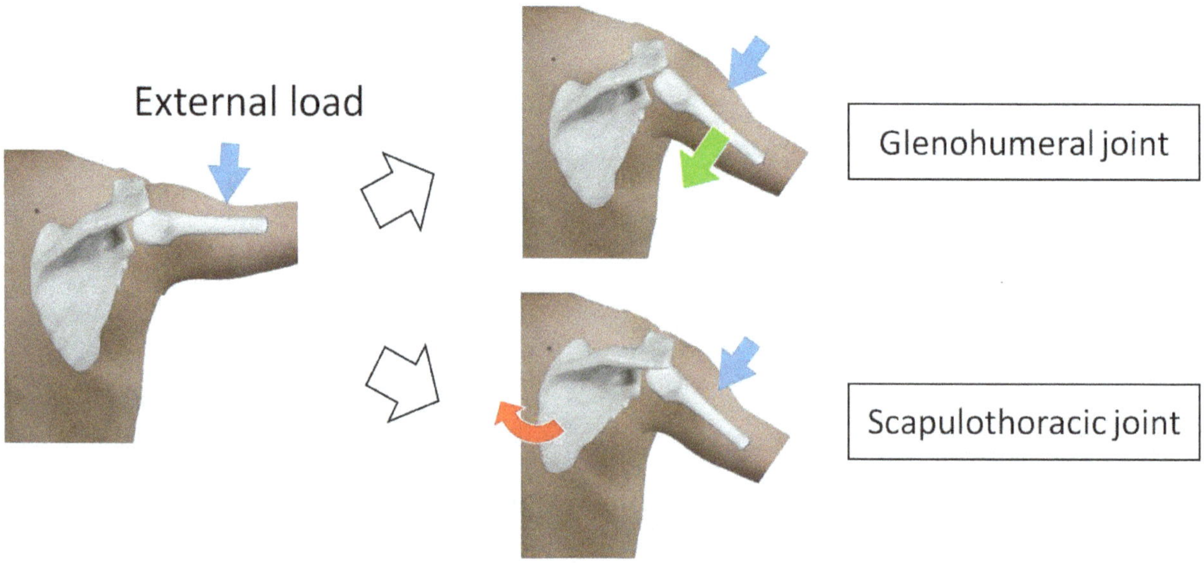

Figure 6. Muscle weakness on shoulder complex. Muscle weakness occurred either on glenohumeral joint or on scapulothoracic joint.

Muscle activity was measured during isometric shoulder abduction, internal rotation, and external rotation in the sitting position. Surface electromyography (EMG; MQ-8, Kissei Comtec, Japan) was used to collect raw EMG data during the task. EMG was reported in 3 s and the signal was recorded at a sampling rate of 1000 Hz. The measurement position of shoulder abduction was configured at shoulder 45° abduction and internal rotation and external rotation were at shoulder 0° abduction (**Figure 7**). The external load was set at three weights in order to evaluate the change with different loads using a handheld-dynamometer (Mobie, SAKAI Medical Co., Japan). The external load during abduction and internal rotation was set at 5, 10, and 15% of each subject's body weight and external rotation was set at 3, 5, and 10%. The target muscles at scapulothoracic joint of abduction task were the serratus anterior, upper, and lower trapezius. Those of internal and external rotation were serratus anterior and middle trapezius. The EMG electrode position was set according to previous studies by Ekstrom et al. and Delagi and Perotto [12, 13]. The integrated EMG (IEMG) was obtained for 3 s in the stable wave during each task and was counted per second. The IEMG per second was normalized by the IEMG at each starting position without an external load. Relative IEMGs were used for statistical comparison of each load in the same muscle. The Friedman test was used to determine whether a load condition had a statistically significant effect on relative IEMG for each muscle. Post hoc analysis was then applied for specific comparisons among the three loads and determined for individual effect differences.

2.3.2. Results

The results of raw waveform are shown in **Figure 8**. Typical raw wave was shown on internal and external rotation. During isometric shoulder internal rotation, the muscle activity of serratus anterior was high and middle trapezius was slightly high. In an opposite way, during isometric shoulder external rotation, the muscle activity of middle trapezius was high and serratus anterior was slightly high. During isometric shoulder abduction, all muscle activities, serratus anterior, upper trapezius, and lower trapezius, were high.

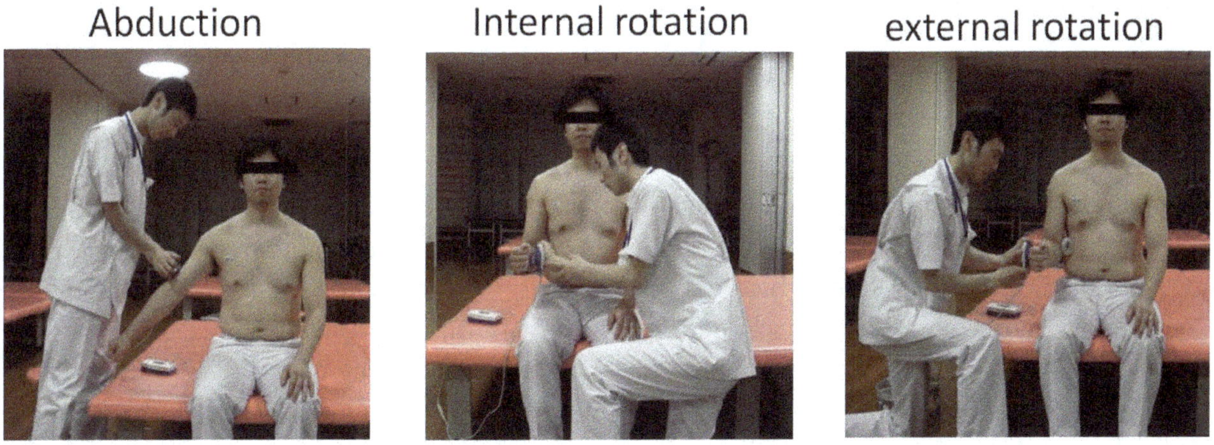

Figure 7. Measurement position regarding shoulder isometric contraction. The measurement position of shoulder abduction was configured at shoulder 45° abduction and internal rotation and external rotation were at shoulder 0° abduction. The external load was set at three weights using a handheld-dynamometer.

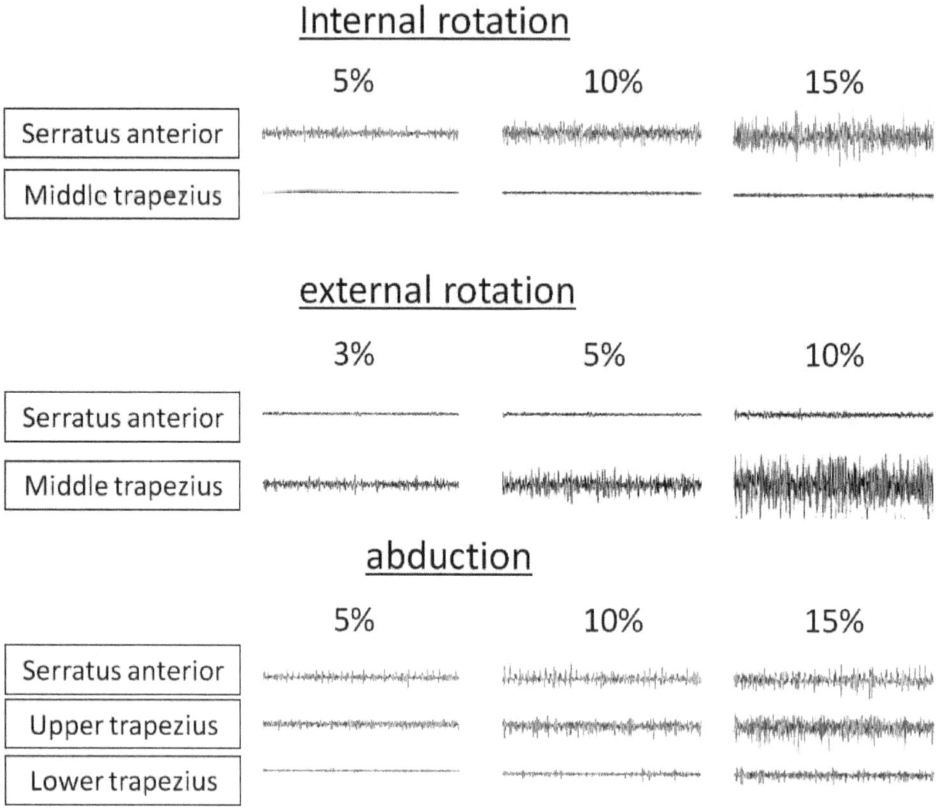

Figure 8. The results of raw waveform during isometric contraction. During isometric shoulder internal rotation, the muscle activity of serratus anterior was high and middle trapezius was slight. In an opposite way, during isometric shoulder external rotation, the muscle activity of middle trapezius was high and serratus anterior was slight. During isometric shoulder abduction, all muscle activities, serratus anterior, upper trapezius, and lower trapezius were high.

Next, relative IEMG was focused (**Table 3**). The relative IEMGs of all muscles were significantly increased at 15% compared to 5 and 10% during abduction and internal rotation. In a similar way, the relative IEMGs of all muscles were significantly increased at 10% compared to 3 and 5% during external rotation. Basically, all muscle activities increased with increasing external load during all trials.

2.3.3. Discussion

From the result of internal and external rotation, it was shown that the amount of muscle activities was unequal during isometric contraction on all scapular muscles. Some muscles have high activities, others have low. But the relative EMGs of all muscle were increased with increasing external load, so these muscles which have low activities were also necessary during isometric contraction. I inferred which muscle had high activity from this and previous studies. If the muscle has the same function with the scapular movement being comprised within the shoulder motion, the muscle must have high activity. In particular, internal rotation includes scapular protraction, which is the function of serratus anterior, and external rotation includes scapular retraction, which is the function of middle trapezius. It is just the same as the result of the studies about strengthening scapular muscles. About isometric shoulder abduction task, serratus anterior, upper trapezius, and lower trapezius have relation to scapular upward rotation, so all

	Serratus anterior	Middle trapezius
5%	4.9 ± 2.4	1.4 ±0.300
10%	8.4 ± 4.300 *	1.8 ± 0.600 *
15%	12.8 ± 7.300	2.7 ± 1.300

*:p<0.05

Internal rotation

	Middle trapezius	Serratus anterior
3%	10.5 ± 9.3	1.8 ± 0.800
5%	16.1 ± 12.700 *	2.6 ± 1.400 *
10%	29.6 ± 23.400	4.7 ± 2.700

*:p<0.05

External rotation

	Serratus anterior	Upper trapezius	Lower trapezius
5%	2.6 ± 0.7	2.5 ±1.000	2.4 ± 1.500
10%	3.7 ± 1.500 *	4.0 ± 2.400 *	4.5 ± 3.100 *
15%	5.7 ± 2.600	6.8 ± 3.400	7.6 ± 5.500

*:p<0.05

Abduction

Table 3. The results of relative IEMG.

muscles might have high activities. As can be seen, it suggested that not all scapular muscles have high activity during isometric contraction and the changes in scapular muscle activity by movement direction are analogous to the case of isotonic contraction. So, for example, when we improve the ability of the endurance to the collision in athletes, we have to consider which direction the force is added and predict which muscle is actively higher. When this is done, the good rehabilitation program will be provided to the patients.

Additionally, considering the result of unequal scapular muscle activities, we can infer the mechanism about scapula stability. Generically, the theory that the scapula was stabilized by "fixation to thorax" has been heard. If something is to fix the scapula to the thorax, the scapula needs to be pulled by the same tension from side to side and up and down. Co-contraction with scapular muscle is needed. Scapula does not fix the thorax if the only unilateral scapular muscle has high activity. So, from this study, the scapula is stabilized not by the fixation to thorax, but by individualized scapular muscle activity to counteract the external load. Individualized scapular muscle activity must contribute to maintain the scapular position. In other words, these scapular muscles which have high activities have the function of resisting external load as the agonist at glenohumeral joint. These muscles may be called the agonist at scapulothoracic joint. Scapular muscles may be classified the agonist and the antagonist like other joint muscles. From this study, it is predicted that the agonist at scapulothoracic joint has the function of countering the external load and the antagonist at scapulothoracic joint has the function of adjusting the scapular position.

2.4. The changes of muscle activity on shoulder joint during maximum isometric contraction by the difference of muscle-weakness region

As above, it was suggested that scapular muscle reacts individually and has the function of counteracting the external load. In clinical situation, therapists usually evaluate the scapular stability using the assessment of whether or not scapular downward rotation occurred during shoulder abduction manual muscle testing. And therapists evaluate whether the muscle strength of shoulder abduction is increased with manual fixation against scapular downward rotation (**Figure 9**). From this assessment, therapists calculate the policy about scapular stability. Considering previous studies, it is predicted that we can use this evaluation at all directions as shoulder abduction. And if the patients have the scapula instability, the scapula will be swaying during the test. Wherein, I verified whether or not this phenomenon occurs in the patients with shoulder disease. Additionally, I measured the scapular muscle activities using electromyography during the muscle testing.

2.4.1. Materials and methods

Two patients with shoulder disease participated in this study. One had muscle weakness mainly at glenohumeral joint (Patient A) and the other had muscle weakness mainly at scapulothoracic joint (Patient B). Additionally, a healthy man without shoulder disease was measured and compared to the patients (Subject C). Patient A was affected with dislocated shoulder and dislocation was reduced. The muscle strength is shown in **Figure 10**. On manual muscle testing,

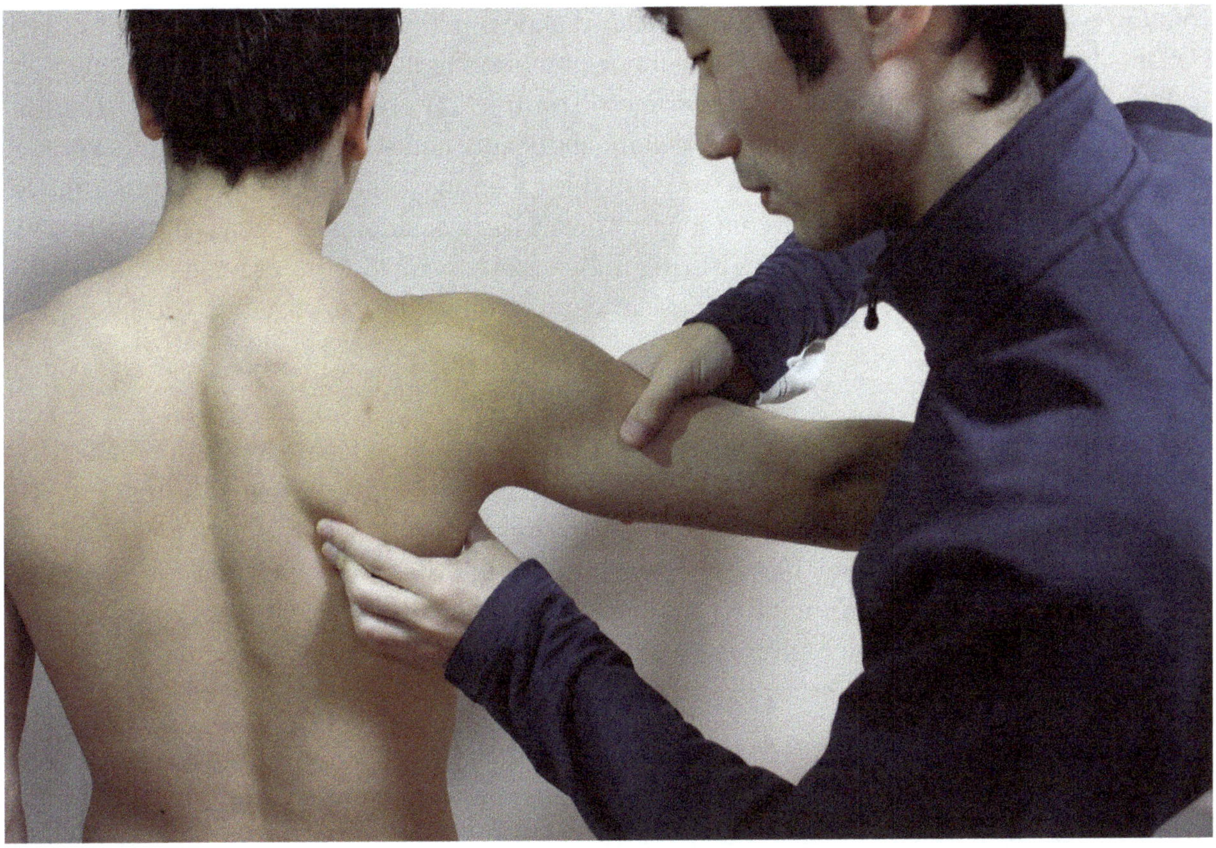

Figure 9. Evaluation about the change of muscle strength by scapular manual fixation. Therapists evaluate whether the muscle strength of shoulder abduction is increased with manual fixation against scapular downward rotation.

scapular protraction and protraction/downward rotation were indicated as level 4, but shoulder external rotation and internal rotation were indicated as level 3. Patient A had muscle weakness mainly at glenohumeral joint. Patient B was affected with humeral head fracture. The muscle strength was that shoulder abduction and external rotation were indicated as level 3 and internal rotation was level 4, but scapular retraction/downward rotation and protraction/upward

Patient A

MMT	Non-affected side	Affected side
Shoulder flexion	5	4
Shoulder abduction	5	4
Shoulder external rotation	5	3
Shoulder internal rotation	5	3
Scapular elevation	5	5
Scapular retraction	5	4
Scapular retraction/ depression	4	4
Scapular protraction/upward rotation	5	4

Patient B

MMT	Non-affected side	Affected side
Shoulder flexion	5	4
Shoulder abduction	5	3
Shoulder external rotation	5	3
Shoulder internal rotation	5	4
Scapular elevation	5	4
Scapular retraction	5	3
Scapular retraction/ depression	5	2
Scapular protraction/upward rotation	5	2

Figure 10. Muscle strength of two patients. Patient A had the muscle weakness at glenohumeral joint and Patient B had the weakness at scapulothoracic joint.

rotation were level 2. Patient B had the muscle weakness mainly at scapulothoracic joint. Two patients had no pain and had comfortable range of motion to measurement. The measurement task was set as three kinds of maximum isometric contraction: shoulder flexion at 90° shoulder flexion, shoulder internal rotation at 0° shoulder abduction, and shoulder external rotation at 0° shoulder abduction. The subjects were measured for the muscle activities and scapular movement during three tasks with external load to break their position slightly. The muscles that were predicted to have high activities during these tasks consulted from previous studies were measured. I assessed the change in the muscle activities when the external load was given.

2.4.2. Results

The result in Subject C, which was healthy man, was shown first. Please look at the raw wave (**Figure 11**). On shoulder flexion, not only just anterior deltoid but also serratus anterior, upper trapezius, middle trapezius, and lower trapezius had high activities that corresponded with the external load. In a way like that, infraspinatus, middle trapezius, and lower trapezius had high activities on external rotation, and pectoralis major and serratus anterior on internal rotation. In other words, the high muscle activities appeared not only at glenohumeral joint but also at scapulothoracic joint by external force.

Next, the result in Patient A, which had the muscle weakness at glenohumeral joint, was shown. On shoulder flexion, the muscle activity of anterior deltoid was increased. But serratus anterior, upper trapezius, middle trapezius, and lower trapezius were not increased like anterior deltoid.

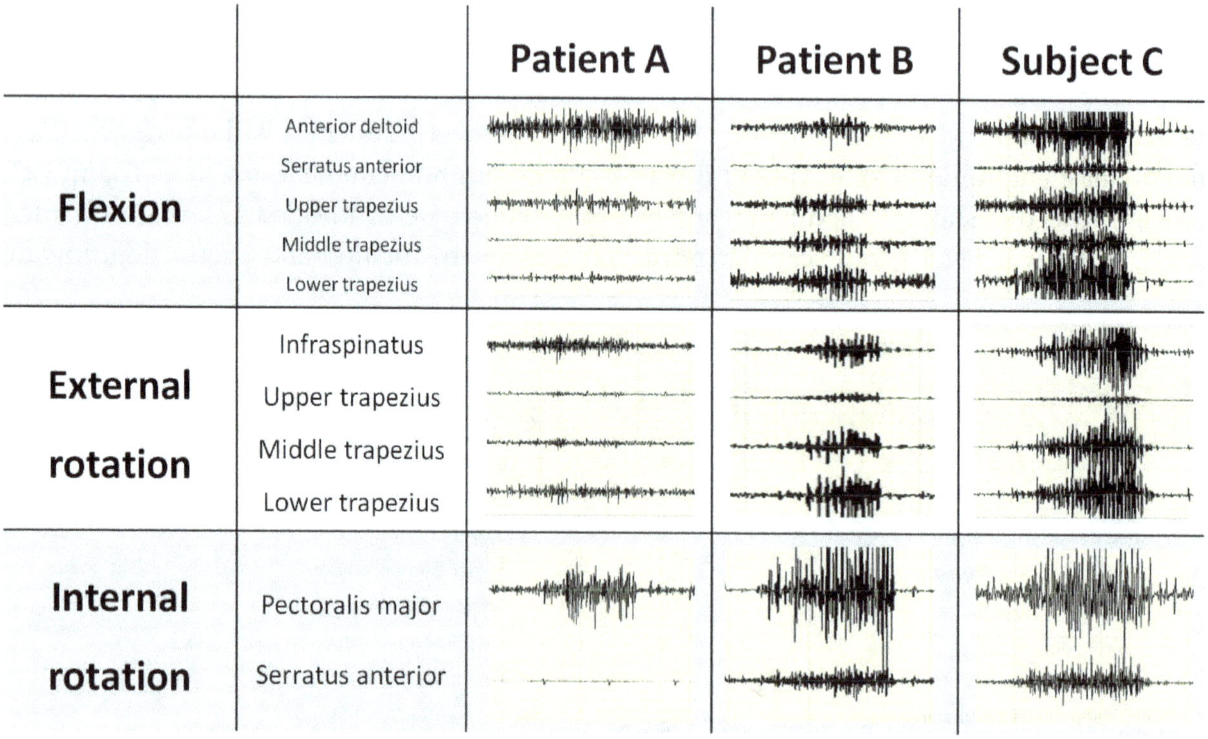

Figure 11. Raw wave in each subject. The result in Patient A was that the muscle activity at glenohumeral joint was high corresponding to the external load but that at scapulothoracic joint was modest in size. In Patient B and Subject C, muscle activities at glenohumeral joint and scapulothoracic joint were increased together.

On external rotation, the muscle activity of infraspinatus was increased in a measure, but those of upper trapezius, middle trapezius, and lower trapezius which were increased in Subject C were not changed. On internal rotation, the muscle activity of pectoralis major was increased by external load and serratus anterior had little change. When taken together, the result was that the muscle activity at glenohumeral joint was high corresponding to the external load but that at scapulothoracic joint was modest in size. From the movie, which was filmed for the scapular stability at the same time, the scapular swaying did not appear by external load.

Lastly, the result in Patient B, which had weakness at scapulothoracic joint, was shown. On shoulder flexion, the muscle activities of anterior deltoid, upper trapezius, middle trapezius, and lower trapezius were increased by external load. On external rotation, not only infraspinatus but also upper trapezius, middle trapezius, and lower trapezius had high activities. On internal rotation, pectoralis major and serratus anterior had high activities. On the whole, muscle activities at glenohumeral joint and scapulothoracic joint were increased together like Subject C. And the movies showed that the scapular movement occurred by external load, the task of flexion; scapular downward rotation, external rotation; scapular protraction, internal rotation; scapular retraction.

2.4.3. Discussion

As can be seen, there were different results between Patient A and Patient B. Now, let us think about these results with the inclusion of previous studies. First, I had indicated that the muscle weakness at scapulothoracic joint causes the muscle weakness on whole shoulder joint. In Patient B, because he had the scapular muscle weakness and the scapular movement occurred by external load, the reason for the whole shoulder muscle weakness will be the weakness at scapulothoracic joint. By the electromyographic wave, scapular muscles had high activities and it is predicted that their activities appeared to resist the external force. So, it is thought that the external force to upper limb reached scapulothoracic joint through glenohumeral joint because the muscle strength at glenohumeral joint was maintained for some level, and the scapular muscles had the activities to resist the external force. But the upper limb was moved causing scapular movement because the muscle strength at scapulothoracic joint was not enough (**Figure 6**). The reason is the weakness at scapulothoracic joint.

On the other hand, in Patient A, it is predicted that the external load did not reach scapulothoracic joint because he had muscle weakness at glenohumeral joint and humerus was moved by external load. So, scapular muscles did not have activities and scapular sway might not appear. The important factor is that the load did not reach scapulothoracic joint.

From this, we will be able to calculate which joints have weakness for improvement by observing the scapular movement during muscle testing with every movement direction not only abduction (**Figure 12**). And it is important that this scapular movement during muscle testing is anticipated movement direction. If the scapular movement appears seriously, we have to provide the exercise for scapular muscle. We can evaluate the responsible region by understanding which muscle should have high activities and analyzing the motion to see the swaying region.

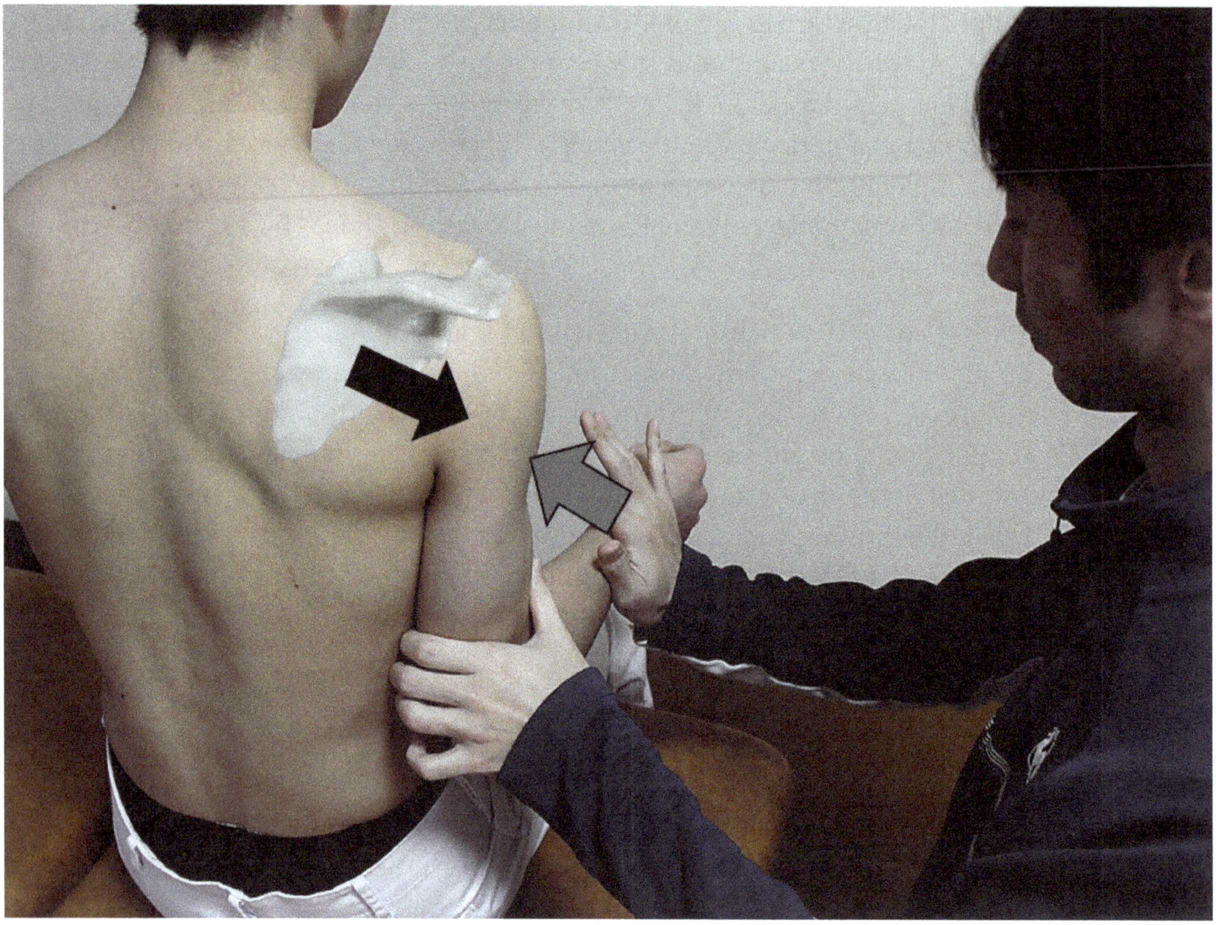

Figure 12. Evaluation regarding scapular movement during muscle testing. We will be able to calculate which joints have weakness for improvement by observing the scapular movement during muscle testing with every movement direction. For example, during muscle testing of external rotation, if scapular protraction appears serious, the responsible region of shoulder muscle weakness will be at scapulothoracic joint.

2.5. The study about the order of activity in scapular muscles

In previous studies, I have shown that there is high activity of scapular muscle and little activity of scapular muscle during shoulder isometric contraction, and these muscles are changed by movement direction. And the muscle strength of scapular muscle influences the muscle strength of whole shoulder joint. From these facts, I have described that we will classify the scapular muscles into the agonist and the antagonist, and the agonist at scapulothoracic joint will have the function of resisting the external load. I thought that if the agonist at scapulothoracic joint has the function of resisting the external load like the agonist at glenohumeral joint, the time of starting the muscle activity of the agonist at scapulothoracic joint will be the same as the agonist at glenohumeral joint. In other words, I thought that the hypothesis about the classification of scapular muscles will be able to be verified by examination in the timing of scapular muscle activity during shoulder motion. However, as the muscle activity of transversus abdominis muscle starts before the motion of upper limb, therapists sometimes regard that scapular stability by scapular muscle activity is established before humeral motion. In this case, scapular muscle activity must start before the muscle activity at glenohumeral joint. Which pattern appeared? So, I examined the order of muscle activities during shoulder motion.

2.5.1. *Materials and methods*

Seventeen healthy men participated in this study. The mean anthropometric characteristics of 15 subjects were age, 25.5 ± 2.2 years; height, 169.4 ± 5.6 cm; and weight, 62.8 ± 7.8 kg. The trials were isometric works against external load in shoulder internal and external rotation at 0° shoulder abduction. And two conditions were set that was and was not informed of the timing of obtaining external load. Then, we measured the time to start activities in the agonist at GHJ and the agonist and antagonist at STJ in these trials.

The subjects were measured in sitting position. A cord of 1.5-kg plumb bob was tightly fastened at the end to the subject's end of the forearm. The cord was set on the level run on the same height-adjusted device. The internal and external rotation directional external load was given to the subject by dropping the plumb bob using trochlear fundamental (**Figure 13**). Electrical switch was set to the subject's forearm and the starting movement was measured by this switch. To measure the muscle activities during the task, electrodes of electromyography were applied to pectoralis major, infraspinatus, serratus anterior, and middle trapezius. The task was tried in two conditions: one was to inform the timing of obtaining external load

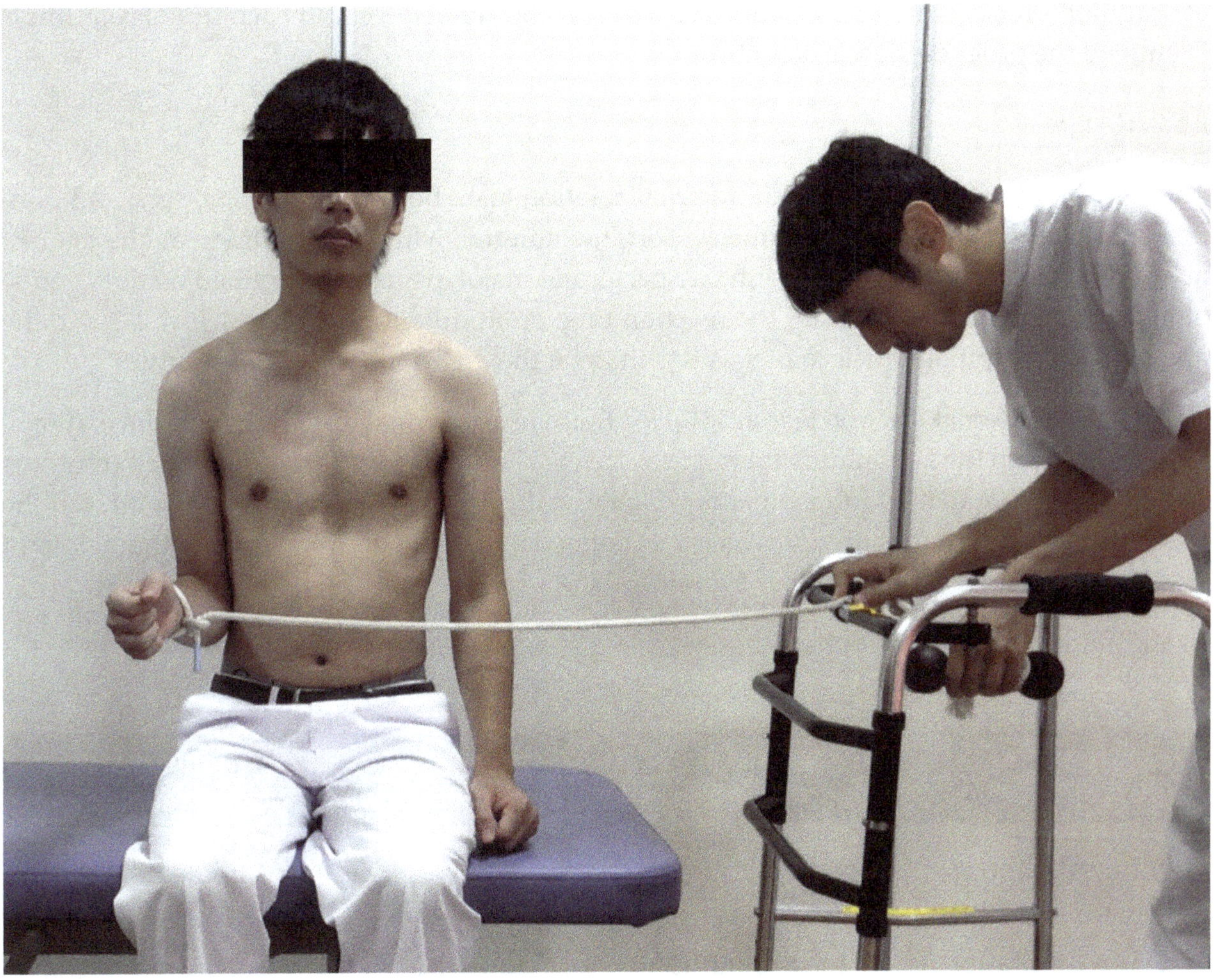

Figure 13. The method of the measurement. A cord of 1.5-kg plumb bob was tightly fastened on the end to the subject's end of the forearm. The cord was set on the level run on the same height-adjusted device. The internal and external rotation directional external load was given to the subject by dropping the plumb bob using trochlear fundamental.

(informational task) and the other was uninformed (non-informational task). The order of the tasks was random.

I calculated the time from starting the motion to starting each muscle activities. Starting the motion was judged by the electrical switch. The definition of starting muscle activity was decided by the time point that recorded amplitude over twice of maximum amplitude in 500 ms before the task. And I classified the measured muscle into the agonist at glenohumeral joint, the agonist at scapulothoracic joint, and the antagonist at scapulothoracic joint on each movement direction (**Figure 14**). First, in shoulder internal rotation at 0° shoulder abduction, the agonist at glenohumeral joint was the pectoralis major. The agonist at scapulothoracic joint was set as the serratus anterior because scapular protraction is by shoulder internal rotation. The antagonist at scapulothoracic joint was defined as the middle trapezius because it has the opposite function of the serratus anterior. The agonist at glenohumeral joint for the external rotation task at 0° shoulder abduction was set as infraspinatus. The middle trapezius was defined as the agonists at scapulothoracic joint because scapular retraction is achieved by external rotation. Serratus anterior was defined as the antagonist at scapulothoracic joint.

The reaction times were compared between the agonist at glenohumeral joint, the agonist at scapulothoracic joint, and the antagonist at scapulothoracic joint in each trial. From this, I examined the order of muscle activities.

2.5.2. Results

The result is shown in **Figure 15** in internal rotation task. Both informational task and non-informational task, the reaction time on serratus anterior which was defined as the agonist at scapulothoracic joint was the same as pectoralis major which was defined as the agonist at glenohumeral joint. However, the reaction time on middle trapezius which was set to the antagonist at scapulothoracic joint was late than on these two muscles significantly.

The result in external rotation was as follows. Both informational task and non-informational task, the reaction time on middle trapezius which was the agonist at scapulothoracic joint was not different from that on infraspinatus which was the agonist at glenohumeral joint. But the reaction time on serratus anterior which was defined as the antagonist at scapulothoracic joint was late than on these two muscles significantly.

In all, similar results were obtained.

	Agonist at glenohumeral joint	Agonist at scapulothoracic joint	Antagonist at scapulothoracic joint
Internal rotation	Pectoralis major	Serratus anterior	Middle trapezius
External rotation	Infraspinatus	Middle trapezius	Serratus anterior

Figure 14. Classification about the agonist and the antagonist. I classified the measured muscle into the agonist at glenohumeral joint, the agonist at scapulothoracic joint, and the antagonist at scapulothoracic joint on each movement direction by scapular movement during the shoulder motion.

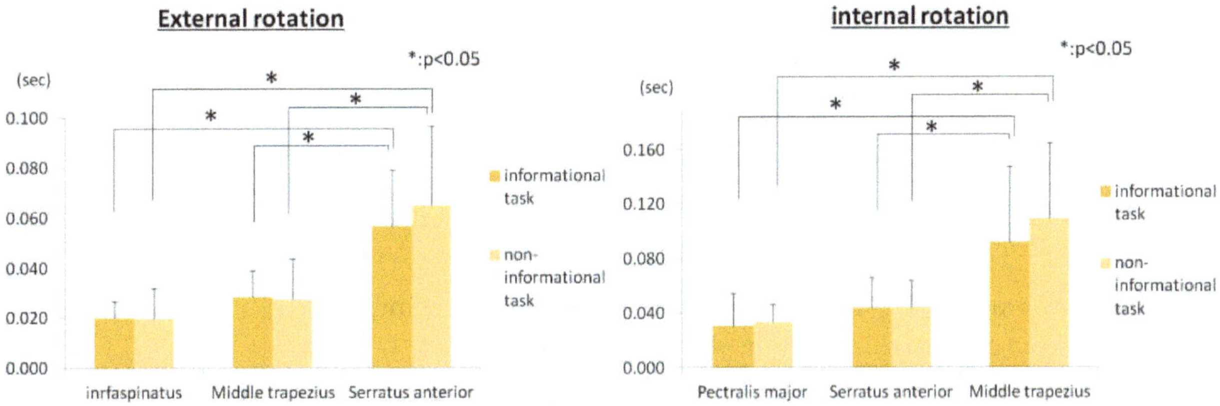

Figure 15. The reaction time of each muscle. The reaction time of the agonist at scapulothoracic joint was the same as that of the agonist at glenohumeral joint. However, the reaction time of the antagonist at scapulothoracic joint was significantly delayed than that of these two muscles.

2.5.3. Discussion

In all trials, the reaction time of the agonist at scapulothoracic joint was the same as that of the agonist at glenohumeral joint. However, the reaction time of the antagonist at scapulothoracic joint was significantly delayed than that of these two muscles.

The study about the relationship between agonist and antagonist was tested a lot for other joints. It is common knowledge that the training for agonist leads to bigger torque at the joint and be able to maintain the joint against stronger external load. On the other hand, regarding antagonist, the muscle activity was examined at the knee, elbow, and glenohumeral joint and the slight muscle activity comes in during isometric, isotonic, and isokinetic contraction [14–16]. And it was known that the muscle activity of antagonist increases on unstable condition at the lower leg. From these facts, it is known that the antagonist has the function about the control of the joint movement caused by agonist and the contribution to the joint stability by co-contraction with agonist [17, 18]. Additionally, Hase et al. reported the result of the measurement about muscle activity at wrist joint during catching of a falling ball dropped on the palm [19]. The maximal muscle activity of the antagonist appeared after that of the agonist slightly and the antagonist had persistent muscle activity before catching. It was concluded that the antagonist will work for the fixation of the joint. Compared to my studies with the previous studies about antagonist on other joints, it was founded that these are some similar points. In my previous studies, the exercise for the agonist at scapulothoracic joint led to an increase in the muscle strength of whole shoulder joint. And the study about the measurement of muscle activities during isometric contraction showed that the antagonist at scapulothoracic joint had slight muscle activity. These results are the same as the other joint studies. Additionally, in this study, the reaction time of the antagonist at scapulothoracic joint was significantly delayed than that of the agonist at glenohumeral joint and scapulothoracic joint. This result has similarity in part as the previous study of wrist joint. By the way, although I did not indicate this report, the same result, the reaction time of the antagonist at scapulothoracic joint was significantly delayed than that of the agonist at glenohumeral joint and scapulothoracic joint, was demonstrated in my study of the task about starting the movement for oneself. As just described, the studies about scapular muscles indicate very similar result to the studies regarding agonist and antagonist at other joints, so we must be able to consider the scapular muscles using the classification as agonist and antagonist. It is conceivable that the agonist at scapulothoracic joint has the function of resisting the external load and the antagonist works for controlling the scapular position.

3. Summary

I had shown some studies about scapular muscles. Summarizing from all studies, we have to discuss the next content during clinical rehabilitation.

First, we do not integrate scapular muscles when thinking about scapular stability. For example, there is the athlete who has poor upper limb ability for endurance to contact by other athlete during sports situation and he/she has scapular instability on these occasions. In this case, we will give him/her the exercise for scapular muscles. However, when the exercise is considered, we have to discuss which muscle especially needs to be strengthened, not gather scapular muscle together. I mean it is important to calculate which direction the external load is absorbed, which direction the athlete have to exert muscle force, and which muscle has the highest muscle activity. The ability for endurance to contact by other athlete must be advanced effectively by strengthening the muscle intensively. We have to consider the impairment using mechanics about scapulothoracic joint.

Next, it is also important that we examine the responsible joint, glenohumeral joint or scapulothoracic joint carefully in every direction when a patient has shoulder muscle weakness. Therapists usually judge this in shoulder flexion and abduction, but we must try in shoulder internal rotation, external rotation, horizontal abduction, and horizontal adduction. The technique of judgment is to observe scapular instability during shoulder muscle testing. Let us check for sure during muscle testing.

Lastly, we have to understand that it is not true that the subject exerts muscle power at glenohumeral joint after scapular stability. The power on shoulder joint is exhibited by working harmoniously with glenohumeral joint and scapulothoracic joint at once. This is very important to think about scapular stability. It is whether scapula stabilizes for external load and weight of the arm. The rehabilitation order that first the scapular position is adjusted and second glenohumeral joint is exercised is not pertinence. Furthermore, in turn, we have to examine the affect for the motion by assessment to glenohumeral joint and scapulothoracic joint at once.

Taking these points into consideration, it should be clear how the scapular is concerned with the motion. From this, the policy will be definitude and we can provide more effective rehabilitation program. Please make good use for clinical reasoning.

Author details

Tomohito Ijiri

Address all correspondence to: tomohito316@hotmail.co.jp

Department of Rehabilitation, Kiba Hospital, Medical Corporation, Juzankai, Osaka, Japan

References

[1] Ludewig PM, Reynolds JF. The association of scapular kinematics and glenohumeral joint pathologies. J Orthop Sports Phys Ther. 2009;**39**:90–104.

[2] Michener LA, Sharma S, Cools AM, Timmons MK. Relative scapular muscle activity ratios are altered in subacromial pain syndrome. J Shoulder Elbow Surg. 2016;**25**:1861–1867.

[3] Cools AM, Witvrouw EE, Declercq GA, Vanderstraeten GG, Cambier DC. Evaluation of isokinetic force production and associated muscle activity in the scapular rotators during a protraction-retraction movement in overhead athletes with impingement symptoms. Br J Sports Med. 2004;**38**:64–68.

[4] Mottram SL. Dynamic stability of the scapula. Man Ther. 1997;**2**(3):123–131.

[5] Ludewig PM, Hoff MS, Osowski EE, Meschke SA, Rundquist PJ. Relative balance of serratus anterior and upper trapezius muscle activity during push-up exercises. Am J Sports Med. 2004;**32**:484–493.

[6] Turuike M, Ellenbecker TS. Serratus anterior and lower trapezius muscle activities during multi-joint isotonic scapular exercises and isometric contractions. J Athl Train. 2015;**50**(266):199–210.

[7] Zhang M, Zhou JJ, Zhang YM, Wang JH, Zhang QY, Chen W. Clinical effectiveness of scapulothoracic joint control training exercises on shoulder joint dysfunction. Cell Biochem Biophys. 2015;**72**:83–87.

[8] Cools AM, Struyf F, De Mey K, Maenhout A, Castelein B, Caqnie B. Rehabilitation of scapular dyskinesis: from the office worker to the elite overhead athlete. Br J Sports Med. 2014;**48**:692–697.

[9] Decker MJ, Hintermeister RA, Faber KJ, Hawkins RJ. Serratus anterior muscle activity during selected rehabilitation exercises. Am J Sports Med. 1999;**27**(6):784–791.

[10] Moseley JB Jr, Jobe FW, Pink M, Perry J, Tibone J. EMG analysis of the scapular muscles during a shoulder rehabilitation program. Am J Sports Med. 1992;**20**:128–134.

[11] Andrews JR, Wilk KE. The athlete's shoulder. America: Churchill Livingstone; 1994. 453–457.

[12] Ekstrom RA, Donatelli RA, Soderberg GL. Surface electromyographic analysis of exercise for the trapezius and serratus anterior muscles. J Orthop Sports Phys Ther. 2003;**33**:247–258.

[13] Delagi EF, Perotto A. Anatomic guide for the electromyographer—the limbs. Springfield: Thomas; 1980.

[14] Bazzucchi I, Sbriccoli P, Marzattinocci G, Felici F. Coactivation of the elbow antagonist muscles is not affected by the speed of movement in isokinetic exercise. Muscle Nerve. 2006;**33**(2):191–199.

[15] Kronberg M, Németh G, Broström LA. Muscle activity and coordination in the normal shoulder. An electromyographic study. Clin Orthop Relat Res. 1990;**257**:76–85.

[16] Remaud A, Cornu C, Guével A. Agonist muscle activity and antagonist muscle co-activity levels during standardized isotonic and isokinetic knee extensions. J Electromyogr Kinesiol. 2009;**19**(3):449–458.

[17] Humphrey DR, Reed DJ. Separate cortical systems for control of joint movement and joint stiffness: reciprocal activation and coactivation of antagonist muscles. Adv Neurol. 1983;**39**:347–372.

[18] Bazzucchi I, Riccio ME, Felici F. Tennis players show a lower coactivation of the elbow antagonist muscles during isokinetic exercises. J Electromyogr Kinesiol. 2008;**18**(5): 752–759.

[19] Hase K. Motor control of the forearm muscles during catching of a falling ball. Jpn J Rehabil Med. 1997;**34**:218–225.

11

Manual Lymphatic Drainage in the Treatment of Chronic Venous Disease

Rute S.S. Crisóstomo and
Paulo A.S. Armada-da-Silva

Additional information is available at the end of the chapter

Abstract

Chronic venous disease (CVD) is a chronic condition that is associated with venous hypertension, vein's valves damage, venous obstruction, and calf muscle pump impairment. This blood circulatory condition is also characterized by important inflammatory changes affecting the skin, the subcutaneous tissue and the muscles, which are probably triggered by blood stasis and venous edema. With disease progression, severe ulcerative skin damage might occur, which when present represent the more severe stage of this condition. CVD has a significant economic, social and health impact, mostly due to raised morbidity and chronicity.

The treatment of patients with CVD might focus on both the symptoms and secondary changes of the disease, such as edema, skin and subcutaneous changes or ulcers. Usually, initial treatment of CVD patients involves a non-invasive, conservative treatment to reduce symptoms, treat secondary changes, and help prevent the development of secondary complications and the progression of the disease. Complementary, some interventional or surgical treatments can be undertaken.

There are several conservative treatments to treat and prevent complications associated with CVD that have been described in the literature, like manual lymphatic drainage (MLD) and compression, physical exercise, intermittent pneumatic pressure, kinesio taping, electrical muscle stimulation, transcutaneous electrical nerve stimulation, hydrotherapy, and health education. Most of these techniques are complementary to compression therapy or pharmacological treatment.

This chapter will address the role of physical therapists in the management of CVD. The chapter will begin by reviewing the basic physiopathology of CVD, including the role of calf muscle pump. The CEAP classification system and the chronic venous severity score will be presented, as these are main tools for clinical assessment of CVD severity. In the remainder of the chapter will address the physiological effects and recommendations for treating CVD of MLD, based on our clinical experience and own research.

Keywords: chronic venous disease, edema, calf muscle pump, manual lymphatic drainage

1. Introduction

The term chronic venous disease (CVD) has been used to describe morphological and functional abnormalities of the venous system of extended duration that are manifested themselves by symptoms and/or signs that indicate the need for evaluation and care by health professionals [1].

Usually, symptoms of leg heaviness, fatigue, and pain are the first complaints referred by patients, which together with varicose veins are present both in mild and severe cases of CVD. These complaints combined with structural changes in superficial, visible veins strongly contribute to a negative self-esteem that also characterizes this disease [2–8]. The diminished health-related quality of life (HRQL) seen in CVD is well studied [2, 8–10]. This negative impact is so important that the previous view of this condition as an aesthetic problem has been abandoned for years.

The socioeconomic burden of CVD is very high. The indirect costs are substantial and are associated with the symptoms, functional impairment, emotional disturbances and negative impact in HRQL [11]. The direct costs of CVD treatment are almost entirely related to its high prevalence, morbidity, and chronicity [11, 12]. In developed countries, around 1–3% of the health costs are due to CVD [13]. However, when patients with less severe stages of the disease are diagnosed and treated early, the physiopathology course of the disease can be prevented or even receded [14].

The severity of CVD is nowadays evaluated based on a multifactorial concept of the disease and using the standardized CEAP (Clinical Etiological, Anatomical and Pathological) classification system. Having a good knowledge of this system is very important to all physical therapist and it is important that health professionals use the same nomenclature so that CVD severity can be accurately assessed and the best treatment delivered [15].

The treatment of patients with CVD might focus on both the symptoms and secondary changes of the disease, such as edema, skin and subcutaneous changes or ulcers. Usually, initial treatment of CVD patients involves a non-invasive, conservative treatment to reduce symptoms, treat secondary changes, and help prevent the development of secondary complications and the progression of the disease. Complementary, some interventional or surgical treatments can be undertaken [15].

Manual lymphatic drainage (MLD) is a low-pressure form of skin-stretching massage, described as a conservative treatment for CVD [16] and as a coadjutant of other treatments, like stockings and surgery [17, 18]. This technique has been proposed for the treatment of venous lymphedema associated to CVD [19, 20], before CVD surgery, or to relief symptoms [17, 18, 21]. It is suggested by the literature that this physical therapy technique should be applied taking into account venous anatomy and that it should increase deep and venous flow [22, 23]. Despite controversial evidence regarding the ability of MLD to reduce edema or lymphedema, this technique when associated with other treatments, the so-called "lymphatic decongestive therapy", that also includes compression, exercise, and education, may have an important role for improving health and functional status in patients with edema associated to sport injury or related to breast cancer surgery, just to mention two common situations [21, 24–26].

This chapter will address the role of physical therapists in the management of CVD. The chapter will begin by reviewing the basic physiopathology of CVD, including the role of calf muscle pump. The CEAP classification system and the chronic venous severity score will be presented, as these are main tools for clinical assessment of CVD severity. In the remainder of the chapter, we will address the physiological effects of MLD on venous circulation and the recommendations for its use in treating CVD.

2. Health and social impact of CVD

2.1. Epidemiology

Chronic venous insufficiency, represents the most severe cases of CVD, and its physiopathology is associated with venous hypertension, vein valve damage, venous obstruction, calf muscle pump impairment, inflammation of tissues (skin, subcutaneous tissue, and muscle) and veins, alteration of veins morphology and function. This disease is characterized by abnormal venous reflux, venous edema, and changes of the skin and subcutaneous tissue, with ulcer representing the most severe stage of this condition, and is classified between C_0 (no signs) and C_6 (active ulcer) CEAP classes [13, 27–32]. Despite some controversies, CVD might exist without the presence of signs [3, 13, 33].

The estimated prevalence of CVD varies according to its severity, being around 10, 9, 1.5, and 0.5% for CEAP clinical levels C_3 (venous edema), C_4 (hyperpigmentation or eczema, lipodermatosclerosis, or atrophie blanche), C_5 (healed venous ulcer), and C_6 (active venous ulcer), respectively [33]. The more advanced stages of venous disease, (C_3–C_6), appear to affect about 5% of the population [1]. Milder CVD conditions, like telangiectasiae and reticular veins (C1 class), have been reported to affect up to 80% of the population, while the incidence of varicose veins (C2 class) has been reported as ranging from 20% to 64% [1].

Despite its frequency in the population, the prevalence of CVD is still underestimated. Epidemiological data estimate a wide range of CVD prevalence, varying between 1-17% in men and 1-40% in women [34]. In the USA alone, approximately 2.5 million people suffer from CVD [2]. Variation in estimations of CVD prevalence are likely explained by differences in gender, age, ethnic group, risk factors and variations in diagnostic criteria and methods [1, 34]. A study where 91545 participants were evaluated, found a CVD prevalence of 83.6%, with 63.9% of the subjects classified as C1-C6, and 19.7% as C0. Regarding CVD prevalence according to gender, this study showed higher number of men in C0 class, higher number of women in C1-C3 classes and equal number of men and women in the more severe groups (C4-C6 class) [35]. Considering only the cases of varicose veins (C2), prevalence has been shown to vary in the range 7-40% in men and 25-32% in women [34].

2.2. Functional and HRQL implications of CVD

Patients with CVD display impaired functional capacity [2, 36] and diminished HRQL [9, 10, 37, 38]. The severity of CVD, HRQL scores, the clinical signs, and venous ultrasound findings of the disease are usually correlated [39].

The impact of CVD on HRQL is primarily seen in the physical items and in the emotional domain, but in its severest stages (presence of venous ulcers) the mental dimension might also become involved [9]. The impact of severe CVD in HRQL is similar to that of other chronic diseases, such as diabetes, cancer, chronic pulmonary disease, and heart failure [9].

Most of chronic leg ulcers are venous in origin [40]. Patients with venous ulcer present severe pain, which is in relationship with impaired tissue healing ability, diminished HRQL, lowered self-esteem, and poor social interactions [2]. The psychological effects of CVD may be not strictly related with ulceration itself but can else be associated with the symptoms caused by this type of wound (80.5-69.4%), altered appearance and esthetical concerns (66.7%), lack of sleep (66.6%), functional impairment (58.3%), and disappointment with treatment outcomes (50%) [2]. Also, patients with uncomplicated varicose veins often have severe symptoms that adversely affect their HRQL, irrespectively of the severity of the disease, refuting the view that this disease is mostly an aesthetic problem [8]. Estimates indicate that near 30% of patients with symptomatic varicose veins, who may not have had their clinical venous condition diagnosed or treated, display symptoms suggestive of a depressive illness [41].

In this disease, 49% of men and 62% of women have symptoms related to CVD [33], like pain, itching, tingling, cramps, restless legs, swelling, heaviness, and fatigue [3, 8]. A recent survey reveals that 14.9% of the general Greek population refers symptoms and/or present signs related to CVD [42].

The number of symptoms reported by patients with CVD varies but are usually several [4, 5, 8]. Importantly, the number and severity of symptoms are not strictly related to CVD severity and, sometimes, strong symptoms, and those that have the largest impact on HRQL, are present in less severe cases [8]. Nevertheless, despite possible indication for surgery, some studies suggest that the majority of the symptoms in patients with varicose veins are nonvenous related [5]. Indeed, it seems very difficult to separate venous from nonvenous causes of symptoms in CVD [6].

Several studies show the presence of both neuropathic and nociceptive pain in patients with CVD [4, 43]. Nevertheless, patients with CVD may present other comorbidities that make it difficult to isolate the CVD-related pain [43, 44].

Approximately one-third of people with CVD report to be a burden going out of home and participating in social events, and that they avoid wearing clothes exposing their legs or going on vacations to very warm places [42]. According to self-reports, functional status is diminished in these patients [36, 39] also because of some physical dysfunctions, like abnormalities in gait [45], impaired balance, peripheral neuropathy [43, 46] weak leg muscles (plantar flexion and dorsiflexion muscles) [29, 30, 45], or diminished ankle range of motion [10, 30, 47]. These dysfunctions are also associated with impaired muscle pump function in the lower extremity [43], an important risk factor for venous ulceration [48].

2.3. Socioeconomic impact of CVD

Severe CVD has a significant economic impact, mostly due to raised morbidity. Over the last decade, neither CVD-associated and inflation-adjusted mean hospital charge, nor length of hospital stay decreased, possibly as a result of poor advancements in prevention and treatment of this disease [49]. It is estimated that 4.6 million of working days per year are lost as a result of CVD [40]. Painful leg ulcers, the odor, the dressing, the frequent need for treatment, with their associated restrictions and social isolation result in a heavy psychosocial burden [50]. In severe CVD, venous ulcers require wound care, compression, chemical and mechanical debridement, and, in frequent cases, antibiotic therapy [49]. While ulcer treatment is usually done in outpatient settings, in some particularly critical situations it may require hospitalization [40]. Western European countries spend 1.5-2% of their annual health budget in the treatment of this disease [51]. The economic burden is not just associated with clinical visits and outpatient treatments, but also with travel time, loss of work hours for patients and family, and physiological impairment related to analgesic and antibiotic use [49]. Limb amputation is a radical outcome of this disease, although in many of cases these are also related to comorbidities, for instance diabetes and arterial vascular disease [49]. Other important complications, such as hemorrhage, thrombosis and pulmonary embolism, also compound the unhealthy profile of these patients [42]. Deep venous thrombosis may cause chronic conditions like post-thrombotic syndrome and CVD, increasing the costs of the treatment [49]. Preventing deep venous thrombosis and complications is one of the most important aims for reducing socio-economic burden associated to CVD [49].

The chronic nature of the problem results in long-term costs and the frequent recurrences, together with the poor effectiveness of current treatments, further expand the cost of this disease [40].

Despite its cost, the efficacy of the pharmacological treatment of CVD is usually poor, and should be combined with other strategies, such as the use of elastic garment compression [33]. Similar procedures are recommended following surgery and sclerotherapy, in which cases post-operative compression therapy and health education are crucial for treatment success

[42, 52]. There are several risk factors associated with CVD that patients should be informed of by the health professionals, like the use of hormonal contraceptives by women, daily routines (sitting or standing), pregnancy, age, obesity and heredity factors (i.e., family history) [1, 37, 42, 49, 53]. Also important, advice regarding behavioral changes, engaging in so-called venous exercises and the proper use of the health care services, should be offered to CVD patients [42]. Getting the right advice from health care professionals is an important measure for preventing and managing CVD [42].

Because of the wide spectrum of factors that cause functional impairment in these patients and the high costs of treatment [2, 3, 8], the prevention of CVD by educational and prophylactic interventions has been shown to be clinically cost-effective, by avoiding disease progression to the last stages [49, 54].

3. Pathophysiology of CDV

Near 60% of blood volume flows is in the venous system, the majority of it in the lower limbs and in the cutaneous circulation, and near 20-25% occupies the splanchnic circulation [55]. The venous system returns the blood to the heart and is a low-pressure, slow-velocity, large-volume and low-resistance vascular system [1]. Venous return results from the interaction of diverse mechanisms, like a central pump (respiratory cycle and heart), a pressure gradient, a peripheral venous pump, and veins valvular system [43]. The venous volume in the lower limb is the result of the interaction between these mechanisms and reflects the balance between blood inflow and outflow [1].

CVD is caused by venous hypertension, valvular insufficiency, and/or blood reflux [56–58]. Venous hypertension might be accompanied by outflow obstruction [57] and can affect the superficial, perforator, and deep veins [3, 58]. Insufficient lymphatic drainage or a dysfunction of calf muscle pump are very often associated with this disease [59]. Venous hypertension is related to structural (veins and valves), hemodynamic (obstruction, reflux, stasis), biomechanical (calf muscle pump strength and ankle range of motion) and biochemical factors (leucocyte-endothelial process inflammation) [57, 58].

The exact mechanisms behind the development of CVD are not clear yet [57, 60]. The major hypothetical sequence of events places venous hypertension as the trigger, causing inflammation of the veins' wall and of vein valves, with inflammation, as the condition aggravates, spreading to the skin and the muscles, causing dermal changes, like hyperpigmentation, subcutaneous tissue fibrosis (lipodermatosclerosis), and tissue necrosis and ulceration [20, 51, 57, 59] in the most severe cases [60].

Venous obstruction occurs because of the triad: blood stasis, changes in the vessel wall, and hypercoagulability [61]. This may occur as a phlebitis (obstructions of superficial venous system) or as deep venous thrombosis (obstructions of deep venous system), and can be diagnosed as acute or chronic [12]. The acute deep venous thrombosis may cause nociceptive pain, swelling and tenderness, and both phlebitis and deep venous thrombosis must be confirmed by venous ultrasonography [57]. The ensuing venous hypertension then opposes venous return, leading to luminal hypoxemia and vein wall distension, which impairs perfusion and causes endothelial hypoxia and leukocyte invasion of the vein's media [61]. A progressive remodeling process is then triggered consisting of hypoxemia-related venous/capillary wall injury, leukocytes accumulation and adhesion, progressive blockage of capillary blood flow, and ongoing damage of subcutaneous tissues and skin (lipodermosclerosis and skin ulceration) [62].

Usually, venous reflux and obstruction occur together [57]. Following obstruction, venous recanalization occurs and blood flow through the vein is restored [61]. However, lysis of the clot or thrombus is usually only partial and the residual thrombus might undergo fibrosis that may completely obstruct the lumen of the vein, for example involving leaflets [61]. Collateral blood circulation may develop in these cases and obstruction may be overcome [57]. Sometimes, calf perforating veins may be an important collateral venous path when the popliteal vein is involved, causing CVD of a secondary etiology [57].

The initial hypertension in CVD may also be caused by valvular incompetence alone [60]. Varicose veins may result from endothelial changes (reduced elastin and smooth muscle content, together with increased collagen) associated with hypoxia, causing weakened venous tone [60]. Other changes include downregulated apoptosis [63], decrease energy for cell metabolism and increased lysossomal activity [64].

3.1. Etiology and anatomical location of CVD

The etiology of CVD can be described as primary, secondary (post-thrombosis) or congenital [13]. Although reflux is the major hemodynamic alteration in CVD, in secondary venous disease most of the cases present a mix of reflux and obstruction [58]. It seems that 80% of cases of CVD have a secondary etiology of post-thrombotic pathology, and 20% are of primary cause, as a result of valvular incompetence [57].

In the superficial system, the insufficiency is most often the result of a primary preexisting weakness in the vessel wall or valve, as a consequence of a direct injury, excessive venous distention caused by hormonal effects or high hydrostatic pressure, or secondary to venous obstruction (i.e., phlebitis) [33, 59, 65, 66]. Failure in valve functioning (superficial veins) may increase superficial venous pressure, resulting in venous dilatation and varicose veins [59]. Although the primary mechanism of valvular incompetence in superficial veins is not fully known [57], it appears that first changes in the mechanical properties of the vein wall caused by increased collagen content and decreased amount of elastin and smooth muscle, leading to vessel enlargement occur and next, valvular insufficiency develops [57].

The perforating veins can also become insufficient by primary incompetence of vein valves or secondary to venous obstruction [67]. In these cases, there is reflux from deep to superficial venous system: with valve incompetence the reflux to saphenous veins may allow the re-entry of venous blood to the deep venous system [67]. In the case of secondary incompetence, the high intravascular pressures are transmitted to superficial veins, causing the enlargement of dermal capillaries and increasing filtration to the interstitial space [57, 67].

Deep veins insufficiency has been suggested to be the consequence of deep veins thrombosis in the majority of cases, i.e., from secondary etiology [59]. However, primary deep venous incompetence is also common (8-22% of the cases [12]) but is usually compensated by a strong muscle [12, 57]. It seems that outflow obstruction and reflux caused by valve damage may cause deep vein thrombosis and these two alterations together increase the probability of the development of post-thrombotic syndrome [12, 61].

Deep venous thrombosis may also occur because of an intrinsic venous process, such as a previous deep venous thrombosis episode with inadequate recanalization or venous stenosis, or because of extrinsic compression, as in May-Thurner syndrome [66]. Also, it can be caused by venous agenesis, such as in the Klippel-Trenaunay syndrome, trauma, surgical mishap, and tumors [57].

Congenital CVD, in which case the condition is already present at birth, also exist. However, this might be recognized only later in life, such as in the cases of the Klippel-Trenaunay (varicosities and venous malformations, capillary malformation, and limb hypertrophy) [33] and Parkes-Weber (venous and lymphatic malformations, capillary malformations, and arteriovenous fistulas) syndromes [66].

4. Venous edema and Lymphedema

CVD is the most common cause of edema with age 50 and over [68]. The venous edema is a very common clinical manifestation of CVD, particularly in C3 to C6 classes [68–72]. The chronic venous edema may blunt the metabolic and immunological capacity of tissues, thus contributing to the risk of venous ulcer [72]. Venous edema occurs when there is an imbalance between vascular filtration and reabsorption and lymphatic reabsorption [19]. About 90% of capillary filtration (proteins, plasma, and other components) is reabsorbed back to the blood, and the remaining 10% is reabsorbed by the lymphatic circulation [20, 73]. In CVD, blood filtration is increased due to the higher intravascular hydrostatic pressure and raised endothelial permeability due to inflammation [19, 73]. In these conditions, venous edema may occur [19, 20]. This is a pitting edema that gets worse through the day and improves during sleeping because of the lying position and leg elevation. Usually, this edema is accompanied by venous symptoms and signs [19, 20]. Clinically, venous edema is perceived as an increase in fluid volume of the skin and subcutaneous tissue, characteristically diminished by pressure [13]. Venous edema usually occurs around the ankle region, but may extend to the leg and foot [13].

The principal physiological function of the lymphatic circulation is to guarantee homeostasis between the vascular and interstitial fluid compartments [74] and this requires that the lymphatic system compensates the excessive blood filtration at the blood capillary level [19]. Any failure in this process will result in accumulation of a protein rich fluid in the interstitial space, which is associated with an inflammatory reaction, fibrosis, overgrowth of adipose and connective tissue, and other symptoms that characterize the lymphedema [74]. There is some evidence of lymphatic failure in venous disease. For example, studies with lymphoscintigraphy, reveal that in post thrombotic syndrome the subfascial lymphatic drainage is reduced that may explain edema and lipodermatoesclerosis seen in this situations. Also, patients with ulcer have reduced lymphatic drainage, suggesting that lymphedema is a contributing factor to ulceration [19]. Approximately 20- 30% of individuals with CDV have mix edema (with venous and lymphatic component), because of fluid overload or recurrent cellulitis [70].

Based on the cause, the lymphedema may be classified as primary (congenital or hereditary) and secondary (acquire) forms [74]. Over one third of patients with CVD will have secondary lymphatic dysfunction but when edema is present in these patients, there is the tendency to misdiagnosis it as primary lymphedema [20].

When edema is at the dorsum of the foot, it is associated to squaring of the toes, thick skin, and is of non-pitting edema type [33]. In these cases, it is assumed that a lymphatic compromise exists [33]. The lymphatic circulation may compensate for the excessive filtration, but lymph vessels also suffer damaged with time (microlymphoangiopathy), because of chronic inflammation and accompanying subcutaneous and skin lesions [20, 66]. Therefore, venous edema becomes compound with signs of lymphedema, with non-pitting edema and with hyperkeratosis, papillomatosis, most in retro and post malleolar regions an in the lateral border of the foot [19]. Clinically, this secondary lymphedema may decrease with limb elevation initially, but with time patients will refer aggravation of swelling in the morning and after the night sleep because an increased osmotic pressure in the interstitial space caused by protein blood extravasation [19].

5. Muscle Pump Function and dysfunction

The venous return from the periphery to the heart via the venous system is linked to the action of a central pump (heart and respiratory cycle), periphery venous pump, a pressure gradient, and competent veins and/or venous valves [43, 75].

The muscle pump refers to the hemodynamics effect of limb muscles contractions and ambulation on venous circulation, which is twofold: (I) to enhance venous return from the lower extremity, and (II) to stimulate local blood flow and raise muscle perfusion during muscle contractile activity [43, 57]. The calf muscle pump has an important role for the effective venous return and relies on dynamic interaction between the ankle joint, muscle fascia, muscles of the calf and venous valves [43, 57].

During muscle contractions, the venous blood is forced in direction to the heart and the valves prevent reflux during relaxation [27, 48, 76]. As deep veins are tethered to surrounding tissues, muscle relaxation causes the veins to open, lead to a sudden drop in pressure within these vessels [58, 77, 78]. The large pressure gradient caused by the drop in deep veins hydrostatic pressure enhances blood flow from superficial to deep veins trough perforator veins, decreasing superficial venous pressure and enhances arterial inflow [43, 57].

The basic concept of muscle pump operation is that the steep increase in intramuscular pressure that accompanies contraction compresses the deep inner muscle veins and veins in the nearby inter-compartmental spaces, expressing the blood across the unidirectional vein valves. During muscle relaxation, intravascular pressure drops but venous blood backflow is prevented by the rapid closure of vein valves. Vein walls are tethered to the surrounding muscles and, therefore, veins are forced to open during muscle relaxation, resulting in large dropping of hydrostatic pressure inside the deep veins, causing aspiration of the blood flowing the superficial system through the perforator veins. The decreased venous pressure due to the muscle pump action also raises perfusion pressure, thus leading to an increase in blood flow across the limb. Despite the simplicity of this model, the efficacy of the muscle pump relies on multiple factors and shows wide variation even among people free from venous dysfunction [79].

Ambulatory venous pressure (AVP) and air plethysmography are gold standard methods for evaluating muscle pump function (usually the foot and calf pumps together) [80, 81]. For ambulatory venous pressure, the conventional procedure measures the intravascular hydrostatic pressure inside a dorsal foot vein, which is then taken as proxy of the pressure in the veins of the lower extremity. The percentage decrease in AVP shows large variability even in healthy control subjects. In a group of CVI participants, AVP decreased by approximately 75% at the end of ten tiptoe exercise compared to basal values, with no differences in the magnitude of AVP decrease between people with different CVI severities [80]. However, compared to healthy groups (CEAP C0 class), CVI groups show a percentage AVP decrease that on average is only approximately 35% in CEAP classes C4…C5, a value that is half of that for participants in C0 class [79]. Surely, the percentage AVP decrease plus the basal venous hydrostatic pressure at foot level determine the ambulatory drop in hydrostatic pressure in dorsal foot veins. In healthy people, the large percentage fall in AVP combines with normal basal hydrostatic venous pressure, so that in such cases mean AVP lowers to around 30 mmHg, contrasting with mean AVP values >55 mmHg in C4-C6 clinical groups [79]. The AVP pressure has a fairly good relationship with venous incompetence, with the risk of ulceration increasing linearly with ambulatory venous hypertension. According to Nicolaides et al. [82], in a cohort of 220 CVI patients the incidence of venous-related ulcers was 0% when AVP levels were <30 mmHg and attained 100% with AVP >90 mmHg.

The magnitude of decrease in AVP is determined by the amount of blood expressed by the muscular contractions but also by the rate of refilling. The time taken to elevate the pressure back to 90% of basal standing levels, a standard measure of recovery time (RT90), is negatively correlated with venous insufficiency severity, being on average >20 s in healthy people and in those with mild venous disease, lowering to approximately 2 s in severe clinical cases [79, 80]. Like for AVP, RT90 values are also predictive of the risk of ulceration [79]. Data obtained with air plethysmography also confirms the presence of muscle pump deficiency in CVI. Standard measures of air plethysmography include the ejection fraction, the venous filling index to 90% of the basal volume, the residual volume fraction, and the venous volume [80, 83][9,12].

These muscle pump function effects have the potential to alleviate symptoms and counteract disability associated with chronic venous disease. The action of the muscle pump in moving venous blood centrally is well described and relies on an imbricate relationship between anatomical and biophysical/physiological factors of at least three separate muscle pumps: the foot, the calf, and the thigh muscle pumps thigh [57, 84]. The calf pump is the most important of the three, as a result of its larger capacitance and highest pressure-generating ability. Together, the foot, calf, and thigh muscle pumps assure near 90% of the venous return in the deep venous system of the leg [85].

5.1. Thigh muscle pump

The calf muscles, and possibly the thigh muscles, act as a pump, also called as "peripheral heart", which can generate pressures of up to 300 mm Hg during exercise [86]. Nevertheless, it has been suggested that thigh muscle pump has a minor effect in venous return, compared to calf muscle pump [43, 57, 84].

The thigh muscle pump may be separated in a posterior division that includes mostly the semimembranous muscle, and an anterior division made up by veins from the quadriceps femoris muscle [32]. The veins inside the semimembranous muscle form longitudinal plexus that are connected in the lower part of the muscle with the popliteal vein and with the deep femoral vein upwards. The quadriceps femoris' veins drain into a large trunk that often join the deep femoral vein to end into the common femoral vein near the root of the thigh. The venous valves of thigh veins may not be entirely competent thus allowing variations in the volume of the thigh venous reservoir to occur with posture changes [84].

5.2. Calf muscle pump

The calf muscle pump is in sequence with the foot pump is the most important muscle pump in the human circulatory system [27, 87]. The calf muscle pump is associated with the strong triceps surae muscle and can be separated in two units: a first unit that includes the soleus muscle (leg pump) and its veins, and a second unit situated in the upper leg region and composed by the gastrocnemius muscle and respective veins (popliteal pump) [88]. The veins in the soleus are organized in a lateral larger group and in a medial one. The lateral veins are larger, run vertically and drain into the fibular veins near the superior border of the soleus muscle. The majority of the medial veins drain horizontally into the posterior tibial veins at different heights of the leg but few course vertically and laterally to join the fibular veins. The gastrocnemius veins take their origin from the calf perforators at the lower part of the muscle then giving origin to a number of pedicles that run upwards through the calf to terminate in a single collector draining into the popliteal vein. Through this collector the gastrocnemius pump powerfully ejects the blood into the popliteal vein, and anatomical variations in this collector are linked to differences in calf pump efficacy [88]. Calf muscles contraction can elevate the pressure to approximately 140 mm Hg and increase venous blood flow through the popliteal and the femoral veins [32]. In competent veins, the centrifugal component during muscle relaxation lasts approximately 200 to 300 milliseconds and represents the physiological reflux, in incompetent veins the duration exceeds 500 milliseconds [32].

Less efficient calf muscle pump function (CMPF) (involving especially the gastrocnemius and soleus muscles) has also been related with muscle inflammation, reduced muscle oxygen supply, muscle necrosis, myofibril atrophy (muscle fibers type I and II) and muscle denervation [28, 29]. A study by Araki et al. [89] concluded that venous insufficiency cannot fully explain venous ulceration, pointing to deficient calf muscle pump as a primary factor in CVD-related skin and tissue damage. Several studies show that early treatment, by exercising the muscle pump, can prevent the most severe forms of CVD [14, 90]. The important role of CMPF on the progression of CVD is well established, but in many individual cases impaired calf pump function may go undetected until most severe changes become evident [91]. Therefore, assessable, accurate and non-invasive methods to evaluate CMPF are needed [30, 59, 90–92].

5.3. Foot muscle pump

The deep venous system of the foot forms a venous plexus that is composed by a lateral vein, a medial vein, and a deep plantar arch. The lateral and medial plantar veins are usually doubled and course either intramuscularly or in between the plantar muscles from a lateral position distally to a medial position near the ankle, where they drain into the paired posterior tibial veins [93]. The deep plantar arch and the lateral and medial plantar veins receive blood from superficial veins located in the sole of the foot and from the metatarsal veins [85, 93]. The plantar deep venous system is connected with the superficial veins on the dorsum of the foot via several perforator veins. The link between these two venous systems is specially well developed between the medial plantar vein and the medial marginal vein , forming what has been named the "medial functional unit", which possesses the unique feature of blood flow being directed from deep to superficial vessels [85, 94].

The physiology of the foot pump is still not totally clear. The anatomical design of the deep plantar system, characterized by the presence of paired veins flanking an artery and joined together by connective tissue, and by the close relation between these veins, the plantar muscles and the metatarsophalangeal joints, is well suited to enhance venous blood flow during weight bearing and ambulation. These imply that the foot pump expels the blood through a double mechanism: contact of the foot with the ground, resulting in extension of the tarsal arch and metatarsophalangeal joints associated with compression of the deep veins and the calcaneous plexus, and by contraction of the plantar muscles surrounding the blood reservoir of the deep venous system [88, 93–95]. The foot pump empties during the stance phase of the gait, as a result of weight-bearing, and pushing off action, and refills during the swing phase, when the foot is cleared from ground contact. Through its mechanisms, this pump moves 25–30 mL of blood, equal to the capacity of the deep medial and lateral plantar veins [94]. Individual differences in plantar support and in the pattern of the foot muscles contraction during the stance phase of the gait cycle have the potential to modify the efficacy of the foot pump [96].

These two mechanisms (weight bearing and muscle contraction), however, do not work synchronously, with plantar compression acting first then followed by the action of the muscle contractions at the foot [93]. These two different foot pump mechanisms may both be present during the stance phase of the gait cycle, but would be active ats [93]. Also, certain clinical conditions of CVD could be explained by a conflict between the mechanisms of the foot pump and the leg pumps [97]. The knowledge about the interaction of the lower limb muscle pumps during contraction/relaxation as a mechanism for venous return is still quite poor [57].

5.4. Impairment of calf muscle pump and functional capacity

Calf muscle pump dysfunction might be caused by weakness of calf muscles but may also be related to decreased range of motion around the ankle joint during walking and other movements [30, 75, 78, 98], neuropathy, muscle denervation or muscle atrophy, or gait abnormalities [29, 36, 43].

Ankle function plays an important role in mobility [36]. Distal leg muscles may exhibit reductions in strength and power with aging, and these affects walking, balance, and increases the risk of falling [99]. Impaired ankle muscles strength has been associated with falls [100]. The power output by dorsiflexion muscles has been found to be closely associated with function in community-dwelling older women in terms of their ability to get up from and sit down on a chair and climb stairs [100]. Plantarflexion strength has been shown to be positively related to both preferred gait speed and fast gait speed [100].

Patients with CVD present limited ankle range of motion [36, 45, 47, 78, 98]. Diminished ankle mobility tends to aggravate as CVD progresses and in parallel with increasing severity of symptoms, thus further contributing to a poor CMPF [78, 98]. Together with decreased ankle range of motion, there is also decreased muscle strength of dorsi and plantarflexors [30, 75], with decreased peak torque, power ability [36], muscle resistance (number of heel rises) [45], and total work performed by the ankle plantarflexors [75]. Other functional alterations associated with CVD include decreased gait speed [36, 45], decreased number of steps per week (in venous ulcer patients) [101], and generally impaired functional capacity and mobility [36]. Also, changes in ankle function alters foot pressure distribution during gait that becomes higher at the midfoot and lower at the toes [43].

These functional alterations, specially the decreased strength of the calf muscles and reduced ambulation, contribute to venous hypertension [30, 43, 46, 47, 57, 98]. Dysfunction of the muscle pumps leads to venous blood not being effectively emptied out of the distal extremity [30]. This rarely occurs as a "primary" disorder in neuromuscular conditions or muscle wasting syndromes; however, clinically significant muscle pump dysfunction often occurs in severe reflux or obstruction [92]. Muscle pump dysfunction appears to be a major mechanism for the development of superficial venous incompetence and its complications, such as venous ulcers, and around 70% of patients with venous ulcer present calf muscle pump dysfunction [48, 66, 89, 91, 102].

Venous blood flow increases during calf muscle contractions in individuals with or without CVD. Popliteal peak flow volume is maximal during the first contraction of the tip-toe set of ten repetitions when the venous reservoir is full [103]. In the CVD patients, but not in the healthy subjects, venous flow augmentation was seen to diminish during the ten tip-toe exercise [104]. Such apparent calf pump dysfunction might be related to weak calf muscles in CVD patients [29, 30] and is compatible with a lower ejection volume, such as has been measured before in this population with air-plethysmography [92]. In addition, abnormal venous blood reflux from deep to superficial venous system through incompetent perforator veins may blunt blood flow through the popliteal vein [104].

Nonetheless, it seems that calf muscle size is not a strong indicator of the efficacy of muscles to pump venous blood during contractions in patients with venous ulcer [105]. Also, gastrocnemius thickness and some other muscle architectural features, like pennation angle, are similar in patients with low to moderate CVD severity and healthy participants, and seem unrelated with the severity of CVD [104]. Despite this fact, for the medial gastrocnemius, a few morphological parameters (like higher muscle fascicle length, and pennation angle) are associated with the degree of increase in peak flow velocity in the popliteal vein during tip-toe movement [104].

6. Clinical and functional assessment of CVD (CEAP classification, VCSS)

6.1. CEAP Classification

Health professionals-reported outcomes, such as VCSS and CEAP classification, are convenient, easily evaluated, and relevant [15].

The CEAP classification was created to facilitate communication about CVD severity and for scientific research [13]. The CEAP classification was based on 1) clinical manifestations (C), 2) etiologic factors (E), described as congenital, primary, secondary (post-thrombotic), 3) anatomical distribution of disease (A), that can be located at superficial, perforator or deep veins, and 4) underlying pathophysiological findings (P), such as reflux, obstruction or both reflux and obstruction [13]. Subscripts are applied to designate S (symptomatic) from A (asymptomatic) limbs [65]. According to CEAP, there are six CVD categories that range from C0 to C6 [13, 65]. Also, the N subscript indicates no evidence of disease and is applicable to E, A, and/or P of CEAP [13, 65].

The C_0 represents those individuals with objective evidence of venous disease (i.e., E, A, and/or P), but with no clinical manifestations. The C_1 is characterized by the presence of telangiectasia or reticular veins (< 3mm in diameter). In the C_2 class varicose veins (> 3 mm in diameter) are present. The C_3 distinguishes itself from the preceding categories by the presence of edema of venous etiology. In the C_4 class, there are now skin trophic changes, like C_{4a}, for pigmentation and/or eczema, and C_{4b}, for lipodermatosclerosis and/or white atrophy. Classes C_5 and C_6 are associated with the occurrence of venous ulcers: the C_5 corresponds to cases of prior ulceration that healed, and C_6 to cases with active venous ulcers [13, 65].

Reticular veins, also called blue veins, subdermal varices, and venulectasies, are dilated subdermal veins, usually 1 mm to less than 3 mm in diameter and with tortuous paths [13].

Telangiectasias, also called spider veins, hyphen webs, and thread veins, represent the confluence of dilated intradermal venules less than 1 mm in caliber [13].

According to the guidelines, varicose veins (also called varix, varices, and varicosities [13]) should be palpable in an upright position and represent abnormal veins with at least 3 mm in diameter, [3, 13, 33]. Varicose veins can be present as a result of hypertension caused by reflux and/or obstruction, as discussed before [12, 57].

The development of varicose veins most frequently involves the saphenous veins, saphenous tributaries, or nonsaphenous superficial leg veins [13]. Varicose veins are usually tortuous, but tubular saphenous veins with demonstrated reflux may be classified as varicose veins [13]. Corona phlebectatica, also called malleolar flare and ankle flare, is commonly viewed as an early sign of CVD, and designates the accumulation of numerous small intradermal veins packed together on the medial or the lateral aspects of the ankle and foot [13].

The venous edema is a pitting edema that get worse through the day and static positions and improves at night with decrease hydrostatic pressure , accomplished for example in supine position and lower limb elevation, and usually is accompanied with venous symptoms and signs [19, 20].

The presence of pigmentation means that the skin becomes darker and brownish [13]. This results from extravasation of red blood cells into the interstitial space [57]. Blood extravasation and skin pigmentation is most noticed around the ankle, but may also be visible in the leg and foot [13, 106].

Atrophie blanche (white atrophy) is an induration of tissues This skin alteration, that should not be confused with healed venous ulcers, is usually well localized. and has the shape of a circular white and atrophic skin surrounded by dilated capillaries and sometimes by hyperpigmentation [13, 106].

Lipodermatosclerosis is also clinical sign of tissue induration, characterized by local chronic inflammation and fibrosis of skin and subcutaneous tissues at the lower region of the leg (also compromising the Achilles tendon), sometimes preceded by diffuse inflammatory edema of the skin, which may be painful and which often is referred to as hypodermitis [13, 106]. Clinically, lipodermatosclerosis must be differentiated from lymphangitis, erysipelas, or cellulitis by their characteristically different local signs and systemic nature characteristics [13].

The eczema is an inflammation process, erythematous dermatitis, which may progress to blistering, weeping, or scaling eruption of the leg skin, and may be located anywhere in the leg [13, 106]. Eczema is very frequent in uncontrolled CVD, but may also be associated to sensitization to local therapy [13].

Venous ulcers are the worst clinical sign of CVD and represent the loss of integrity of the skin, with a full-thickness defect and occur most frequently near the ankle region [13], at the site of major perforating veins and the greatest hydrostatic pressure [66]. Venous ulcers are also characterized by failure to heal spontaneously and are sustained by CVD [13].

The CEAP classification is the gold standard for classification of chronic venous disorders today and its use is recommended by the relevant guidelines [33]. Nevertheless, for proper use of CEAP some facts have to be taken into account: the CEAP classification is limited as a severity classification, C_2 summarizes all kinds of varicose veins, in C_3 it may be difficult to separate between venous and other reasons for edema, and corona phlebectatica is not included in the classification [107]. Further revisions of the CEAP classification may help to overcome the still-existing deficits [107]. Complementary to this classification system, some concepts were defined to give consistency to the scientific terms, like the CVD concept that designates any venous disorder associated to every clinical class, and the concept of chronic venous insufficiency, which represents the more severe stages of the disease (C_{3-6}) [13, 65].

The CEAP classification is the gold standard for classification of chronic venous disorders today, and its use is recommended by the relevant guidelines [33]. Nevertheless, when using the CEAP system a few issues must be acknowledged: as a classifications system the CEAP has limitation. For example in C_3, it may be difficult to separate between venous edema from edema with other causes [106].

6.2. Venous clinical severity score (VCSS)

The Venous clinical severity score (VCSS) was developed to supplement the CEAP classification and to give an additional weight to the more severe consequences of CVD [108]. The VCSS score has shown good intra- and inter-observer reliability and responsiveness to change [108–110]. This is a score that quantifies 10 items using the range: 0 (none), 1 (mild), 2 (moderate), and 3 (severe), with a total range score of 0–30 (best to worth) [106, 108–110]. In CEAP classes C_0 to C_6, the VCSS score is reported to range between of 3–18 [111]. A worthwhile clinical improvement for patients with CVD can be observed with a relative improvement of 70% in VCSS score [110] or with an absolute improvement of 4 points [7]. Differences between clinical classes are 1–2 points of VCSS below C_3, and 2–5 points above C_3 [111]. The items of the VCSS are:

- Pain or discomfort; (i.e., aching, heaviness, fatigue, soreness, burning, with presumed venous origin), patients are asked to describe for each leg the category that best describes this item;
- Varicose veins (with diameter ≤ 3 mm in standing position);
- Venous edema (presumed venous origin, i.e., pitting edema present every day and with significant changes by standing/limb elevation or evidence of venous etiology, like varicose veins or history of deep vein thrombosis) - clinical staff must exam both legs and should ask patients about the extent of edema experienced;
- Skin pigmentation (presumed of venous origin and not including focal pigmentation over varicose veins or pigmentation due to other chronic diseases) - clinical staff must exam each leg;
- Inflammation (more than just recent pigmentation, like erythema, cellulitis, venous eczema, dermatitis);
- Induration (presumed of venous origin with secondary skin and subcutaneous changes, such as chronic edema with fibrosis, hypodermitis, white atrophy, and lipodermatoesclerosis);

- Active ulcers number
- Active ulcers duration (patients are referred to describe the duration of the longest unhealed ulcer);
- Active ulcers size (score according the size of the largest active ulcer);
- Use of compression therapy (patients should be asked about their compliance to compression therapy).
- The assessment of the items of VCSS score should be carried out for both legs.

Despite their relevance, VCSS and CEAP evaluation can be biased by observer expectations and because patient-reported outcomes are recognized by medical authorities as the ultimate outcome for health-care interventions, self-reported assessment of symptoms and HRQL is recommended for CVD as well [15, 112]. The most comprehensively validated scales for assessing HRQL in CVD include the chronic venous insufficiency questionnaire (CIVIQ), for population with CVD and without ulcer; the Aberdeen varicose vein questionnaire (AVVQ), for population with varicose veins; and the venous insufficiency epidemiological and economic study on quality of life (VEINES-QOL), for population with CVD of all classes [113].

7. Conservative treatment of CVD

The main goals of conservative treatment for CVD, used as an adjunctive treatment or in isolation, focus on both the symptoms and secondary changes of the disease, such as for instance, edema, skin and subcutaneous changes or ulcers [33], and the prevention of secondary complications, like venous thrombosis [114]. Usually, initial treatment of CVD involves a non-invasive conservative treatment to reduce symptoms and help prevent the development of secondary complications and the progression of the disease [66]. Complementary, or posteriorly, some interventional or surgical treatments can be undertaken [33, 66].

Behavioural education, like giving advices to raise the legs to minimize edema and reducing intra-abdominal pressure, about the right exercises, for using compressive stockings and proper care of the skin and wounds, together with pharmacological therapy, is the most common referred conservative treatments [33, 66]. The conservative pharmacological treatment with venoactive drugs may be indicated for patients with pain and edema and should be implemented in association with compression for healing venous ulcers [33]. If conservative treatment is unsuccessful or provides an unsatisfactory response, then further treatment, including surgery, should be considered based on anatomic and pathophysiological features [66].

Interventional treatments, like sclerotherapy, ablative therapy with endovenous radiofrequency and laser, endovascular therapy, are less invasive than surgery for treating CVD [66]. It has been recommended to use these techniques to treat superficial incompetence (endovenous thermal ablation, as laser and radiofrequency) and varicose veins (sclerotherapy) [33].

Surgical treatments are recommended in severe forms of CVD, like venous ulcers that did not heal after 6 months of treatment [66]. There are several surgical procedures described in the literature, like ligation, stripping and venous phlebectomy, subfascial endoscopic perforator surgery or valve reconstruction [66].

In CVD, compression, like that provided by stockings, is recommended as a primary treatment, except when patients are candidates for vein ablation, in which case compression is also suggested as an adjuvant treatment, particularly to prevent ulcer recurrence [33]. Compression therapy is recommended as a complement to surgery (like stripping), and to venoactive drug treatment, in order to control edema and pain, and to enhance venous ulcer healing [33].

The severity of the disease is related with the difficulty of the peripheral venous system to evacuate the venous blood from the periphery in the direction of the heart [33], resulting in venous stasis [33, 115]. Furthermore, it is assumed that there is a strict relation between blood flow velocity and secondary deep vein thrombosis [114]. The prevention of stasis is a main goal in CVD treatment and decisive in preventing venous complications and is frequently done through conservative approaches. Conservative CVD treatment might include intermittent pneumatic compression [116], compression stockings and bandages [77, 117, 118], and muscle pump activation using electrical muscle stimulation [77, 119], transcutaneous electrical nerve stimulation [119], or active and passive movements [103, 119]. In this regard, MLD maneuvers may be an alternative treatment to enhance venous flow [21–23]. Nevertheless, this intervention needs specialized professionals and could be an expensive health care treatment. Teaching caregivers or patients simple lymphatic drainage, despite the lower efficacy showed in the treatment of lymphedema, when compared with MLD applied by professionals [25], could be an alternative.

The important role played by the ankle range of motion and calf muscle strength in the efficacy of CMPF is now widely recognized [30, 36, 43, 45, 90]. Likewise, altered CMPF seems to play a key role in the physiopathology of CVD [30, 36, 43, 45]. Physical exercise is nowadays widely recommended for CVD management [90, 120]. In previously conducted randomized controlled trials, exercise training in patients with CVD [90] or with post-thrombotic syndrome [120] was shown to improve calf muscles' peak torque at slow (60º/s) and fast (120º/s) speeds [90], maximal heel rise repetitions [120], CMPF [90], and HRQL [120]. However, the role of physical exercise in ameliorating the measures of clinical severity of CVD or in improving few performance features, such as joint range of motion or work and power ability of ankle plantarflexors could not be clearly demonstrated [90, 120].

8. Manual lymphatic drainage

There are four recognized techniques of MLD: the Földi [121], Vodder [122], Casley-Smith [123] and Leduc [124].

The four methods of MLD show some differences, but the major basic principles are very similar. In short, the maneuvers should be applied softly (with specific exceptions), should consist of a skin-stretching form of massage (not sliding), should comply with the direction of lymph flow, should be done using the entire hand or exceptionally with fingers, and should begin at the proximal regions of the extremity [122–126].

MLD is used as a conservative treatment of lymphedema, independently of the specific method [127]. In the case of the Leduc method, MLD consists of a skin-stretching [127] form of massage that applies low pressure (<40 mm Hg) to the underlying tissues [124] along the anatomical distribution of the superficial lymphatic vessels and ganglions, stimulating lymph flow [128, 129] and the reabsorption of interstitial fluid and macromolecules through the lymphatic circulation [124, 128, 129]. At the lower extremity, the call-up maneuver, a technique belonging to the Leduc method initiates with inciting (or call-up) maneuvers in the inguinal region (ganglionar stimulation) and then progresses distally along the lower extremity down to the edematous region, again employing call-up maneuvers, in order to stimulate lymph flow by enhancing the contractility of lymphagions of lymph collectors, [128, 129]. The reabsorption maneuver, another Leduc technique, is then applied over the edema to drain the interstitial fluid and soluble macromolecules through the lymphatic circulation [128–130] by stretching the leak filaments (connections between connective tissue to endothelial cell of lymphatic capillaries) when the skin is mobilized [128–130]. The whole procedure ends with a second round of call-up maneuvers, which are then applied in the reverse direction, ending at the groin region, in the case of the lower limb [128, 129]. Technically, the call-up maneuver initiates with the most proximal part of the hand and ends with the hands touching the skin while producing skin-stretching and is applied to promote the increase of lymph flow [128, 129]. The reabsorption maneuver initiates with the most distal part of hand and ends with hands touching the skin while applying skin-stretching [128, 129].

8.1. Contraindications/Precautions

There are several contraindications and precautions for MLD and decongestive lymphatic therapy. It is suggested that cardiac, pulmonary and renal functions should be monitored because of temporary increase in blood flow and circulatory loading [73]. As for the contraindications, the literature describes erysipelas, lymphatic systemic infection and lymphangitis, meaning inflammation of the lymphatic system, as absolute contraindications for MLD and decongestive lymphatic therapy [131]. Severe renal and heart failure are also contraindications for the use of multilayer bandages and intermittent pneumatic compression [132], whereas caution should be enforced when employing MLD in patients with severe cardiac insufficiency [128, 131, 132]. Unstable hypertension, thyroid dysfunction, hepatic cirrhosis with abdominal fluid (ascites), superior vena cava obstruction, untreated tuberculosis or malaria, are also contraindications for physical treatment [131, 132]. If swelling occurs for a long time after initial breast surgery, medical examination should be sought and any physical treatment will be stopped if inflammation occurs [132]. Also, Crohn disease, recent surgery, and diabetes are some additional clinical conditions that may be monitored for precaution [73].

8.2. Manual Lymphatic Drainage in Lymph edema

There are several indications for the use of MLD other than lymphedema, like CVD, post-thrombotic syndrome, chronic wounds, traumatic edema (iatrogenic, postsurgical, and musculoskeletal injury), complex regional pain syndrome, and lymphedema [73].

The evidence of MLD for the treatment of edema (related to cancer or traumatic during sport activity, or other orthopedic injuries) [25, 26, 133] and in improving functional status (related to total knee arthroplasty) [24] is unclear but has been considered somehow effective, but more research is needed. Nevertheless, MLD might have an important role in CVD by improving HRQL, symptoms [134, 135], and range of motion [24] when edema/lymphedema is present. In palliative treatment, MLD improves pain and dyspnea [25].

Based on a systematic review, the importance of MLD for preventing the incidence of lymphedema is unclear [25]. A meta-analysis shows that MLD does not provide further therapeutic benefit in reducing lymphedema related to breast cancer, when compared to the standard treatment or with compression therapy [25], but another study has demonstrated a benefit when employing MLD in these cases [136]. However, the small benefit of MLD must be evaluated together with its cost in terms of time and money spent by patients and health care systems and such cost-benefit evaluation favours the option for compression therapy by using multilayer bandages or compression hosiers and adding MLD only if the response to treatment is unsatisfactory [136].

Lymphatic drainage employing a simpler sequence, but using the same principles as MLD, in a way that can be applied by patients as a self-drainage [137, 138] is less effective than MLD in reducing limb volume or lymphedema related to breast cancer but can be used as a more economical MLD option [25].

It has been also suggested that MLD, despite the augmentation of lymph flow (increasing lymphagion contraction and lymphatic reabsorption), might also be responsible for increasing arteriolar blood flow, redirection of flow toward collateral vessels, anastomoses, and perhaps stimulating angionesis, but these hypothetical effects of MLD need scientific evidence [73].

Younger patients, those heavier in weight and higher in body mass index are more likely to show poor lymphedema treatment outcome after intensive decongestive therapy [25]. When an elastic sleeve and multilayer bandaging are associated to MLD, there is a higher chance that the lymphedema treatment is successful [139].

Decongestive lymphatic therapy is the physical treatment for lymphedema by combining MLD with other treatments, like low-stretch bandaging and compression garments, exercise, and skin care, and sometimes also with intermittent pneumatic compression [30, 127, 140]. This method may reveal itself as effective in the treatment of lymphedema of the lower limb as it is for that affecting the upper limb as a result of cancer [135, 141].

Most often, decongestive lymphatic therapy is applied along two phases: the first is the edema reduction and intensive one, and the second one is the maintenance phase [127, 142, 143].

Decongestive lymphatic therapy is often prescribed for patients with venous ulcer and when CVD are associated with mixed edema (lymphatic and venous origin), now combining MLD, compression bandages, and stocking, physical therapy to improve calf muscle performance, and in few cases, intermittent pneumatic compression [16]. In the case of CVD, wearing compression garments is essential for treatment efficacy [16, 143].

8.3. Manual lymphatic drainage in CVD

8.3.1. The technique

The manual technique of MLD is not usually described in the literature. Nevertheless, based on research [21–23], the hands of the physical therapist must do the maneuvers producing a low pressures form of skin stretching. The pressure applied by the hands onto the skin and underlying soft tissues should be carefully adjusted to remain soft and just enough to stretch the skin for at least 4 s. When both legs are treated, the whole session take approximately 40–45 min [17, 18, 21]. The duration and the number of sessions at the studies assessing the role MLD in CVD patients [17, 18] are similar, during 2–5 weeks, patients should complete 10–14 sessions of MLD.

The sequence of the maneuvers follows that commonly used for lymphedema, first, moving from proximal to distal and, second, moving from distal to proximal [128, 129]. The maneuvers can be applied in the following sequence: inguinal region (10 MLD maneuvers), progressing downwards through the thigh, (30 MLD maneuvers at medial and 30 at lateral aspect of thigh), the popliteal region (10 MLD maneuvers applied immediately above the popliteal fossa and another 10 times maneuvers performed immediately below the popliteal fossa), downwards to the leg (30 MLD maneuvers at medial and lateral aspect of leg), and finishing in the dorsal aspect of the foot 30 MLD maneuvers). Next, the maneuvres should be carried out in the reverse order upwards: 15 maneuvers on the dorsal aspect of the foot, 15 maneuvers both on lateral and medial aspect of the leg, 5 maneuvers both below and above popliteal fossa, 15 maneuvers above both the lateral and above the medial aspect of the thigh, 5 MLD maneuvers on the inguinal region (**Figure 1**)[21]

8.3.2. Physiological effects in venous hemodynamic

Some studies suggest that MLD has an effect on blood flow in superficial veins, especially through the call-up maneuver [144]. Also the real impact of MLD in hemodynamics has been suggested to be insignificant [128]. One study concluded that 5 to 15 minutes of MLD does not

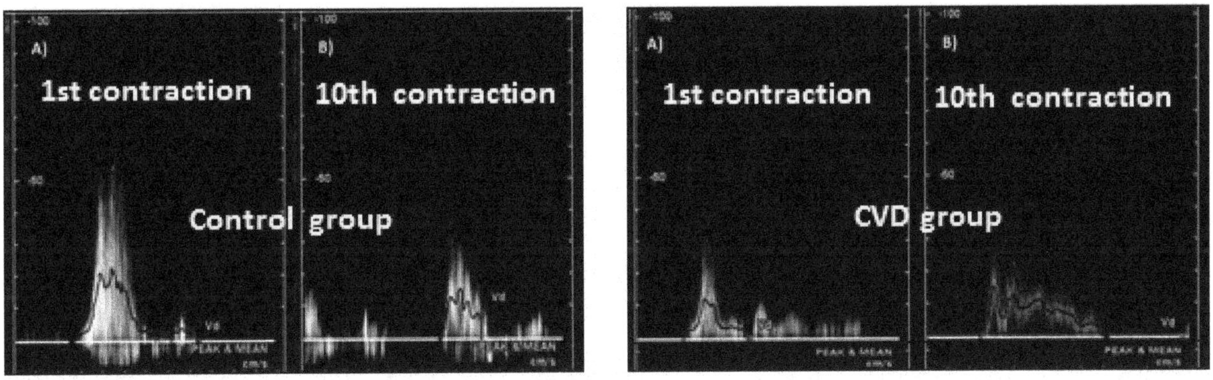

Figure 1. Venous ultrasound assessment at popliteal vein during 1st and 10th calf contraction. Venous ultrasound assessment at popliteal vein during 1st (A) and 10th (B) calf contraction, during tiptoe movement for both control (no CVD) and CVD (C_0–C_4) groups.

change cardiac output in patients with heart failure despite the near 100% increase in venous return after 5 minutes of MLD [128]. Nevertheless, recent studies reveal that in real-time the blood flow in superficial and deep veins increase, despite the presence or absence of venous pathology [22, 145].

Current concepts regarding MLD indicate that each maneuver should take around 4 s from beginning to end [22, 23, 129]. MLD techniques, which are based on manual stretching of the skin and underlying soft tissues, increase venous blood flow along the superficial veins, as has already been suggested [144], but also along the deep venous system, which course beneath the deep fascia. As commonly taught, the call-up maneuver is applied in a proximal to distal direction and enhances venous blood flow. The reabsorption maneuver instead begins distally and then moves proximally, stimulating lymph flow and fluid reabsorption [129]. One study does not substantiate such differential effects between the two maneuvers [22]. In fact, the two maneuvers enhanced venous blood flow to a similar extent and in both deep (femoral vein) and superficial (great saphenous vein) veins.

The amount of strain applied to the skin and deeper tissues by MLD is not known. Although studies using radiolabelled tracers demonstrate the efficacy of MLD in stimulating lymph flow, the exact mechanisms by which these techniques work are not fully elucidated [121, 130]. Skin and deep fasciae are connected by ligamentous structures at the level of the thigh, knee, popliteal fossa, and leg, which give stability to the skin and act like an anchor during lower limb movements [146]. The skin stretching applied during MLD might produce enough increase in pressure upon underlying structures to enhance venous flow in superficial and deep veins, as occurs during the physiological stretching of the skin during limb movement [147].

MLD must take into account venous anatomy and venous blood flow direction just like the lymphatic anatomy and the lymph flow directions, particularly when applied to larger body segments (like the course of GSV), such as the thigh, to be more effective in increasing venous flow [23, 128, 129, 145, 148].

The increased blood flow in the superficial veins would result in higher blood flow across perforating veins and into the deep veins, thereby raising blood flow in the deep venous system as well. In addition, the pressure applied to the skin, as said before, would probably reach the muscles underneath, and pressure would also increase in deep seated structures including veins, further stimulating blood flow. Also, muscle tone might increase during the time MLD techniques are being applied, induced by the manual stimulation, or in response to the movement of the lower extremity, which could have contributed to the observed increase in venous blood flow.

8.3.3. Therapeutic efficacy of manual lymphatic drainage for treatment of patients with chronic venous disease

MLD has also been used as a conservative treatment for CVD, [16], mostly when venous lymphedema is present [19, 20]. MLD applied before surgery in patients with CVD improves the clinical class of CEAP classification, HRQL, depression, anxiety, edema, and symptoms

[17, 18, 21]. Nevertheless, foot volumetry and reflux volume index only improve when MLD is associated to surgery and compression stockings [17, 18].

Previous studies show that MLD (10 sessions in 2 weeks) used in CVD patients who were referred to vascular surgery is effective in diminishing pain and edema and in improving HRQL [17]. When employed for a longer period of time (14 sessions in 5 weeks), MLD also seems to effectively contribute, together with surgery, to improve CVD severity [18]. However, such effect of MLD could be explained by faster recovery during the post-operative time. However, a recent study reveals that MLD (4-weeks period of MLD treatment, comprising ten 40 to 45 min-duration of each of 10 sessions) has a real effect in improving CVD-related symptoms, pain-HRQL and clinical severity (mostly related to venous edema), independently from vascular surgery, with the positive outcomes of MLD persisting after 1 month follow-up [21]. Nonetheless, MLD seems to be ineffective in changing leg volume, ankle muscles strength, ankle active range of motion, and the physical, social or psychological components of HRQL of CIVIQ [21].

There is no evidence that MLD treatment may significant change ankle muscles performance (either during plantarflexion or during dorsiflexion) and ankle range of motion. However, the role of physical exercise in ameliorating the measures of clinical severity of CVD or in improving some performance features, such as joint range of motion or work and power ability of ankle plantarflexors, could not be clearly demonstrated [90, 120].

However, the possibility that MLD might improve ankle function during more natural activities, such as gait, has not been assessed yet.

MLD increases peripheral venous blood flow in superficial and deep veins in normal limbs and in those with CVD and may be an important conservative treatment for prevent blood stasis and its complications [21–23, 125]. The prevention of stasis, by increase venous return, is a main goal in CVD treatment and decisive in preventing venous complications, and there are several conservative approaches [114]. During the application of the MLD maneuver (with pressure <40 mmHg), the volume of venous blood outflow from deep and superficial veins increases substantially without collapsing the veins [22, 23].

Studies suggested that despite the increase of venous flow during MLD being similar in healthy and CVD groups (C_{1_5}), in most severe cases of this disease this augmentation might not occur [22, 23]. CVD causes significant damage to the skin and underlying tissues. Persistent inflammation of the skin leads to disease complications such as lipodermatosclerosis, characterized by fibrosis and microcirculatory changes [149], leg edema [27] may interfere with the movement of the skin and underlying soft tissues essential to MLD efficacy.

The adherence to compressive stockings is usually decisive to manage symptoms and complications of CVD and venous stasis [150]. Some studies refer the importance of wearing compression stocking during the application of MLD [17, 18]. In one study, 23 out of the 41 patients did not wear compression stockings and only four participants fully adhere to this treatment, with no influence on MLD efficacy. However two patients in the control group (no MLD treatment) were excluded during the study because they present deep venous thrombosis and coincidently these two participants did not comply with the use of compression stoking [21].

8.4. Recommendations for treating CVD with MLD

MLD should be applied as a low pressure, manual skin-stretching form of massage applied from distal to proximal throughout the lower limb, with the two hands of the physical therapist placed side by side and respecting the anatomy and flow of venous vessels, in order to increase venous return from the lower limb in subjects with or without CVD (C_{1_5}).

MLD treatment for CVD should be applied during 2–5 weeks; patients should complete 10–14 sessions (45 min duration for both legs) of MLD. The sequence of MLD maneuvers should be applied proximal to distal, followed by a sequence in reverse direction (i.e., from distal to proximal) such as recommended for lymphedema [124, 128]. Because inflammation may be present in these patients, direct manual skin-stretching should be avoided over the edema, as for local inflammation in lymphedema. Although there is no evidence of the efficacy of MLD in treating venous ulcer (C_6), it can be applied in these patients as long as no contraindications are present [21].

Despite no evidence that MLD prevent secondary complications associated to venous stasis, like venous thrombosis, the use of MLD may be an option to increase superficial and deep venous flow [23, 104]. In particular, MLD is recommended before venous surgery and should be complemented with compression stockings [17, 18].

It is recommended to use MLD to relief edema, symptoms, severity of disease, and ameliorate HRQL. These effects are more consistent when MLD is used as a coadjutant treatment of compression stocking [17, 18, 21]. When adherence to compression treatment is difficult, MLD can be an option to relief symptoms and improve HRQL in patients with CVD [21].

Compromised muscle pump function, low muscle strength, and limited ankle range of motion can be addressed with other conservative approaches, like physical exercise.

9. Conclusion

CVD is a very common disease across the world. Despite the cosmetic issues, there are very important dysfunctions associated with this pathology, like muscle pump dysfunction, symptoms like pain, limitation of range of motions and muscle strength, gait alterations, Lymph(edema), higher risk of deep venous thrombosis, among other. Physical therapists may have an important role in assessing (using a uniformed procedure with other health professionals) and treating these dysfunctions using a wide number of strategies, like exercise, Kinesio taping, and others. MLD may be an alternative coadjutant conservative treatment of patients with CVD, previous or not to surgery. Although there is already information about the importance of MLD as a treatment choice for CVD, further research is warrant to determine the best way to combine this approach with the existing CVD treating tools.

Author details

Rute S.S. Crisóstomo[1]* and Paulo A.S. Armada-da-Silva[2]

*Address all correspondence to: crisostomo.rute@gmail.com

1 Instituto Politécnico de Castelo Branco – Escola Superior de Saúde Dr. Lopes Dias

2 Universidade de Lisboa – Faculdade de Motricidade Humana

References

[1] Writing C, Wittens C, Davies AH, Bækgaard N, Broholm R, Cavezzi A, et al., Editor's choice—Management of chronic venous disease. Clinical practice guidelines of the European society for vascular surgery (ESVS). European Journal of Vascular and Endovascular Surgery. 2015;**49**:678-737

[2] Koupidis SA, Paraskevas KI, Stathopoulos V, Mikhailidis DP. Impact of lower extremity venous ulcers due to chronic venous insufficiency on quality of life. The open cardiovascular medicine journal. 2008;**2**:105-109

[3] Eklof B, Perrin M, Delis KT, Rutherford RB, Gloviczki P, American Venous F, et al. Updated terminology of chronic venous disorders: The VEIN-TERM transatlantic interdisciplinary consensus document. Journal of Vascular Surgery. 2009;**49**(2):498-501

[4] Boisseau MR. Leukocyte involvement in the signs and symptoms of chronic venous disease. Perspectives for therapy. Clinical Hemorheology and Microcirculation. 2007;**37**(3):277-290

[5] Bradbury A, Evans C, Allan P, Lee A, Ruckley CV, Fowkes FG. What are the symptoms of varicose veins? Edinburgh vein study cross sectional population survey. British Medical Journal/British Medical Association. 1999;**318**(7180):353-356

[6] Campbell WB, Decaluwe H, Boecxstaens V, MacIntyre JA, Walker N, Thompson JF, et al. The symptoms of varicose veins: difficult to determine and difficult to study. European Journal of Vascular Surgery. 2007;**34**(6):741-744

[7] Cesarone MR, Belcaro G, Rohdewald P, Pellegrini L, Ledda A, Vinciguerra G, et al. Improvement of signs and symptoms of chronic venous insufficiency and microangiopathy with Pycnogenol: A prospective, controlled study. Phytomedicine. 2010;**17**(11):835-839

[8] Darvall KA, Bate GR, Adam DJ, Bradbury AW. Generic health-related quality of life is significantly worse in varicose vein patients with lower limb symptoms independent of CEAP clinical grade. European Journal of Vascular Surgery. 2012;**44**(3):341-344

[9] Andreozzi GM, Cordova RM, Scomparin A, Martini R, D'Eri A, Andreozzi F, et al. Quality of life in chronic venous insufficiency. An Italian pilot study of the Triveneto Region. International Angiology: A journal of the International Union of Angiology. 2005;**24**(3):272-277

[10] Furtado K, Pina E, Moffatt CJ, Franks PJ. Leg ulceration in Portugal: Quality of life. International Wound Journal. 2008;**5**(1):34-39

[11] Lamping DL, Schroter S, Kurz X, Kahn SR, Abenhaim L, Evaluation of outcomes in chronic venous disorders of the leg: Development of a scientifically rigorous, patient-reported measure of symptoms and quality of life. Journal of Vascular Surgery. 2003;**37**(2):410-419

[12] Labropoulos N, Gasparis AP, Pefanis D, Leon LR, Jr., Tassiopoulos AK. Secondary chronic venous disease progresses faster than primary. Journal of Vascular Surgery. 2009;**49**(3):704-710

[13] Eklof B, Rutherford RB, Bergan JJ, Carpentier PH, Gloviczki P, Kistner RL, Revision of the CEAP classification for chronic venous disorders: Consensus statement. Journal of Vascular Surgery. 2004;**40**(6):1248-1252

[14] Nullen H, Diagnosis and treatment of varicose veins: Part 1: definition, epidemiology, etiology, classification, clinical aspects, diagnostic and indications. Der Chirurg; Zeitschrift für alle Gebiete der operativen Medizen. 2010;**81**(11):1035-46

[15] Guex JJ. Importance of patient-reported outcomes in chronic venous disorders. Phlebology. 2012;**27**(Suppl 1):136-138

[16] Steins A, Jünger, M. Physical therapy in patients with chronic venous insufficiency. Phlebologie. 2000;**29**:48-53

[17] Molski P, Kruczynski J, Molski A, Molski S. Manual lymphatic drainage improves the quality of life in patients with chronic venous disease: A randomized controlled trial. Archives of Medical Science. 2013;**9**(3):452-458

[18] Molski P, Ossowski R, Hagner W, Molski S. Patients with venous disease benefit from manual lymphatic drainage. International Angiology: A Journal of the International Union of Angiology. 2009;**28**(2):151-155

[19] Mortimer PS. Implications of the lymphatic system in CVI-associated edema. Angiology. 2000;**51**(1):3-7

[20] Raju S, Furrh JBt, Neglen P. Diagnosis and treatment of venous lymphedema. Journal of Vascular Surgery. 2012;**55**(1):141-149

[21] dos Santos Crisóstomo RS, Costa DS, de Luz Belo Martins C, Fernandes TI, Armada-da-Silva PA. Influence of manual lymphatic drainage on health-related quality of life and symptoms of chronic venous insufficiency: A randomized controlled trial. Archives of Physical Medicine and Rehabilitation. 2015;**96**(2):283-291

[22] Dos Santos Crisóstomo RS, Candeias MS, Ribeiro AM, da Luz Belo Martins C, Armada-da-Silva PA. et al. Manual lymphatic drainage in chronic venous disease: A duplex ultrasound study. Phlebology. 2014;**29**(10):667-676

[23] Crisóstomo RSS, Candeias MS, Armada-da-Silva PAS. Venous flow during manual lymphatic drainage applied to different regions of the lower extremity in people with and without chronic venous insufficiency: A cross-sectional study. Physiotherapy, 2016

[24] Ebert JR, Joss B, Jardine B, Wood DJ. Randomized trial investigating the efficacy of manual lymphatic drainage to improve early outcome after total knee arthroplasty. Archives of Physical Medicine and Rehabilitation. 2013;**94**(11):2103-2111

[25] Huang TW, Tseng SH, Lin CC, Bai CH, Chen CS, Hung CS, et al. Effects of manual lymphatic drainage on breast cancer-related lymphedema: A systematic review and meta-analysis of randomized controlled trials. World Journal of Surgical Oncology. 2013;**11**:15

[26] Vairo GL, Miller SJ, McBrier NM, Buckley WE. Systematic review of efficacy for manual lymphatic drainage techniques in sports medicine and rehabilitation: An evidence-based practice approach. The Journal of Manual and Manipulative Therapy. 2009;**17**(3):e80-e89

[27] Meissner MH, Moneta G, Burnand K, Gloviczki P, Lohr JM, Lurie F, et al. The hemodynamics and diagnosis of venous disease. Journal of Vascular Surgery. 2007;**46**(Suppl S):4S-24S

[28] Yamaki Nozaki M, Sakurai H, Soejima K, Kono T, Hamahata A. Advanced chronic venous insufficiency is associated with increased calf muscle deoxygenation. European Journal of Vascular Surgery. 2010;**39**(6):787-794

[29] Qiao T, Liu C, Ran F, The impact of gastrocnemius muscle cell changes in chronic venous insufficiency. European Journal of Vascular Surgery. 2005;**30**(4):430-436

[30] Panny M, Ammer K, Kundi M, Katzenschlager R, Hirschl M. Severity of chronic venous disorders and its relationship to the calf muscle pump. VASA. Zeitschrift für Gefässkrankheiten. 2009;**38**(2):171-176

[31] Rowland TW, The circulatory response to exercise: role of the peripheral pump. International Journal of Sports Medicine. 2001;**22**(8):558-565

[32] Simka M, Calf muscle pump impairment and delayed healing of venous leg ulcers: Air plethysmographic findings. The Journal of Dermatology. 2007;**34**(8):537-544

[33] Gloviczki P, Comerota AJ, Dalsing MC, Eklof BG, Gillespie DL, Gloviczki ML, et al. The care of patients with varicose veins and associated chronic venous diseases: Clinical practice guidelines of the society for vascular surgery and the american venous forum. Journal of Vascular Surgery. 2011;**53**(5 Suppl):2S-48S

[34] Robertson L, Evans C, Fowkers F. Epidemiology of chronic venous disease. Phlebology. 2008;**23**:103-11

[35] Rabe E, Guex JJ, Puskas A, Scuderi A, Fernandez Quesada F, Coordinators V. Epidemiology of chronic venous disorders in geographically diverse populations: results from the Vein Consult Program. International Angiology. 2012;**31**(2):105-115

[36] de Moura RM, RM, Gomes Hde A, da Silva SL, Britto RR, Dias RC. Analysis of the physical and functional parameters of older adults with chronic venous disease. Archives of Gerontology and Geriatric. 2012;**55**(3):696-701

[37] Beebe-Dimmer JL, Pfeifer JR, Engle JS, Schottenfeld D. The epidemiology of chronic venous insufficiency and varicose veins. Annals of epidemiology. 2005;**15**(3):175-184

[38] Vasquez MA, Munschauer CE. Venous clinical severity score and quality-of-life assessment tools: Application to vein practice. Phlebology. 2008;**23**(6):259-275

[39] Passman MA, McLafferty RB, Lentz MF, Nagre SB, Iafrati MD, Bohannon WT, et al. Validation of venous clinical severity score (VCSS) with other venous severity assessment tools from the American Venous Forum, National Venous Screening Program. Journal of Vascular Surgery. 2011;**54**(6 Suppl):2S-9S

[40] Lal BK. Venous ulcers of the lower extremity: Definition, epidemiology, and economic and social burdens. Seminars in Vascular Surgery. 2015;**28**(1):3-5

[41] Sritharan K, Lane TRA, Davies AH, The burden of depression in patients with symptomatic varicose veins. European Journal of Vascular and Endovascular Surgery: The Official Journal of the European Society for Vascular Surgery. 2012;**43**(4):480-44

[42] Dimakakos E, Syrigos K, Scliros E, Karaitianos I. Prevalence, risk and aggravating factors of chronic venous disease: An epidemiological survey of the general population of Greece. Phlebology. 2013;**28**(4):184-190

[43] Shiman MI, Pieper B, Templin TN, Birk TJ, Patel AR, Kirsner RS. Venous ulcers: A reappraisal analyzing the effects of neuropathy, muscle involvement, and range of motion upon gait and calf muscle function. Wound Repair and Regeneration: official publication of the Wound Healing Society [and] the European Tissue Repair Society. 2009;**17**(2):147-152

[44] Reinhardt F, Wetzel T, Vetten S, Radespiel-Troger M, Hilz MJ, Heuss D, Peripheral neuropathy in chronic venous insufficiency. Muscle Nerve. 2000;**23**(6):883-887

[45] van Uden CJ, van der Vleuten CJ, Kooloos JG, Haenen JH, Wollersheim H. Gait and calf muscle endurance in patients with chronic venous insufficiency. Clinical Rehabilitation. 2005;**19**(3):339-344

[46] Newland MR, Patel AR, Prieto L, Boulton AJ, Pacheco M, et al. Kirsner RS. Neuropathy and gait disturbances in patients with venous disease: A pilot study. Archives of Dermatology. 2009;**145**(4):485-486

[47] Dix FP, Brooke R, McCollum CN. Venous disease is associated with an impaired range of ankle movement. European Journal of Vascular Surgery. 2003;**25**(6):556-561

[48] Kan YM, Delis KT, Hemodynamic effects of supervised calf muscle exercise in patients with venous leg ulceration: A prospective controlled study. Archives of surgery. 2001;**136**(12):1364-1369

[49] Tsai S, Dubovoy A, Wainess R, Upchurch GR, Jr., Wakefield TW, Henke PK. Severe chronic venous insufficiency: Magnitude of the problem and consequences. Annals of Vascular Surgery. 2005;**19**(5):705-711

[50] Domingues EA, Cavalcanti MC, Costa PC, Lopes MH, Monteiro I, Alexandre NM. et al. Pain prevalence, socio-demographic and clinical features in patients with chronic ulcers. Journal of Tissue Viability. 2016;**25**(3):180-184

[51] Sandor T, Pathomechanism of chronic venous insufficiency and leg ulcer. Acta physiologica Hungarica. 2004;**91**(2):131-145

[52] Bobridge A, Sandison S, Paterson J, Puckridge P, Esplin M. A pilot study of the development and implementation of a 'best practice' patient information booklet for patients with chronic venous insufficiency. Phlebology. 2010;**26**(8):338-343

[53] Carpentier PH, Maricq HR, Biro C, Poncot-Makinen CO, Franco A. Prevalence, risk factors, and clinical patterns of chronic venous disorders of lower limbs: A population-based study in France. Journal of Vascular Surgery. 2004;**40**(4):650-659

[54] Allegra C, Chronic venous insufficiency: The effects of health-care reforms on the cost of treatment and hospitalisation-an Italian perspective. Current medical research and opinion. 2003;**19**(8):761-769

[55] Greaney JL, Farquhar WB, Why do veins stiffen with advancing age? Journal of Applied Physiology. 2011;**110**(1):11-12

[56] Lim CS, Davies AH. Pathogenesis of primary varicose veins. The British journal of surgery. 2009;**96**(11):1231-1242

[57] Meissner MH, Gloviczki P, Bergan J, Kistner RL, Morrison N, Pannier F, et al. Primary chronic venous disorders. Journal of Vascular Surgery. 2007;**46**(Suppl S):54S-67S

[58] Ibegbuna V, Delis KT, Nicolaides AN. Haemodynamic and clinical impact of superficial, deep and perforator vein incompetence. European Journal of Vascular Surgery. 2006;**31**(5):535-541

[59] Sandor T. Chronic venous disease. A state of art. Orvosi Hetilap. 2010;**151**(4):131-139

[60] Bergan JJ, Pascarella L, Shmid-Schonbein GW. Pathogenesis of chronic venous disease: Insight from animal model of venous hypertension. Journal of Vascular Surgery. 2008;**47**:183-192

[61] Lopez JA, Kearon C, Lee AY. Deep venous thrombosis. Hematology/the Education Program of the American Society of Hematology, 2004;439-456

[62] Malone PC, Agutter PS. To what extent might deep venous thrombosis and chronic venous insufficiency share a common etiology? International Angiology: A Journal of the International Union of Angiology. 2009;**28**(4):254-268

[63] Ascher E, Jacob T, Hingorani A, Tsemekhin B, Gunduz Y. Expression of molecular mediators of apoptosis and their role in the pathogenesis of lower-extremity varicose veins. Journal of Vascular Surgery. 2001;**33**(5):1080-1086

[64] Stvrtinova V, Ferencikova J, Lysosomal enzymes and superoxide production in polymorphonuclear leukocytes of patients with primary varicose veins. Cor et vasa. 1992;**34**(3):255-264

[65] Padberg FT, Jr. CEAP classification for chronic venous disease. Disease-a-month: DM. 2005;**51**(2-3):176-182

[66] Eberhardt RT, Raffetto JD. Chronic venous insufficiency. Circulation. 2005;**111**(18): 2398-2409

[67] Delis KT. Perforator vein incompetence in chronic venous disease: A multivariate regression analysis model. Journal of Vascular Surgery. 2004;**40**(4):626-633

[68] Ely JW, Osheroff JA, Chambliss ML, Ebell MH. et al. Approach to leg edema of unclear etiology. Journal of the American Board of Family Medicine : JABFM. 2006;**19**(2):148-160

[69] Hirai M, Iwata H, Miyazaki K, Koyama A, Ikeda K, Hukiage M, et al. Effect of gaiters on muscle pump activity in healthy volunteers. Phlebology, 2012

[70] Raju, S, Furrh JBt, Neglen P. Diagnosis and treatment of venous lymphedema. Journal of vascular surgery. 2012; 55(1):141-9.

[71] Piller N. Phlebolymphoedema/chronic venous lymphatic insufficiency: An introduction to strategies for detection, differentiation and treatment. Phlebology. 2009;**24**(2):51-5

[72] Fernandez AP, Miteva M, Roberts B, Ricotti C, Rouhani P, Romanelli P. Histopathologic analysis of dermal lymphatic alterations in chronic venous insufficiency ulcers using D2–40. Journal of the American Academy of Dermatology. 2011;**64**(6):1123 e1-1123 e12

[73] Morgan CL. Medical management of lymphedema. In: Tretbar LI, Lee B-B, Blondeau B, Morgan CL, Simonian SJ, editors. Lymphedema: Diagnosis and Treatment. London: Springer, 2008, pp. 43-54

[74] Cueni LN, Detmar M. The lymphatic system in health and disease. Lymphatic Research and Biology. 2008;**6**(3-4):109-122

[75] Yang D, Vandongen YK, Stacey MC. Changes in calf muscle function in chronic venous disease. Cardiovascular Surgery (London, England). 1999;**7**(4):451-456

[76] Recek C. Calf pump activity influencing venous hemodynamics in the lower extremity. The International Journal of Angiology: Official Publication of the International College of Angiology, Inc. 2013;**22**(1):23-30

[77] Clarke Moloney M, Lyons GM, Breen P, Burke PE, Grace PA. Haemodynamic study examining the response of venous blood flow to electrical stimulation of the gastrocnemius muscle in patients with chronic venous disease. European Journal of Vascular Surgery. 2006;**31**(3):300-305

[78] Cavalheri G, Jr, de Godoy JM, Belczak CE. Correlation of haemodynamics and ankle mobility with clinical classes of clinical, aetiological, anatomical and pathological classification in venous disease. Phlebology. 2008;**23**(3):120-124

[79] Eifell RK, Ashour HY, Lees TA. Comparison of new continuous measurements of ambulatory venous pressure (AVP) with conventional tiptoe exercise ambulatory AVP in relation to the CEAP clinical classification of chronic venous disease. Journal of Vascular Surgery. 2006;**44**(4):794-802

[80] Neglen P, Raju S. Ambulatory venous pressure revisited. Journal of Vascular Surgery. 2000;**31**(6):1206-1213

[81] Neglen P, Raju S. Differences in pressures of the popliteal, long saphenous, and dorsal foot veins. Journal of Vascular Surgery. 2000;**32**(5):894-901

[82] Nicolaides AN, Hussein MK, Szendro G, Christopoulos D, Vasdekis S, Clarke H. The relation of venous ulceration with ambulatory venous pressure measurements. Journal of Vascular Surgery. 1993;**17**(2):414-419

[83] Katz ML, CA., Kerr R. Air plethysmography (APG): A new technique to evaluate patients with chronic venous insufficency. The Journal of Vascular Technology. 1991;**1991**:23-27

[84] Ludbrook J. The musculovenous pumps of the human lower limb. American Heart Journal. 1966;**71**(5):635-641

[85] Black CM. Anatomy and physiology of the lower-extremity deep and superficial veins. Techniques in Vascular and Interventional Radiology. 2014;**17**(2):68-73

[86] Gaweesh AS, Impeded venous drainage: Novel view of chronic venous disease pathophysiology. Medical Hypotheses. 2009;**73**(4):548-552

[87] Alimi YS, Barthelemy P, Juhan C. Venous pump of the calf: A study of venous and muscular pressures. Journal of Vascular Surgery. 1994;**20**(5):728-735

[88] Uhl JF, Gillot C. Anatomy of the veno-muscular pumps of the lower limb. Phlebology. 2015;**30**(3):180-193

[89] Araki CT, Back TL, Padberg FT, Thompson PN, Jamil Z, Lee BC, et al. The significance of calf muscle pump function in venous ulceration. Journal of Vascular Surgery. 1994;**20**(6):872-877; discussion 8–9

[90] Padberg FT, Jr, Johnston MV, Sisto SA. Structured exercise improves calf muscle pump function in chronic venous insufficiency: A randomized trial. Journal of Vascular Surgery. 2004;**39**(1):79-87

[91] Bradbury AW. Epidemiology and aetiology of C_{4-6} disease. Phlebology. 2010;**25**(Suppl 1):2-8

[92] Nicolaides AN. Investigation of chronic venous insufficiency: A consensus statement (France, March 5-9, 1997). Circulation. 2000;**102**(20):E126-E163

[93] Corley GJ, Broderick BJ, Nestor SM, Breen PP, Grace PA, Quondamatteo F, et al. The anatomy and physiology of the venous foot pump. Anatomical record (Hoboken, NJ: 2007). 2010;**293**(3):370-8

[94] Uhl JF, Gillot C. Anatomy of the foot venous pump: Physiology and influence on chronic venous disease. Phlebology. 2012;**27**(5):219-230

[95] Broderick BJ, Corley GJ, Quondamatteo F, Breen PP, Serrador J, Ólaighin G. Venous emptying from the foot: Influences of weight bearing, toe curls, electrical stimulation, passive compression, and posture. Journal of Applied Physiology (1985). 2010;**109**(4):1045-1052

[96] Saggini R, Bellomo RG, Iodice P, Lessiani G. Venous insufficiency and foot dysmorphism: Effectiveness of visco-elastic rehabilitation systems on veno-muscle system of the foot and of the calf. International Journal of Immunopathology and Pharmacology. 2009;**22**(3 Suppl):1-8

[97] Ricci S, Moro L, Antonelli Incalzi R. The foot venous system: Anatomy, physiology and relevance to clinical practice. Dermatologic Surgery: Official Publication for American Society for Dermatologic Surgery [et al.]. 2014;**40**(3):225-233

[98] Back TL, TL, Padberg FT, Jr., Araki CT, Thompson PN, Hobson RW, 2nd. Limited range of motion is a significant factor in venous ulceration. Journal of Vascular Surgery. 1995;**22**(5):519-23

[99] Webber SC, Porter MM. Reliability of ankle isometric, isotonic, and isokinetic strength and power testing in older women. Physical Therapy. 2010;**90**(8):1165-1175

[100] Suzuki T, Bean JF, Fielding RA. Muscle power of the ankle flexors predicts functional performance in community-dwelling older women. Journal of the American Geriatrics Society. 2001;**49**(9):1161-1167

[101] Clarke-Moloney M, Godfrey A, O'Connor V, Meagher H, Burke PE, Kavanagh EG, et al. Mobility in patients with venous leg ulceration. European Journal of Vascular Surgery 2007;**33**(4):488-93

[102] O'Brien J, Edwards H, Finlayson K, Kerr G. Understanding the relationships between the calf muscle pump, ankle range of motion and healing for adults with venous leg ulcers: A review of the literature. Wound Practice and Research. 2012;**20**(2)

[103] Staubesand J, Heisterkamp T, Stege H. Use of duplex sonography to investigate the effect of active and passive movement at the ankle joint for promoting venous return. Clinical Anatomy. 1995;**8**(2):96-101

[104] Crisostomo RS, Candeias MS, Armada-da-Siva PA. The use of ultrasound in the evaluation of the efficacy of calf muscle pump function in primary chronic venous disease. Phlebology. 2014;**29**(4):247-256

[105] Moloney MC, Lyons GM, Egan M., Wallis F, Burke PE. Does size matter? The impact of calf muscle volume on venous return in patients with venous leg ulcer. Phlebology. 2007;**22**:65-9

[106] Vasquez MA, MA, Rabe E, McLafferty RB, Shortell CK, Marston WA, Gillespie D, Revision of the venous clinical severity score: Venous outcomes consensus statement: Special communication of the American Venous Forum Ad Hoc Outcomes Working Group. Journal of Vascular Surgery. 2010;**52**(5):1387-96

[107] Rabe E, Pannier F. Clinical, aetiological, anatomical and pathological classification (CEAP): Gold standard and limits. Phlebology. 2012;**27**(Suppl 1):114-118

[108] Rutherford RB, Padberg FT, Jr., Comerota AJ, Kistner RL, Meissner MH, Moneta GL. Venous severity scoring: An adjunct to venous outcome assessment. Journal of Vascular Surgery. 2000;**31**(6):1307-1312

[109] Ricci MA, Emmerich J, Callas PW, Rosendaal FR, Stanley AC, Naud S, et al. Evaluating chronic venous disease with a new venous severity scoring system. Journal of Vascular Surgery. 2003;**38**(5):909-915

[110] Kakkos SK, Rivera MA, Matsagas MI, Lazarides MK, Robless P, Belcaro G, et al. Validation of the new venous severity scoring system in varicose vein surgery. Journal of Vascular Surery. 2003;**38**(2):224-8

[111] Lozano Sanchez FS, Carrasco Carrasco E, Diaz Sanchez S.,, Gonzalez Porras JR, Escudero Rodriguez JR, Marinello Roura J, Chronic venous disease in Spain: Doctor-patient correlation. European Journal of Vascular Surgery. 2012;**44**(6):582-6

[112] Catarinella FS, Nieman FH, Wittens CH. The relation between clinical scores and quality-of-life in long-term follow-up. Phlebology. 2016;**31**(1 Suppl):99-105

[113] Launois R, Review article: Health-related quality-of-life scales specific for chronic venous disorders of the lower limbs. Journal of Vascular Surgery: Venous and Lymphatic Disorders. 2015;**3**:219-27.e3

[114] Morris RJ, Woodcock JP, Evidence-based compression: Prevention of stasis and deep vein thrombosis. Annals of Surgery. 2004;**239**(2):162–71

[115] Lurie F, Pevec WC, Ultrasound estimates of venous valve function in screening for insufficiency and following patients with chronic venous disease. The International journal of angiology: official publication of the International College of Angiology, Inc. 2000;**9**(4):246-9

[116] Lurie F, Scott V, Yoon HC, Kistner RL. On the mechanism of action of pneumatic compression devices: Combined magnetic resonance imaging and duplex ultrasound investigation. Journal of Vascular Surgery. 2008;**48**(4):1000-6

[117] Downie SP, Raynor SM, Firmin DN, Wood NB, Thom SA, Hughes AD, et al. Effects of elastic compression stockings on wall shear stress in deep and superficial veins of the calf. American journal of physiology. Heart and circulatory physiology. 2008;**294**(5):H2112-20

[118] Partsch H, Menzinger G, Borst-Krafek B, Groiss E. Does thigh compression improve venous hemodynamics in chronic venous insufficiency? Journal of Vascular Surgery. 2002;**36**(5):948-952

[119] Izumi M, Ikeuchi M, Mitani T, Taniguchi S, Tani T. Prevention of venous stasis in the lower limb by transcutaneous electrical nerve stimulation. European Journal of Vascular Surgery. 2010;**39**(5):642-5

[120] Kahn SR, Shrier I, Shapiro S, Houweling AH, Hirsch AM, Reid RD, et al. Six-month exercise training program to treat post-thrombotic syndrome: A randomized controlled two-centre trial. Canadian Medical Association Journal. 2011;**183**(1):37-44

[121] Tan IC, Maus EA, Rasmussen JC, Marshall MV, Adams KE, Fife CE, et al., Assessment of lymphatic contractile function after manual lymphatic drainage using near-infrared fluorescence imaging. Archives of Physical Medicine and Rehabilitation. 2011;**92**(5):756-764 e1

[122] Kasseroller RG, The Vodder School: The Vodder method. Cancer. 1998;**83**(12 Suppl American):2840-2842

[123] Casley-Smith JR, Boris M, Weindorf S, Lasinski B. Treatment for lymphedema of the arm – The Casley-Smith method: A noninvasive method produces continued reduction. Cancer. 1998;**83**(12 Suppl American):2843-2860

[124] Leduc O, Leduc A, Bourgeois P, Belgrado JP. The physical treatment of upper limb edema. Cancer. 1998;**83**(12 Suppl American):2835-9

[125] Foldi E. The treatment of lymphedema. Cancer. 1998;**83**(12 Suppl American):2833-4

[126] Foldi E. Treatment of lymphedema and patient rehabilitation. Anticancer Research. 1998;**18**(3C):2211-2

[127] Koul R, Dufan T, Russell C, Guenther W, Nugent Z, Sun X, et al. Efficacy of complete decongestive therapy and manual lymphatic drainage on treatment-related lymphedema in breast cancer. International journal of radiation oncology, biology, physics. 2007;**67**(3):841-6

[128] Leduc O, Crasset V, Leleu C, Baptiste N, Koziel A, Delahaie C, Impact of manual lymphatic drainage on hemodynamic parameters in patients with heart failure and lower limb edema. Lymphology. 2011;**44**(1):13-20

[129] Lee BB, Bergan J, Rockson SG, editors. Lymphedema: A Concise Compendium of Theory and Practice. New York: Springer; 2011

[130] Leduc O, Bourgeois P, Leduc AM. Manual Lymphatic drainage: scintigraphic demonstration of its efficacy on colloidal protein reabsorption. In: Partsh, editor. Progress in Lymphology IX. Excerpta Medica, Amsterdam: Elsevier; 1988

[131] Lymphoedema Framework. Management of Lymphoedema. International Consensus. London: MEP Ltd.; 2006

[132] Leduc O. European consensus: Rehabilitation after breast cancer treatment. The European Journal of Lymphology. 2008;**XIX**(55):13-20

[133] Majewski-Schrage T, Snyder K. The effectiveness of manual lymphatic drainage in patients with orthopedic injuries. Journal of Sport Rehabilitation. 2016;**25**(1):91-7

[134] Kim YB, Hwang JH, Kim TW, Chang HJ, Lee SG. Would complex decongestive therapy reveal long term effect and lymphoscintigraphy predict the outcome of lower-limb lymphedema related to gynecologic cancer treatment? Gynecologic Oncology. 2012;**127**(3):638-42

[135] Lasinski BB, McKillip Thrift K, Squire D, Austin MK, Smith KM, Wanchai A, A systematic review of the evidence for complete decongestive therapy in the treatment of lymphedema from 2004 to 2011. PM & R: The Journal of Injury, Function, and Rehabilitation. 2012;**4**(8):580-601

[136] McNeely ML, ML, Peddle CJ, Yurick JL, Dayes IS, Mackey JR. Conservative and dietary interventions for cancer-related lymphedema: A systematic review and meta-analysis. Cancer. 2011;**117**(6):1136-48

[137] Williams AF, Vadgama A, Franks PJ, Mortimer PS. A randomized controlled crossover study of manual lymphatic drainage therapy in women with breast cancer-related lymphoedema. European journal of cancer care. 2002;**11**(4):254-1

[138] de Godoy JM, Torres CA, Godoy MF. Self-drainage lymphatic technique. Angiology. 2001;**52**(8):573-4

[139] Ezzo J, Manheimer E, McNeely ML, Howell DM, Weiss R, Johansson KI, et al. Manual lymphatic drainage for lymphedema following breast cancer treatment. The Cochrane Database of Systematic Reviews. **2015**(5):CD003475

[140] Foeldi E, Foeldi M, Clodius L. The lymphedema chaos: A lancet. Annals of Plastic Surgery. 1989;**22**:505-15

[141] Devoogdt N, Van Kampen M, Geraerts I, Coremans T, Christiaens MR. Different physical treatment modalities for lymphoedema developing after axillary lymph node dissection for breast cancer: A review. European Journal of Obstetrics, Gynecology, and Reproductive Biology. 2010;**149**(1):3-9

[142] Fialka-Moser V, Korpan M, Varela E, Ward A, Gutenbrunner C, Casillas JM, et al. The role of physical and rehabilitation medicine specialist in lymphoedema. Annals of Physical and Rehabilitation Medicine. 2013;**56**(5):396-410

[143] The diagnosis and treatment of peripheral lymphedema: 2013 consensus document of the international society of lymphology. Lymphology. 2013;**46**(1):1-11

[144] Leduc A, Leduc O. Drenagem linfática – teoria e prática. 2nd ed. Brasil: Manole; 2000. pp. 33-62

[145] Crisóstomo RS, Candeias MS, Armada-da-Silva, PA. Venous flow during manual lymphatic drainage applied to different regions of the lower extremity in people with and without chronic venous insufficiency: a cross-sectionl study. Physiotherapy. 2016.

[146] Nash LG, Phillips MN, Nicholson H, Barnett R, Zhang M. Skin ligaments: Regional distribution and variation in morphology. Clinical Anatomy. 2004;**17**(4):287-93

[147] Benjamin M, The fascia of the limbs and back-a review. Journal of Anatomy. 2009;**214**(1):1-18

[148] Martin ML, Hernandez MA, Avendano C, Rodriguez F, Martinez H. Manual lymphatic drainage therapy in patients with breast cancer related lymphoedema. BMC Cancer. 2011;**11**:94

[149] Smith PC, The causes of skin damage and leg ulceration in chronic venous disease. The International international journal of lower extremity wounds. 2006;**5**(3):160-8

[150] Ziaja D, Kocelak P, Chudek J, Ziaja K. Compliance with compression stockings in patients with chronic venous disorders. Phlebology. 2010;**26**(8):353-60

Permissions

All chapters in this book were first published in CPT, by InTech Open; hereby published with permission under the Creative Commons Attribution License or equivalent. Every chapter published in this book has been scrutinized by our experts. Their significance has been extensively debated. The topics covered herein carry significant findings which will fuel the growth of the discipline. They may even be implemented as practical applications or may be referred to as a beginning point for another development.

The contributors of this book come from diverse backgrounds, making this book a truly international effort. This book will bring forth new frontiers with its revolutionizing research information and detailed analysis of the nascent developments around the world.

We would like to thank all the contributing authors for lending their expertise to make the book truly unique. They have played a crucial role in the development of this book. Without their invaluable contributions this book wouldn't have been possible. They have made vital efforts to compile up to date information on the varied aspects of this subject to make this book a valuable addition to the collection of many professionals and students.

This book was conceptualized with the vision of imparting up-to-date information and advanced data in this field. To ensure the same, a matchless editorial board was set up. Every individual on the board went through rigorous rounds of assessment to prove their worth. After which they invested a large part of their time researching and compiling the most relevant data for our readers.

The editorial board has been involved in producing this book since its inception. They have spent rigorous hours researching and exploring the diverse topics which have resulted in the successful publishing of this book. They have passed on their knowledge of decades through this book. To expedite this challenging task, the publisher supported the team at every step. A small team of assistant editors was also appointed to further simplify the editing procedure and attain best results for the readers.

Apart from the editorial board, the designing team has also invested a significant amount of their time in understanding the subject and creating the most relevant covers. They scrutinized every image to scout for the most suitable representation of the subject and create an appropriate cover for the book.

The publishing team has been an ardent support to the editorial, designing and production team. Their endless efforts to recruit the best for this project, has resulted in the accomplishment of this book. They are a veteran in the field of academics and their pool of knowledge is as vast as their experience in printing. Their expertise and guidance has proved useful at every step. Their uncompromising quality standards have made this book an exceptional effort. Their encouragement from time to time has been an inspiration for everyone.

The publisher and the editorial board hope that this book will prove to be a valuable piece of knowledge for researchers, students, practitioners and scholars across the globe.

List of Contributors

Hitoshi Asai
Department of Physical Therapy, Graduate Course of Rehabilitation Science, School of Health Sciences, College of Medical, Pharmaceutical and Health Sciences, Kanazawa University, Kanazawa, Japan

Elisa Edi Anna Nadia Lioce
School of Physical Medicine and Rehabilitation, University of Torino, Torino, Italy

Matteo Novello and Caterina Guiot
Department of Neuroscience, University of Turin, Corso Raffaello, Torino, Italy

Michaela Tomanova
Brandýs nad Orlicí Rehabilitation Clinic, Brandýs nad Orlicí, Czech Republic

Özlem Çinar Özdemir and Mahmut Surmeli
School of Physical Therapy and Rehabilitation, Abant Izzet Baysal University, Bolu, Turkey

Masanori Ito, Yuki Takahashi, Satoshi Fujiwara and Naoki Kado
Department of Physical Therapy, Kobe College of Rehabilitation and Welfare, Kobe-shi, Hyogo, Japan

Tadashi Ito
Three-dimensional motion analysis room, Aichi Prefecture Mikawa Aoitori Medical and Rehabilitation Center for Developmental Disabilities, Okazaki-shi, Aichi, Japan

Michel Probst
KU Leuven, Department of Rehabilitation Sciences, Belgium

Naruemon Leelayuwat
Department of Physiology, Faculty of Medicine, Khon Kaen University, Khon Kaen, Thailand
Exercise and Sport Sciences Development and Research Group, Khon Kaen University, Khon Kaen, Thailand

Shinichiro Morishita and Atsuhiro Tsubaki
Institute for Human Movement, Medical Sciences, Niigata University of Health and Welfare, Niigata, Japan

Tomohito Ijiri
Department of Rehabilitation, Kiba Hospital, Medical Corporation, Juzankai, Osaka, Japan

Rute S.S. Crisóstomo
Instituto Politécnico de Castelo Branco - Escola Superior de Saúde Dr. Lopes Dias

Paulo A.S. Armada-da-Silva
Universidade de Lisboa - Faculdade de Motricidade Humana

Index

www.ingramcontent.com/pod-product-compliance
Lightning Source LLC
La Vergne TN
LVHW060600210926
848485LV00005B/1348
* 9 7 8 1 6 3 9 8 7 4 2 9 3 *